STUDYING A STUDY
&
TESTING A TEST

SIXTH EDITION

STUDYING A STUDY
&
TESTING A TEST

READING EVIDENCE-BASED HEALTH RESEARCH

Richard K. Riegelman, M.D., M.P.H., Ph.D.

Professor of Epidemiology & Biostatistics, Medicine, and Health Policy
Founding Dean, George Washington School of Public Health and Health Services
The George Washington University

Contributing Author
Michael L. Rinke, M.D., Ph.D. (candidate)

Assistant Professor of Pediatrics
Johns Hopkins University School of Medicine
The Johns Hopkins University

 Wolters Kluwer | Lippincott Williams & Wilkins
Health
Philadelphia · Baltimore · New York · London
Buenos Aires · Hong Kong · Sydney · Tokyo

Acquisitions Editor: Susan Rhyner
Product Managers: Angela Collins & Jenn Verbiar
Marketing Manager: Joy Fisher-Williams
Vendor Manager: Bridgett Dougherty
Manufacturing Manager: Margie Orzech
Designer: Holly Reid McLaughlin
Compositor: S4Carlisle
Sixth Edition

9 8 7 6 5 4 3 2 1

Library of Congress Cataloging-in-Publication Data

Riegelman, Richard K.
Studying a study & testing a test / Richard Riegelman.—6th ed.
p. ; cm.
Studying a study and testing a test
Rev. ed. of: Studying a study and testing a test / Richard K. Riegelman.
Includes bibliographical references and index.
ISBN 978-0-7817-7426-0 (alk. paper)
I. Riegelman, Richard K. Studying a study and testing a test   II. Title.   III. Title: Studying a study and testing a test.
[DNLM: 1. Biometry.   2. Epidemiologic Methods.   3. Evidence-Based Medicine—methods. WA 950]
610'.72—dc23

                                        2012008446

DISCLAIMER
Care has been taken to confirm the accuracy of the information present and to describe generally accepted practices. However, the authors, editors, and publisher are not responsible for errors or omissions or for any consequences from application of the information in this book and make no warranty, expressed or implied, with respect to the currency, completeness, or accuracy of the contents of the publication. Application of this information in a particular situation remains the professional responsibility of the practitioner; the clinical treatments described and recommended may not be considered absolute and universal recommendations.

The authors, editors, and publisher have exerted every effort to ensure that drug selection and dosage set forth in this text are in accordance with the current recommendations and practice at the time of publication. However, in view of ongoing research, changes in government regulations, and the constant flow of information relating to drug therapy and drug reactions, the reader is urged to check the package insert for each drug for any change in indications and dosage and for added warnings and precautions. This is particularly important when the recommended agent is a new or infrequently employed drug.

Some drugs and medical devices presented in this publication have Food and Drug Administration (FDA) clearance for limited use in restricted research settings. It is the responsibility of the health care provider to ascertain the FDA status of each drug or device planned for use in their clinical practice.

To purchase additional copies of this book, call our customer service department at **(800) 638-3030** or fax orders to **(301) 223-2320**. International customers should call **(301) 223-2300**.

Visit Lippincott Williams & Wilkins on the Internet: http://www.lww.com. Lippincott Williams & Wilkins customer service representatives are available from 8:30 am to 6:00 pm, EST.

CONTENTS

PREFACE

WHY "READING EVIDENCE-BASED HEALTH RESEARCH"— A PREFACE TO THE SIXTH EDITION

Studying a Study and Testing a Test was first published more than 30 years ago. The initial and continuing goal is to provide practical and comprehensive tools for everyone who seeks to critically read the health research literature and put the results into practice. During the three decades since the first edition, we have moved from "eminence-based" to "evidence-based" thinking. Today all current and future health professionals need to understand the basics of reading the health research literature.

The momentum has accelerated in recent years. For instance, medical literature reading and evidence-based medicine are being integrated into all three steps of the U.S.M.L.E. of the National Board of Medical Examiners. A wide range of health professions now recognize the importance of evidence-based practice and are incorporating reading the research literature into their curricula and their examinations. The grading of evidence-based recommendations discussed in Chapter 13 has been integrated into health reform legislation and has implications for quality and costs of health care.

The process of formalizing the presentation of evidence has continued since the last edition with the dissemination of a menagerie of new acronyms from MOOSE to STROBE to PRISMA. These guidelines for structuring the reporting of research are making the research literature more consistent and more complete. Understanding these frameworks helps the reader know what to look for and where to look.

Perhaps the biggest change in recent years has been the move to make research relevant to practice. As Dr. Lawrence Green has written, "If we want more evidence-based practice we need more practice-based evidence."(1) As we will explore, the development of translational research is increasing moving the focus from efficacy and safety under carefully controlled research conditions to effectiveness and safety in practice. The sixth edition takes on these challenges by adding new chapters on safety, prediction, and decision rules and translating research into practice.

The sixth edition of *Studying a Study and Testing a Test* is now subtitled "Reading Evidence-Based Health Research" to stress its relevance to everyone who reads the research. The book has been restructured to make it easier to use as a textbook while making every effort to retain its appeal to the individual reader. The book now consists of 14 chapters divided into two units "Studying a Study" and "Testing a Test". New to the sixth edition are "learn more" boxes in each chapter, providing more detailed discussion and examples.

The Web site http://thepoint.lww.com includes interactive practice questions testing your mastery of the material covered in each chapter as well as additional materials to support your efforts to read the research literature. Together the text and the Web site are intended to cover the skills and knowledge needed to read the evidence-based research.

Studying a Study and Testing a Test remains a book you can use on your own to help you read the research or as part of a Journal Club. Journal Clubs are now seen as an important format for learning to read the research. The sixth edition and Web site are designed to be an important part of making this happen.

One warning before you proceed. Reading the health research literature can be habit forming. You may even find it enjoyable.

REFERENCE

1. Green L. Guidelines and categories for classifying participatory research project in health. http://www.lgreen.net/guidelines.html. Accessed February 5, 2012.

ACKNOWLEDGMENTS

The challenges associated with producing the sixth edition of *Studying a Study and Testing a Test* have been made easier by the support and encouragement I have received from students, colleagues, and, of course, the many readers of the previous editions from around the world.

This edition required writing, restructuring, rewriting, and adding new materials to maximize the use of *Studying a Study and Testing a Test* as a textbook while retaining its value for the individual reader. All these benefited from feedback from students at the George Washington University School of Public Health and Health Services as well as the School of Medicine and Health Sciences.

Valuable input was provided by a large number of students and colleagues. Special acknowledgment is due to Erin McIntyre a P.A./M.P.H. student who contributed her ideas to the book in class and read and gave me feedback on every word of the manuscript. The staff of LWW has been essential to the design and production of the sixth edition. The new look of the cover and the content of the book reflect their skills in design. The care that went into every page of the book reflects their attention to detail. If any errors have occurred, the responsibility is mine alone.

The *Studying a Study and Testing a Test* site on thePoint is a joint project with my wife Linda. She has a unique ability to understand what technology can add to the learning process, an intuitive sense of how to make technology work, and the patience to explain it all to me. Writing a sixth edition of a book is an especially enjoyable experience if it means that you get to build upon the past while looking to the future. This has been the case with the sixth edition of *Studying a Study and Testing a Test*. I hope you will enjoy reading it as much as I enjoyed writing it.

Richard Riegelman, M.D., M.P.H., Ph.D.

INTRODUCTION

The traditional course in reading the health literature consists of "Here's *The New England Journal of Medicine*. Read it!" This approach is analogous to learning to swim by the total immersion method. Some persons can learn to swim this way, of course, but a few drown, and many learn to fear the water.

In contrast to the method of total immersion, you are about to embark on a step-by-step, active-participation approach to reading the evidence-based health research. With the tools that you will learn, you will soon be able to read a journal article critically and efficiently. Considerable emphasis is placed on the errors that can occur in the various kinds of studies, but try to remember that not every flaw is fatal. The goal of literature reading is to recognize the limitations of a study and then put them into perspective. This is essential before putting the results into practice.

To make your job easier, we will use a framework, which we will call the M.A.A.R.I.E. framework, to organize our review of each of the types of investigations. Before developing and illustrating the components of this framework, however, let us begin with a flaw-catching exercise. A flaw-catching exercise is a simulated journal article containing an array of errors. Read the following flaw-catching exercise and then try to answer the accompanying questions.

CRIES SYNDROME: CAUSED BY TELEVISION OR JUST BAD TASTE?

A condition known as Cries syndrome has been described as occurring among children of 7 to 9 years old. The condition is characterized by episodes of uninterrupted crying lasting at least an hour per day for three consecutive days. The diagnosis also includes symptoms of sore throat, runny nose, and fever, which precede the onset of the crying and are severe enough to keep the child out of school.

Investigators identified 100 children with Cries syndrome. For each Cries syndrome child, a classmate was chosen for comparison from among those who did not miss school. The study was conducted more than 1 month after the onset of symptoms. The investigators examined 20 variables, which included all the factors they could think of as being potentially associated with Cries syndrome. They collected data on all medication use, number of spankings, hours of television viewing, and number of hours at home, as well as 16 other variables.

Using pictures, they asked the children to identify the medications they had taken while they had Cries syndrome. Their classmates without Cries syndrome were also asked to use the pictures to identify medications taken during the same period. The investigators then asked each child to classify each medication taken as a good-tasting or bad-tasting medication. The data on spankings were obtained from the primary caregiver. The investigators found the following data:

Percentage of children who reported taking bad-tasting medication

Cries syndrome	90%
Controls	10%

Average number of spankings per day

Cries syndrome	1
Controls	2

Average number of television-viewing hours per day

Cries syndrome	8 (range 5 to 12)
Controls	2 (range 0 to 4)

Among the 20 variables, analyzed one at a time, the above were the only ones that were statistically significant using the usual statistical methods. The *P*-values were .05 except for the hours of television, which had a *P*-value of .001. The investigators drew the following conclusions:

1. Bad-tasting medication is a contributory cause of Cries syndrome because it was strongly associated with Cries syndrome.

2. Spanking protects children from Cries syndrome because the controls had an increased frequency of being spanked.

3. Television viewing of at least 4 hours per day is required for the development of Cries syndrome, because all children with Cries syndrome and none of the controls watched television more than 4 hours per day during the period under investigation.

4. Because Cries syndrome patients were nine times as likely to take bad-tasting medication, the investigators concluded that removing bad-tasting medication from the market would eliminate almost 90% of Cries syndrome cases among children similar to those in this investigation.

5. In addition, regular spanking of all children of 7 to 9 years old should be widely used as a method of preventing Cries syndrome.

Now to get an idea of what you will be learning in the "Studying a Study" unit, see if you can answer the following questions:

1. What type of investigation is this?

2. What is the study hypothesis?

3. Is the control group correctly assigned?

4. Are reporting and/or recall biases likely to be present in this study?

5. Does the method of data collection raise issues of precision and accuracy?

6. Is the estimate of the strength of the relationship performed correctly?

7. Is statistical significance testing performed correctly?

8. Is an adjustment procedure needed?

9. Is an association established between the use of bad-tasting medicine and the Cries syndrome?

10. Is it established that the spankings occurred prior to the development of Cries syndrome?

11. Is it established that altering the frequency of spankings will alter the frequency of Cries syndrome?

12. Is it established that television viewing of at least 4 hours per day is a necessary cause of Cries syndrome?

13. Can the investigators conclude that removing bad-tasting medication from the market would reduce the frequency of Cries syndrome by almost 90% among children similar to those in the study?

14. Can the investigators conclude that regular spanking of all children of 7 to 9 years old should be widely used as a method of preventing Cries syndrome?

To see how you have done, go to http://thepoint.lww.com. This is a good time to locate and bookmark this Web site since it provides additional materials that will help you gain hands-on practice using the skills that you will learn throughout *Studying a Study and Testing a Test*.

UNIT I

STUDYING A STUDY

1

Studying a Study: M.A.A.R.I.E. Framework—Method, Assignment, Assessment

Four basic types of investigations which compare groups of people are found in the health research literature (1,2):

- *population comparisons or ecological studies*
- *case-control studies or retrospective studies*
- *cohort studies or prospective studies*
- *randomized controlled trials or randomized clinical trials*

Each type of investigation attempts to address a defined question or hypothesis by comparing one or more study groups with one or more control groups.[1.1]

An organizing framework can be used to evaluate each of these types of investigation. The framework is divided into six components:

- **Method**
- **Assignment**
- **Assessment**
- **Results**
- **Interpretation**
- **Extrapolation**

We call this the **M.A.A.R.I.E.** framework, an acronym using the first letter of each component: **M**ethod, **A**ssignment, **A**ssessment, **R**esults, **I**nterpretation, and **E**xtrapolation. Figure 1.1 outlines the general application of the framework to a research study.

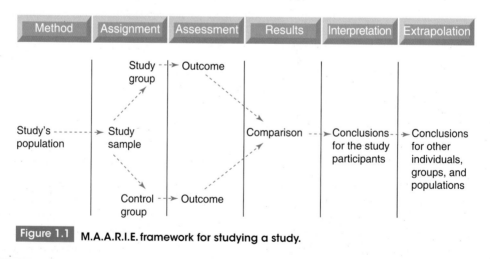

Figure 1.1 M.A.A.R.I.E. framework for studying a study.

[1.1] The investigations discussed in the "Studying a Study" section are sometimes called *analytical studies*. Analytical studies compare one or more study groups with one or more control groups. However, investigations do not always have control groups. *Descriptive studies* obtain data on a group of individuals without comparing them to another group. Sometimes descriptive studies may use data external to the investigation to compare a group in the investigation with other groups or to the same group at an earlier period. These comparison groups are sometimes called *historical controls*.

METHOD QUESTIONS

Method issues are common to all types of health research. They require the investigators to clarify exactly what they are attempting to achieve by defining what they will investigate, who they will investigate, and how many they will investigate. Each of the six components in the M.A.A.R.I.E. framework can be divided into three specific issues. For method, the issues and key questions are as follows:

- **Study hypothesis:** What is the study question being investigated?
- **Study population:** What population is being investigated including the inclusion and exclusion criteria for the participants in the investigation?
- **Sample size and statistical power:** How many individuals are included in the study and in the control groups? Are the numbers adequate to demonstrate statistical significance if the study hypothesis is true?

Before investigators can decide which and how many individuals to include in an investigation, they need to define the study hypothesis. Then they can focus on the question of which individuals from which populations should be included in the investigation.

Health research is not generally conducted by including everyone in the population of interest. Rather, it is performed using only a smaller group, or *sample*, of all individuals who could in theory be included. For all types of health research, choosing whom to include and how many to include in an investigation are basic method issues. Thus, **M**ethod, the first component of the M.A.A.R.I.E. framework, defines the study question and sets the rules for obtaining the study and control samples.

In recent years, ethical issues have been of increasing concern. Much of the attention on research issues in health research has focused on the methods used in randomized controlled trials. However, a number of issues apply to all forms of health research. As part of the methods component it is important to ask the question: Who is the investigator(s) and who is the funder(s) of the research? Potential conflicts of interest are now handled using formal procedures that are based on the belief that full disclosure of potential conflicts is the appropriate strategy for addressing these issues. Thus in high quality journals expect to see extensive information on the potential conflicts of interest of the investigators, the roles that each investigator played in the research, and a prominently placed identification of the funder(s).

The M.A.A.R.I.E. framework continues with the following additional components:

Assignment: Allocation of participants to study and control groups

Assessment: Measurement of outcome(s) or end point(s) in the study and control groups

Results: Comparison of the outcome in the study and control groups

Interpretation: Meaning of the results for those included in the investigation

Extrapolation: Meaning of the results for those not included in the investigation

To illustrate the application of the M.A.A.R.I.E. framework to population comparisons, case-control studies, cohort, and randomized controlled trials, let us outline the essential features of each type of study. We will then see how we can apply each type of investigation to the question of the potential risk of stroke with birth control pill use. The implications of these components of the M.A.A.R.I.E. framework differ slightly according to the type of investigation, as we discuss later in this chapter.

We will discuss each type of investigation by assuming that there is one study group and one control group. However, in all types of studies, more than one study group and more than one control group can be included.

APPLYING THE M.A.A.R.I.E. FRAMEWORK

Population Comparisons

The unique feature of population comparisons or ecological studies is their ability to suggest relationship between risk factors and diseases or other outcomes without having information on any one individual. Population comparisons are designed to compare the rates of events in two or more populations or to investigate changes that have occurred in the same population over a period of time. Alternatively, population comparisons may examine differences between two or more populations at the same point in time (Fig. 1.2).

Population comparisons compare rates in two or more populations without having available information on particular individuals. Population comparisons typically observe the rates of a disease or other outcome and the rates of a risk factor or other characteristic. They often ask whether populations with higher rates of the risk factor also have higher rates of the disease.

To examine the relationship between the use of birth control pills and stroke in young women, the investigator using a population comparison might proceed as follows:

Assignment: Select a study population and measure its rate of strokes among young women and a similar comparison control population and measure its rate of strokes among young women

Assessment: Determine the rate of use of birth control pills among young women in the study population and in the control population

Results: Compare the rates of use of birth control pills with the rates of strokes among young women in the study population and in the control population

Interpretation: Draw conclusions about the meaning of birth control pill use for women included in the investigation

Extrapolation: Draw conclusions about the meaning of birth control pill use for women not like those included in the investigation, such as women who have the option to use newer low-dose birth control pills.

When populations of young women with high rates of strokes also have high rates of use of birth control pills compared with populations of young women with low rates of strokes we say that a *group association* exists. That is, even though we do not know whether the particular women who developed stroke actually used birth control pills, we can conclude that an association exists at the group or population level. Identifying group associations are often the first step in demonstrating a cause and effect relationship, but as we will see group associations often merely suggest hypotheses for further investigation.

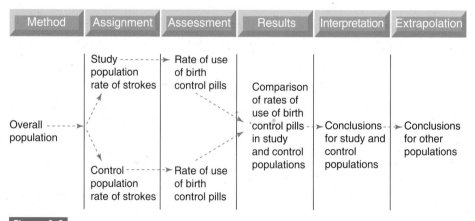

Figure 1.2 M.A.A.R.I.E. framework for a population comparison.

Case-Control Study

The unique feature of case-control studies of disease is that they begin by identifying individuals who have developed or failed to develop the disease or condition being investigated. After identifying those with and without the disease, they look back in time to determine the characteristics of individuals before the onset of disease. In case-control studies, the *cases* are the individuals who have developed the disease, and the *controls* are the individuals who have not developed the disease. To use a case-control study to examine the relationship between birth control pill use and stroke in young women, an investigator might proceed as follows:

> **Assignment:** Select a study group of young women who have had a stroke (cases) and a group of otherwise similar young women who have not had a stroke (controls). Because the development of the disease has occurred without the investigator's intervention, this process can be called *observed assignment.*

> **Assessment:** Determine whether each woman in the case or study group and also in the control group previously took birth control pills. The previous presence or absence of the use of birth control pills is the outcome in a case-control study.

> **Results:** Calculate the chances that the group of women with a stroke had used birth control pills versus the chances that the group of women without stroke had used birth control pills.

> **Interpretation:** Draw conclusions about the meaning of birth control pill use for women included in the investigation.

> **Extrapolation:** Draw conclusions about the meaning of birth control pill use for categories of women not like those included in the investigation, such as women on newer low-dose birth control pills.

Figure 1.3 illustrates the application of the M.A.A.R.I.E. framework to this investigation. Notice that case-control studies unlike population comparisons identify individuals and ask whether there is an association at the individual level between young women with strokes and the use of birth control pills. Thus case-control studies are capable of establishing what we will call an *individual association.*

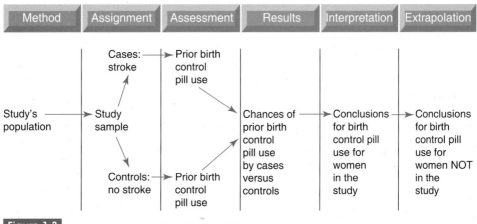

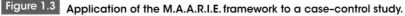

Figure 1.3 Application of the M.A.A.R.I.E. framework to a case-control study.

Cohort Study

Cohort studies of disease differ from case-control studies in that they begin by identifying individuals for study and control groups before the investigator is aware of whether they have developed the disease or other outcome. A *cohort* is a group of individuals who share a common experience. A cohort study begins by identifying a cohort that possesses the characteristics under study as well as a cohort that does not possess those characteristics. Then the frequency of developing the disease in each of the cohorts is obtained and compared. To use a cohort study to examine the relationship between birth control pill use and stroke, an investigator might proceed as follows:

Assignment: Select a study group of women who are using birth control pills and an otherwise similar control group of women who have never used birth control pills. Because the use of birth control pills is observed to occur without the investigator's intervention, this process is also called *observed assignment*.

Assessment: Determine who in the study group and the control group develops strokes. As opposed to a case-control study, the outcome for a cohort study is the subsequent presence or absence of a stroke.

Results: Calculate the chances of developing a stroke for women using birth control pills versus women not using birth control pills.

Interpretation: Draw conclusions about the meaning of birth control pill use for women included in the study.

Extrapolation: Draw conclusions about the meaning of birth control pill use for women not included in the study, such as women on newer low-dose birth control pills.

Figure 1.4 illustrates the application of the M.A.A.R.I.E. framework to a cohort study.

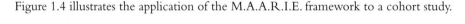

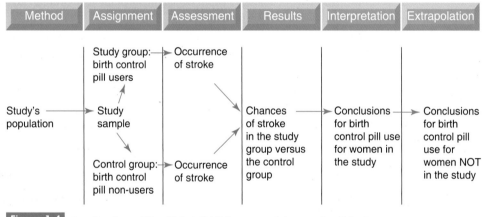

Figure 1.4 Application of the M.A.A.R.I.E. framework to a cohort study.

Randomized Controlled Trial

Randomized controlled trials are also called randomized clinical trials. They are a form of experimental study. As in cohort studies, individuals are assigned to study and control groups before determining who develops the disease or other outcome. The unique feature of randomized controlled trials, however, is the process for assigning individuals to study and control groups. In a randomized controlled trial, participants are randomized either to a study group or to a control group.

Randomization means that chance is used to assign a person to either the study or the control group. This is done so that any one individual has a known, but not necessarily equal, probability of being assigned to the study group or the control group. Ideally, the study participants as well as the investigators are not aware of which participants are in which group. *Double-blind* assignment means that neither the participant nor the investigators know whether the participant has been assigned to the study group or the control group. Single blinding implies that the participants are unaware of their group assignments.

To use a randomized controlled trial to examine the relationship between birth control pill use and stroke, an investigator might proceed as follows:

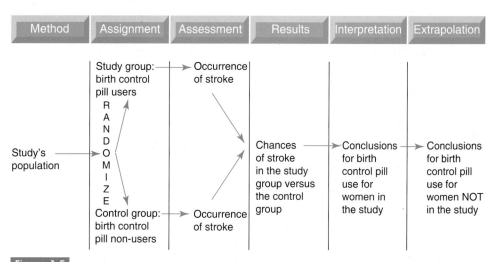

Figure 1.5 Application of the M.A.A.R.I.E. framework to a randomized controlled trial.

Assignment: Using randomization, women are assigned in a double-blind fashion to a study group that will be prescribed birth control pills or to a control group that will not be prescribed birth control pills.

Assessment: Observe these women to determine who subsequently develops stroke. As in a cohort study, in a randomized controlled trial the outcome is the presence or absence of stroke.

Results: Calculate the chances that women using birth control pills will develop a stroke versus women not using birth control pills.

Interpretation: Draw conclusions about the meaning of birth control pill use for women included in the study.

Extrapolation: Draw conclusions about the meaning of birth control pill use for women not included in the study, such as women on new low-dose birth control pills.

Figure 1.5 illustrates the application of the M.A.A.R.I.E. framework to a randomized controlled trial.

ADVANTAGES AND DISADVANTAGES OF THE BASIC STUDY TYPES (3,4,5)

The basic components and key questions we have outlined are common to the four basic types of investigations, the population comparison (or ecological study), case-control (or retrospective study), cohort (or prospective study), and randomized controlled trial (or experimental study). Each type, however, has its own strengths, weaknesses, and roles to play in health research.

Population comparisons have the advantage of not requiring information on specific individuals. They can often be conducted using routinely collected data that may permit the use of large data sets. This makes them relatively inexpensive to perform and rapid to conduct. They often provide a starting point for investigating relationships and generating hypotheses. In addition, once a cause and effect relationship and/or the efficacy of an intervention has been established, population comparisons can often be helpful in determining whether the intervention has effectiveness, that is it works in practice.

Case-control studies have the distinct advantage of being useful for studying rare conditions or diseases. If a condition is rare, case-control studies can detect differences between groups using far fewer individuals than other study designs. Often, much less time is needed to perform a case-control study because the disease has already developed. This method also allows investigators to simultaneously explore multiple characteristics or exposures that are potentially associated with a disease. One could examine, for instance, the many variables that are possibly associated with colon cancer, including diet, surgery, ulcerative colitis, polyps, alcohol, cigarettes, and family history.

Case-control studies are often capable of showing that a potential "cause" and a disease or other outcome occur together more often than expected by chance alone. Thus case-control studies are useful as initial investigations designed to establish the existence of an association at the individual level. Because case-control studies are able to examine rare diseases and rare outcomes, they can be used to investigate rare but serious adverse effects of treatment. The major objection to case-control studies is that they are prone to errors and biases that will be examined in the following chapters.

Cohort studies have the major advantage of demonstrating with greater assurance that a particular characteristic preceded a particular outcome being studied. As we will see, this is a critical distinction when assessing a cause-and-effect relationship. *Concurrent cohort studies or perspective cohort studies,* which follow patients forward over long periods are expensive and time consuming. It is possible, however, to perform a cohort study without such a lengthy follow-up period. If reliable data on the presence or absence of the study characteristic are available from an earlier time, these data can be used to perform a *nonconcurrent cohort study*, often called a *retrospective cohort study*. In a nonconcurrent or retrospective cohort study, the assignment of individuals to groups is made on the basis of these past data. However, the groups are identified without the investigator being aware of whether or not the participants developed the outcomes being assessed. Only after assignment has occurred, can the investigator look at the data on disease occurrence or other outcome.

For instance, if low-density lipoprotein (LDL) readings from a group of adults were available from 15 years before the current study began, those with and those without elevated LDL readings could be used as study and control groups. After establishing the study and control groups, it might be possible to search the database to assess the subsequent development of coronary artery disease, strokes, or other potential consequences of elevated LDL readings that might have occurred. The critical element, which characterizes all cohort studies, is the identification of individuals for study and control groups without knowledge of whether the disease or condition under investigation has developed.

Cohort studies can be used to delineate various consequences that may be produced by a single risk factor. For instance, researchers can simultaneously study the relationship between hypertension and stroke, myocardial infarction, heart failure, and renal disease. Cohort studies can produce more in-depth understanding of the effect of an etiologic factor on multiple outcomes.

Both case-control and cohort studies are *observational studies*; that is, they observe the assignment of individuals rather than impose the characteristics or interventions.

Randomized controlled trials are distinguished from observational studies by the randomization of individuals to study and control groups. Randomization helps to ensure that the study characteristic, and not some underlying predisposition, produces the study results. Randomized controlled trials can be used to study interventions including those that aim to prevent, cure, or palliate disease. They are capable of establishing whether an intervention has *efficacy*; that is, whether it works under carefully controlled research conditions. As we will see, when properly performed, randomized controlled trials are able to demonstrate all three definitive criteria for contributory cause or efficacy: individual association, prior association, and altering the cause alter the effect. The strengths and weaknesses of randomized controlled trials are explored in depth in Chapter 4.

As we have seen, there are three key questions to ask pertaining to the method component of the M.A.A.R.I.E. framework. There are also three key questions to ask regarding each of the other components. These questions are briefly outlined in the following sections. These 15 questions along with the 3 questions from the method component make up what we might call the Questions to Ask when Studying a Study. These questions form the basis for the M.A.A.R.I.E. framework and can serve as a checklist when reading journal articles. We will examine the questions in greater detail in the chapters that follow.

ASSIGNMENT QUESTIONS

The assignment component asks the following three questions about the characteristics of the study and the control groups:

- **Process of assignment:** What method is being used to identify and assign individuals or populations to study and control groups, that is, observed or randomization?
- **Confounding variables:** Are there differences between the study and control groups, other than the characteristic under investigation, that may affect the outcome of the investigation?
- **Masking or blinding:** Are the participants and/or the investigators aware of the assignment to a particular study or control group?

ASSESSMENT QUESTIONS

The process of assessment asks three basic questions about the quality of how the investigation's outcomes were measured:

- **Appropriate:** Does the measurement of an outcome address the study's question?
- **Accurate precise and measurement:** Is the measurement of an outcome an accurate and precise measure of the phenomenon that the investigation seeks to assess?
- **Complete and unaffected by observation:** Is the outcome measurement nearly 100% complete and is it affected by the participants' or the investigators' knowledge of the study group or control group assignment?

RESULTS QUESTIONS

The results component quantitatively compares the measures of outcome obtained in the study group and in the control group. It requires us to ask the following three basic questions:

- **Estimation:** What is the magnitude or strength of the relationship observed in the investigation?
- **Inference:** What statistical technique(s) are used to perform statistical significance testing?
- **Adjustment:** What statistical technique(s) are used to take into account or control for differences between the study group and control group that may affect the results?

INTERPRETATION QUESTIONS

The interpretation component asks us to draw conclusions regarding the participants in the investigation. Initially, it asks us to draw conclusions about cause-and-effect relationships, or what we will call *contributory cause* when we are talking about the etiology of a disease, or *efficacy* when we are asking whether an intervention works to improve outcome. We also ask whether the intervention produces harms and whether it works especially well or not well at all for *subgroups*, that is, those with special characteristics. The three basic questions for interpretation are as follows:

- **Contributory cause or efficacy:** Does the factor being investigated alter the probability that the disease will occur (contributing cause) or work to reduce the probability of an undesirable outcome (efficacy)?
- **Harms:** Are adverse events that impact the meaning of the results identified?
- **Subgroups and interactions:** Do the outcomes in subgroups differ and are there interactions between factors that affect outcome?

EXTRAPOLATION QUESTIONS

Extrapolation of health research studies asks how we can go beyond the data and the participants in a particular investigation to draw conclusions about individuals, groups, and populations that are not specifically included in the investigation. These groups may be your patients, your institution, or your community. These three key questions address extrapolation:

- **To similar individuals, groups, or populations:** Do the investigators extrapolate or extend the conclusions to individuals, groups, or populations that are similar to those who participated in the investigation?
- **Beyond the data:** Do the investigators extrapolate by extending the conditions beyond the dose, duration, or other characteristics of the investigation?
- **To other populations:** Do the investigators extrapolate to populations or settings that are quite different from those in the investigation?

The 6 components and 18 questions put together in the following chart comprise the M.A.A.R.I.E. framework for Studying a Study.

Questions To Ask: Studying a Study

Method—The purpose, population, and study sample for the investigation
1. **Study hypothesis:** What is the study question being investigated?
2. **Study population:** What population is being investigated including the inclusion and exclusion criteria for the participants in the investigation?
3. **Sample size and statistical power:** How many individuals are included in the study and in the control groups? Are the numbers adequate to demonstrate statistical significance if the study hypothesis is true?

Assignment—Allocation of participants to study and control groups
1. **Process:** What method is used to identify and assign individuals or populations to study and control groups?
2. **Confounding variables:** Are there differences between study and control groups, other than the factor being investigated that may affect the outcome of the investigation?
3. **Masking or blinding:** Are the participants and/or the investigators aware of the participants' assignment to a particular study or control group?

Assessment—Measurement of outcomes or end points in the study and control groups
1. **Appropriate:** Does the measurement of outcomes address the study's question?
2. **Accurate and precise:** Is the measurement of outcomes an accurate and precise measure of the phenomenon that the investigators seek to assess?
3. **Complete and unaffected by observation:** Is the outcome measurement nearly 100% complete and is it affected by the participants' or the investigators' knowledge of the study or control group assignment?

Results—Comparison of outcomes in the study and control groups
1. **Estimation:** What is the magnitude or strength of the relationship observed in the investigation?
2. **Inference:** What statistical technique(s) are used to perform statistical significance testing?
3. **Adjustment:** What statistical technique(s) are used to take into account or control for differences between the study group and the control group that may affect the results?

Interpretation—Meaning of the results for those included in the investigation
1. **Contributory cause or efficacy:** Does the factor being investigated alter the probability that the disease will occur (contributory cause) or work to reduce the probability of undesirable outcomes (efficacy)?

Questions To Ask: Studying a Study *(Continued)*

2. **Harms:** Are adverse events that affect the meaning of the results identified?
3. **Subgroups and interactions:** Do the outcomes in subgroups differ and are there interactions between factors that affect outcome?

Extrapolation—Meaning of the results for those not included in the investigation

1. **To similar individuals, groups, or populations:** Do the investigators extrapolate or extend the conclusions to individuals, groups, or populations that are similar to those who participated in the investigation?
2. **Beyond the data:** Do the investigators extrapolate by extending the conclusions beyond the dose, duration, or other characteristics of the investigation?
3. **To other populations:** Do the investigators extrapolate to populations or settings that are quite different from those in the investigation?

The four types of studies that we have now introduced are not the only important types of human research. Learn More 1.1 discusses additional types of human research and the roles that they can play.

LEARN MORE 1.1 ■ OTHER TYPES OF HUMAN RESEARCH ■ Other types of human studies may set the stage for analytical studies by helping to generate ideas. Alternatively they may provide explanations for the observed results of analytical studies. These types of research are said to have roles in exploration and explanation. Two important types of studies that complement analytical studies have been called *qualitative studies* and *descriptive studies*.

Qualitative research is an increasingly important type of research which looks in-depth at a small sample. It is the small size and intensive investigation not its inability to make quantitative measurements that characterizes research as qualitative. Qualitative research may explore the potential determinants of disease. Qualitative research may focus on the process of decision making and provides clues about underlying mechanisms that are useful in evaluating the reasons for successes or failures of interventions.

Focus groups are an increasingly important form of social science research that are being used in marketing, including social marketing as well as in gaining insight into how and why people come to conclusions or hold opinions. The opinions examined increasing go beyond commercial products and opinions of politicians to include use of health services, acceptance of new and existing technology, and speculation about the reasons for diseases and health outcomes. The ideas generated by these types of investigations may generate new hypothesis to be examined using analytical studies. They may also help assess barrier to implementation and suggest new approaches when extrapolating beyond analytical research data as illustrated in the next scenario.

Mini-Study 1.1 ■ A focus group of diabetics identified ease of blood sugar testing as key to their successful control of their blood sugar. Randomized controlled trials of new methods for blood sugar testing confirmed the importance of ease of use. Subsequent evaluation studies followed a small group of users of the new blood sugar testing equipment and found that success with blood sugar testing appeared to be greatest when individuals had a target for fasting and late afternoon blood sugar.

This example illustrates how qualitative research can generate hypotheses that may be investigated using analytical studies including randomized

(Continued)

controlled trials. It also illustrates how qualitative research can be used to help evaluate outcomes. Thus, qualitative research should not be viewed as competitive with quantitative research but rather as complementary often assisting in framing the issues and evaluating the outcomes examined in analytical research.

Descriptive studies usually imply that the goal of the research is not to compare groups or populations but to measure a characteristic of a group or population. Descriptive studies of this type often do not have a hypothesis to test, and they may be used to develop hypotheses. Descriptive studies are usually quantitative and may seek to establish the frequently or prevalence of a condition. The results of descriptive studies may help with allocation of resources and help guide the focus of future research. Thus, descriptive studies like qualitative studies often complement analytical studies.[1,2]

The following scenario illustrates potential uses of descriptive studies for generating hypotheses:

Mini-Study 1.2 ■ Children with hepatoma, a common cancer in much of Asia and Africa, were studied and found to have hepatitis B infection in >90% of cases even when cirrhosis was absent. This data suggested the hypothesis that hepatitis B was associated with and may have a causal relationship to hepatoma.

This investigation did not have a control group and is thus a descriptive study. Nonetheless, investigators are assuming that the 90% of hepatitis B is much greater than would be expected. Descriptive studies may suggest a hypothesis for further study.[1,3]

Now let us take a more in-depth look at how we can combine the use of our basic types of study designs to draw conclusions about contributory cause or alternatively about efficacy.

COMBINING THE BASIC TYPES OF STUDIES

Let us look at the way the basic types of investigations may be used together to establish contributory cause or alternatively to establish efficacy. Contributory cause implies that the following definitive criteria have been established:

- The "cause" is associated with the "effect" at the individual level
- The "cause" precedes in time the "effect"
- Altering the "cause" alters the "effect"[1,4]

[1,2] Descriptive studies may be derived from *surveys* that collect data on a sample of individuals. Surveys may also be used as the basis for a special type of analytical studies known as *cross-section studies* if samples are used to create and compare subgroups with and without a characteristic of interest. Cross-sectional studies may be seen as a special type of observational study in which the independent and the dependent variable are measured at the same point in time. Thus, cross-sectional studies reflect the prevalence of a condition not its incidence.

[1,3] Descriptive studies often are used to describe the clinical course of a disease or condition. In doing this, they utilize measures often called *rates*. Key rates used to describe the course of a disease or condition are the *incidence rate*, the *prevalence*, and the *case-fatality*. The incidence rate is the number of cases divided by the population at risk per year. It is often expressed as number of cases/100,000 population/year. Prevalence is the probability that the disease or condition is present at a particular point in time. Prevalence may be expressed as a probability or percentage. Case-fatality expresses the probability of dying from the disease once it is diagnosed.

[1,4] As we will discuss in a later chapter, the criteria for efficacy, that is, an intervention works under the conditions in which it is investigated, are the same as those required to definitively establish contributory cause. Often it is difficult or unethical to perform investigations needed to definitively establish contributory cause or efficacy. In these situations, ancillary or additional criteria can often be made to make scientific judgments or educated guesses about contributory cause or efficacy. In addition, when we are dealing with communicable diseases, these criteria need to be modified to incorporate information on the communicable nature of the disease.

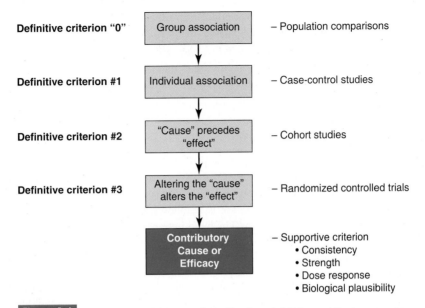

Figure 1.6 Use of multiple types of studies to establish contributory cause or efficacy.

The four basic types of investigations are often combined to fulfill these criteria as illustrated in Figure 1.6. Population comparisons can be often used to generate hypotheses by using data from populations without knowing whether the outcome for particular individuals. Thus, we call the results of population comparisons "criterion 0." They lay the groundwork for subsequent studies by generating hypotheses to be investigated, but they do not in-and-of-themselves establish any of the definitive criteria.

Case-control studies are especially good at definitively establishing criterion #1, the "cause" is associated with the "effect" at the individual level. By association we mean that the "cause" and the "effect" occur together in individuals more often than we expect by chance alone.

Cohort studies are often the definitive method for established criterion #2, the "cause" precedes the "effect." Because cohort studies assemble their study and control groups before the outcomes are known, they are considered more reliable than case-control studies for establishing which came first.

Randomized controlled trials are often needed to definitively establish that altering the cause alters the effect. The randomization process is designed to create very similar study and control groups. The study group is offered an intervention designed to alter the outcome and while the control group is not offered the intervention. If the study group has a better outcome than the control group, we can conclude that the altering the "cause" alters the "effect."

Now that we have outlined the basic types of studies and the components of the M.A.A.R.I.E. framework, let us take a more in-depth look at each of the six components of the M.A.A.R.I.E. framework.

Method

Investigations begin by identifying a study hypothesis as well as study and control samples to investigate a specific question in a defined population. Remember, the three key questions of method are as follows:

- **Study hypothesis:** What is the study question being investigated?

- **Study population:** What population is being investigated including the inclusion and exclusion criteria for the participants in the investigation?
- **Sample size and statistical power:** How many individuals are included in the study and in the control groups? Are the numbers adequate to demonstrate statistical significance if the study hypothesis is true?

Now let us examine these questions one at a time.

Study Hypothesis

The study's hypothesis, or study question, provides the starting point from which an investigation is organized. It defines the purpose of the investigation. Thus, a study hypothesis is essential for all investigations that compare study and control groups. When reading the health research literature, therefore, the first question to ask is as follows: What is the study hypothesis? Investigators should explicitly define a hypothesis. The hypothesis may be an association between a characteristic known as a *risk factor* (e.g., birth control pills) and a disease (e.g., stroke), or between an intervention (e.g., reduction in blood pressure) and an improvement in outcome (e.g., reduced frequency of strokes).[1.5]

To conduct an investigation, it is important to have a specific study hypothesis that is compatible with the type of investigation being conducted. Failure to clarify the hypothesis being investigated makes it difficult for the researcher to choose the study design and the reader to assess its appropriateness. For instance, imagine the following situation:

Mini-Study 1.3 ■ An investigator wishes to demonstrate that birth control pills are a contributory cause of strokes. The investigator conducts a case-control study using very careful methods. The results demonstrate a strong relationship between birth control pills and strokes. The investigator concludes that birth control pills are a contributory cause of stroke.

This investigator has failed to recognize that the use of a case-control study implies that the investigator is interested in demonstrating criterion #1 of contributory cause that is birth control pills are associated with strokes at the individual level. Case-control studies are not capable of completely demonstrating that birth control pills are a contributory cause of strokes.

Hypotheses for investigations may be generated using a number of different approaches. Learn More 1.2 discussed the basic methods that can be used to generate hypotheses.

Study Population

The population being studied must be defined before beginning an investigation. This requires the investigators to define the characteristics of individuals who will be selected for the study group and the control group. The study's populations may or may not represent the population that we are interested in for purposes such as prevention or treatment. This population of interest is called

---

[1.5] The term "risk factor" will be used here as a generic term implying only that at least an association at the individual level has been established. When only an association at the individual level has been established, the term *risk marker* can be used. When an association at the individual level as well as the "cause" precedes the "effect" has been established, the term *risk predictor* may be used.

LEARN MORE 1.2 ■ HYPOTHESIS GENERATION—WHERE DO HYPOTHESES COME FROM? (6) ■ Hypotheses for research investigations can be generated through at least two fundamentally different mechanisms. One is often called *deductive reasoning* and the other *inductive reasoning*. Hypotheses based on deductive reasoning originate in generalizations about biological relationship. These generalizations may come from the basic sciences or from clinical setting. Hypotheses generated from inductive reasoning, however, are based on clinical or population observations or associations that produce ideas or hypotheses that suggest cause and effect relationships or the efficacy of interventions.

Both types of reasoning are common sources of hypotheses for analytical studies. Deductive reasoning may be grounded in generalizations from basic sciences such as genetics, understanding of transport mechanisms, or extracellular receptors, etc. Clinical understandings my produce ideas that have importance in term of the etiology of disease or the efficacy of interventions. At the clinical level, deductive reasoning may rely on physiological principles, anatomical relationships, or understandings of the developmental process. Each of these may provide the basis for producing hypotheses about new situations or new setting.

The use of analogies is a special form of deductive logic, in which we obtain hypotheses directly from what we understand about other clinical or basic science situations. Whenever we study animals and generate hypotheses to investigate in humans we are generating hypotheses by deductive reasoning. Whenever we draw clinical conclusions such as technology that works in the coronary arteries is also likely to work in the carotid, renal, or femoral arteries, we are using deductive reasoning to produce hypotheses for investigation.

As opposed to deductive reasoning, many hypotheses that we investigate using analytical studies are derived from data or observations on similar populations; that is, they are based on inductive reasoning. The process of deriving hypotheses by inductive reasoning uses a series of strategies that rely on clinical and population data. Among the most important of these strategies are the following:

Method of differences: Different rates of occurrence of a factor in different populations that also differ in their rates of disease can suggest a hypothesis. For instance, the higher rates of melanoma in states with warmer temperature and more days of sunshine suggested a relationship between melanoma and sun exposure. The higher rate of human immunodeficiency virus (HIV)/acquired immunodeficiency syndrome (AIDS) in African countries with lower rates of male circumcision suggested the potential for an effective intervention.

Method of agreement: when a factor and a disease occur together in a number of different situations, it may suggest the hypothesis that the factor plays a causal role. For instance, the role that blood exposure plays in transfusions, needle exchange, and treatment for hemophilia led to the hypothesis of blood-borne transmission of HIV.

Method of concomitant variation: When the frequency of a factor increases and decreases before a parallel change in frequency of a disease, it may lead to the hypothesis that the factor plays an etiological role in the disease. A dramatic increase in lung cancer a decade or more after an increase in cigarette smoking among males followed by a similar increase among females after an increase in female cigarette smoking strongly suggested an etiological relationship between cigarettes and lung cancer.

Method of clusters and exceptions: In addition to associations in large populations, hypotheses may be developed based upon data from small-scale clinical observation or *clusters*. Clusters are the occurrence of an unexpected number of rare events in a small geographic area or over a short period. Clusters may result from chance or they may suggest more general hypotheses about etiology or effectiveness. For instance, a handful of cases of an angiosarcoma, a unusual liver tumor, among workers exposed to

(Continued)

polyvinyl chloride in the same factory strongly suggested an etiological relationship. A small number of prostitutes with negative-HIV tests despite multiple exposures to HIV suggested the hypothesis of potential genetic protection from HIV infection.

Unexpected clinical observations are often the basis for hypothesis generation. Adverse events such as those associated with drugs may form the basis for new treatments. In recent years, unexpected hair growth in balding males and unanticipated improvement in erectile dysfunction have been the basis for hypotheses about effectiveness of drugs for these conditions. Similarly, the appearance of a small number of cases of a disease among those at low risk may suggest hypotheses. Investigating exposures of males with breast cancer or females with evidence of testosterone effects may lead to important hypotheses for future investigation.

Thus, both deductive and inductive methods play important roles in hypothesis generation. Neither of the methods can be considered definitive, and hypotheses generated from these methods need to be investigated using the types of analytical methods that are discussed in the future chapters.

the *target population*. More generally, the target population is the large group of individuals to whom we wish to apply the results of the investigation. It is important to appreciate whether the population actually included in an investigation actually reflects the target population, as illustrated in the next example:

Mini-Study 1.4 ■ A vaccine designed for high-risk premature infants in intensive care units was investigated among healthy newborns. The healthy newborns were shown to have a strong antibody response to the vaccine and a high degree of clinical protection.

No matter how well designed this investigation, its implications for high-risk premature infants in the intensive care use will be limited. When the target population for an intervention, whether for prevention or cure is known, it is important that the study's population reflect the target population.

In order to define the study population, investigators need to specify what are called *inclusion criteria* and *exclusion criteria*. Inclusion criteria must be present for an individual to be eligible to participate in an investigation. Even if the inclusion criteria are met, presence of exclusion criteria means that the individual is not eligible for the investigation. Let us see why inclusion and exclusion criteria are needed by looking at the next example:

Mini-Study 1.5 ■ An investigator wanted to study the effect of a new therapy for duodenal ulcers. He selected all available duodenal ulcer patients and found that the treatment, on average, resulted in no improvement in outcome. Later research revealed that the therapy provided a substantial improvement in outcome for recurrent duodenal ulcer patients who did not have an elevated gastrin level.

If this investigation had been conducted by requiring recurrent disease as an inclusion criterion and had used elevated gastrin levels as an exclusion criterion, the results would have been very different. Inclusion criteria serve to identify the types of individuals who should be included in the investigation. Exclusion criteria serve to remove individuals from eligibility because of special circumstances that may complicate their treatment or make interpretation more difficult.

Inclusion and exclusion criteria define the characteristics of the population being studied. In addition, they narrow the group to which the results can be directly applied. For instance, if those with a first diagnosis of duodenal ulcers are not included in the study, the results of the study may not apply to them.

Sample Size and Statistical Power

Having identified the study hypothesis and the study population, the reader of the health research literature should focus on the sample size of individuals selected for study and control groups. The question to ask is

- Is there an adequate number of participants to demonstrate statistical significance if the study hypothesis is true?

The answer to this question is given by the *statistical power* of an investigation. Statistical power is the probability of demonstrating statistical significance if the study hypothesis is true. Research articles often identify the *type II error* rather than statistical power. Type II error is the complement of the statistical power. In other words, type II error is the probability of failing to demonstrate statistical significance if the study hypothesis is true in the larger population from which the study's samples are obtained.

Thus, if the type II error is 10%, the statistical power is 90%; if the type II error is 20%, the statistical power is 80%. Well-designed investigations should include enough individuals in the study and control groups to provide at least an 80% statistical power, or 80% probability of demonstrating statistical significance if the study hypothesis is true in the larger population from which the study's samples are obtained.

As we will see when we further discuss sample size in Chapter 4, statistical power depends on a series of assumptions. In addition, the number of individuals required to obtain the same statistical power is much smaller in case-control studies compared with cohort studies or randomized controlled trials. Failure to appreciate this distinction can lead to the following type of result:

> **Mini-Study 1.6** ■ Investigators wished to study whether birth control pills are associated with the rare occurrence of strokes in young women. The researchers monitored 2,000 women on birth control pills and 2,000 women on other forms of birth control for 10 years. After spending millions of dollars in follow-up, they found two cases of stroke among the pill users and one case among the non–pill-users. The differences were not statistically significant.

In case-control studies of birth control pills and stroke, we are interested in determining whether the use of birth control pills is greater among those with stroke. Birth control pill use may be an overwhelmingly common characteristic of young women who have experienced a stroke. If so, the sample size required to conduct a case-control study may be quite small, perhaps 100 or less in each group.

However, when conducting a cohort study or randomized controlled trial, even if there is a very strong relationship between birth control pill use and stroke, it may be necessary to follow a large number of women who are taking and are not taking birth control pills to demonstrate a statistically significant relationship between birth control pills and strokes. When the occurrence of an outcome such as stroke is rare, say considerably <1%, many thousands of women may be required for the study and control groups in cohort and randomized controlled trials to provide an adequate statistical power to demonstrate statistical significance, even if the study hypothesis is true. In Chapter 4, we explore in more depth the implications of sample size.

Thus, the method component of the M.A.A.R.I.E. framework requires that we consider the study's hypothesis, the study's population being investigated, and the adequacy of the sample size. Equipped with an understanding of these key method questions, we are ready to turn our attention to the next component of our M.A.A.R.I.E. framework, assignment.

Assignment

The second component of the M.A.A.R.I.E. framework is assignment, the selection of participants for the study and control groups. Regardless of the type of investigation, there are three basic assignment questions:

- **Process:** What method is being used to assign participants to study and control groups?
- **Confounding variables:** Are there differences between the study and the control groups, other than the factor being investigated, that may affect the outcome of the investigation?
- **Masking:** Are the participants and/or the investigators aware of the participants' assignment to a particular study or control group?

Process

Population comparisons, case-control, and cohort studies are known as *observational studies*. In an observational study, no intervention is attempted, and thus no attempt is made to alter the course of a disease. The investigators observe the course of the disease among individuals or groups with and without the characteristics being studied. Therefore, the assignment process can be called observed assignment.

In case-control and cohort studies, individual assignment is observed. This term implies that the researcher identifies individuals who meet the inclusion and exclusion criteria to become participants in an investigation. The researcher does not intervene to place the individual into a study or control group. Their assignment is the result of the natural course of events or the impact of clinical decision making as part of the process of health care.

The goal in creating study and control groups is to select participants for each of these groups who are as similar as possible, except for the presence or absence of the characteristic being investigated. Sometimes this goal is not achieved in a particular study because of a flawed method of observed assignment that creates what is called a *selection bias*.

Few terms are less clearly understood or more loosely used than the word "bias." Bias is not the same as prejudice. It does not imply a prejudgment before the facts are known. Bias in assignment occurs when investigators unintentionally allow factors into either the study or the control group that influence the outcome of the study. Differences between the study and control groups, due to method of assignment, which affect the outcome being measured are known as *selection bias*. The elements of selection bias are illustrated in the following hypothetical study:

Mini-Study 1.7 ■ A case-control study of premenopausal breast cancer compared the past use of birth control pills among 500 women who have breast cancer to the past use of the pill among 500 age-matched women admitted to the hospital for hypertension or diabetes. Investigators found that 40% of the women with breast cancer had used birth control pills during the preceding 5 years, whereas only 5% of those with hypertension or diabetes in the control group had used the pill. The authors concluded that a strong association existed between the use of birth control pills and the development of premenopausal breast cancer.

To determine whether a selection bias may have existed, we need to examine how the patients were assigned to the study and the control groups. We should first ask whether the women in the control group were similar to the women in the study group except that they did not have breast cancer. The answer is no. The women in the control group were quite different from the women in the study group because they had been admitted to the hospital for hypertension or diabetes. One must then ask whether these unique characteristics (hypertension or diabetes) were likely to have affected the results under investigation—that is, use of birth control pills.

The answer is yes. Because birth control pills are widely known to increase blood pressure and blood sugar, clinicians generally do not and should not prescribe birth control pills to women with hypertension or diabetes. Thus, the unique health characteristics of these women in the control group most likely contributed to a lower use of birth control pills. This investigation's method of assignment, therefore, created a selection bias; the groups differed in a way that made a difference in outcome.

Selection bias can also occur in a cohort study, as illustrated in the following example:

> **Mini-Study 1.8** ■ The effect of cigarette smoking on the development of myocardial infarctions was studied by selecting 10,000 middle-aged cigarette smokers and 10,000 middle-aged cigar smokers who have never smoked cigarettes. Both groups were observed for 10 years. The investigators found that the cigarette smokers had a rate of new myocardial infarction of 4 per 100 over 10 years, whereas the cigar smokers had a rate of new myocardial infarction of 7 per 100 over 10 years. The results were statistically significant. The investigators concluded that cigarette smokers have a lower risk of myocardial infarctions than cigar smokers do.

Despite the statistical significance of this difference, the conclusion conflicts with the results of many other studies. Let us see if selection bias could have led to this.

The first question is whether the study and control groups differ. The answer is yes: cigar and cigarette smokers differ in a number of ways. For example, men constitute the vast majority of cigar smokers, whereas many more women smoke cigarettes than cigars. To establish the potential for a selection bias, we must also ask whether this difference could affect the outcome being measured. Again, the answer is yes. Middle-aged men have a higher risk of myocardial infarction than middle-aged women do. Thus, both elements of selection bias are present. The study and control groups differ with regard to a particular factor and differences in that factor could affect the outcome being measured. Similarly cigar smokers may be older than cigarette smokers and age greatly affect the risk of coronary artery disease.

Confounding Variables

Even when a study is properly designed so that selection bias is unlikely, difference between groups can occur by chance. This is called *random error*. Thus, either selection bias or chance can produce study and control groups that differ according to certain characteristics that might affect the results of the investigation. When these differences in characteristics affect outcome, regardless of why they occurred, we refer to them as *confounding variables*. Thus, selection bias is a special type of confounding variable, which results from the way the study group or control group subjects are selected.

It is important to compare the study group and the control group subjects to determine whether they differ in ways that are likely to affect the outcome of the investigation even when there is no evidence of selection bias. Most research articles include a table, often the first table in the article, which identifies the characteristics that the investigators know about the study and the control groups. This allows the researcher and the reader to compare the groups to determine whether large or important differences have been identified. These differences may be the result of bias or chance. Regardless of whether they result from bias or chance, these differences need to be recognized and subsequently considered into account or adjusted for as part of the analysis of results.[1.6]

At times confounding variables can be prevented by using methods known as *matching* and *pairing* as discussed in Learn More 1.3.

LEARN MORE 1.3 ■ MATCHING AND PAIRING ■ One method for circumventing the problem of confounding variables is to match individuals who are similar with respect to characteristics that might affect the study's results. For instance, if age is related to the probability of being a member of either the study group or the control group, and if age is also related to the outcome being measured, then the investigator may match for age. For instance, for every 65-year-old in the control group, investigators could choose one 65-year-old for the study group, and similarly with 30-year-olds, 40-year-olds, and so on. If properly performed, the process of matching guarantees that the distribution of ages in each group will be the same.

Matching is not limited to making the groups uniform for age. It may be used for any characteristic related to the probability of experiencing the outcome under study. For example, if one were planning a cohort study addressing the relationship between birth control pills and breast cancer, family history of premenopausal breast cancer would be an important characteristic to consider for matching.

A disadvantage of matching groups is that the investigators cannot study the effect that the "matching characteristic" has on the outcome being measured. For instance, if they match for age and family history of premenopausal breast cancer, they lose the ability to study how age or family history affects the development of breast cancer. Furthermore, they lose the ability to study factors that are closely associated with the matched factor. This pitfall of matching is illustrated in the following example:

Mini-Study 1.9 ■ One hundred patients with adult-onset diabetes were compared with 100 nondiabetic adults to study factors associated with adult-onset diabetes. The groups were matched to ensure a similar weight distribution in the two groups. The authors also found that the total calories consumed in each of the two groups was nearly identical, and concluded that the number of calories consumed was not related to the possibility of developing adult-onset diabetes.

The authors of the study, having matched the patients by weight, attempted to study the differences in calories consumed. Because there is a strong association between weight and calories consumed, it is not surprising that the authors found no difference in consumption of calories between the two groups matched for weight. This type of error is called *overmatching*.

The type of matching used in the diabetes example is called *group matching*. Group matching seeks an equal distribution of matched characteristics in each group. A second type of matching is known as *pairing*. Pairing involves identifying one individual in the study group who can be

(Continued)

[1.6] Note that the reader can evaluate only those characteristics the investigator identifies. Thus, the reader should ask whether there are additional characteristics that would have been important to compare. The investigators can only adjust for difference that they identify. However, randomization, especially when the sample size is large, is capable of eliminating differences the investigator does not recognize. That is, when randomization is used; chance alone tends to produce similar groups when the sample size is large. This is how randomization is capable of eliminating potential confounding variables even those that are unknown to the investigators. We will discuss more about this seemingly magic ability of randomization in Chapter 4.

compared with one individual in the control group. Pairing of individuals using one or a small number of characteristics can be a very effective way to avoid selection bias.

Pairing is a useful technique for preventing selection bias, but it needs to be used sparingly. Although it may in theory be desirable to pair for a large number of characteristics, this may make identification of a control individual to pair with a study individual much more difficult, as illustrated in the next example:

Mini-Study 1.10 ■ A case–control study was conducted of the relationship between lung cancer and exposure to a drug. The investigators attempted to pair the cases with controls matched for pack-year of cigarette smoking and exposure to environmental factors such as radon, age, and gender—all factors that were believed to be related to the chances of developing lung cancer. Unfortunately, the investigators were not able to complete the investigation because they could not identify controls that fulfilled these criteria.

Thus, for practical reasons, it is important to limit matching to very important characteristics that will not prevent identification of enough subjects to use as controls.

This problem can sometimes be circumvented by using a study subject as his or her own control in what is called a *cross-over study*. In a cross-over study, the same individuals are compared with themselves, for instance, while on and off medication. When properly performed, cross-over studies allow an investigator to use the same individuals in the study group and control group, and to then pair their results, thus keeping many factors constant.[1.7]

Cross-over studies must be used with great care, however, or they can produce misleading results, as the following hypothetical study illustrates:

Mini-Study 1.11 ■ A study of the benefit of a new nonnarcotic medication for postoperative pain relief was performed by giving 100 patients the medication on postoperative day 1 and a placebo on day 2. For each patient, the degree of pain was measured using a well-established pain scale. The investigators found no difference between levels of pain on and off the medication.

When evaluating a cross-over study, one must recognize the potential for an effect of time and a carry-over effect of treatment. Pain is expected to decrease with time after surgery, so it is not accurate to compare the degree of pain on day 1 with the degree of pain on day 2. Furthermore, one must be careful to assess whether there may be a carry-over effect in which the medication from day 1 continues to be active on day 2. Thus, the absence of benefit in this cross-over trial should not imply that pain medication on day 1 after surgery is no more effective than a placebo on day 2.

Matching and pairing are two methods for preventing confounding variables that can be helpful techniques, when properly used. It is important to recognize that they are not the only techniques available to address the issues of confounding variables. One can think of inclusion and exclusion criteria as another technique for ensuring that the study and control groups are similar. In addition, adjustment of data as part of the results component can be combined with group matching or pairing to take into account the impact of confounding variables that are present.

[1.7] All types of pairing allow the use of statistical significance tests, which increase the probability of demonstrating statistical significance for a particular size study group. Statistical significance tests used with pairing are called *paired test*, although they are often called *matched tests* even though they cannot be used for data that utilizes group matching.

Finally, randomization can be thought of as the best way to prevent the occurrence of confounding especially when the sample size is large. More than one of these methods for dealing with the possibility of confounding may be and often is used in investigations.

Masking

Masking, or blinding, attempts to remove one source of bias by preventing each study participant and the investigators from knowing whether any one individual was assigned to a study group or to a control group. The term *masking* is considered a more accurate reflection of the actual process and is currently considered the technically correct term, although the term *blinding* is still commonly used.

When masking is successfully conducted as part of the assignment process, we can be confident that knowledge of group assignment did not influence the outcomes that were measured as part of the assessment process. Masking of study subjects is a desirable technique that may be used in a randomized controlled trial. However, it is not usually feasible in either case-control or cohort investigations. In case-control studies, the patients have already experienced the outcome. In cohort investigations, the patients have already experienced the factors being investigated. Thus, in randomized controlled trials in which masking is attempted we need to ask whether masking was successfully achieved. In case-control and cohort studies as well as in randomized controlled trials in which masking was not attempted, it is important to consider whether the knowledge regarding the group assignment influenced the measurement of the outcome performed as part of the assessment. Therefore, we now need to turn our attention to assessment.

Assessment

Assessment is the measurement of outcomes or end points in the study group and in the control group. To understand the meaning of measuring outcomes, we need to remember that in case-control studies, outcomes represent the presence or absence of previous characteristics or risk factors such as use of birth control pills or cigarette smoking. In cohort studies and randomized controlled trials, outcomes refer to the consequences of risk factors such as thrombophlebitis or lung cancer.[1.8]

To assess the results of an investigation, researchers must define the outcome or end point they intend to measure. The measurement of the outcome or end point can be considered valid when it fulfills the following criteria:

Appropriate: The measurement of the outcome addresses the study's question.

Accurate: On average, it has the same numerical value as the phenomenon being investigated. That is, it is free of systematic error or bias.

Precise: Produces nearly identical results when repeated under the same conditions. It has minimum variation as a result of the effects of chance. That is, there is minimum random error. *Precise* may also be referred to as *reproducibility* or *reliability*.

In addition, the implementation of the measurement should not introduce additional potential biases. The implementation should be as follows:

Complete: The outcomes or end points of all participants have been measured.

Unaffected by the process: Neither the participants' nor the investigators' knowledge of the study group or control group assignment affects the measurement of outcome. Also, the process of observation itself doesn't affect the outcome.

Now, let us look at the meaning and implications of each of these criteria.[1.9]

[1.8] Because the term "outcome" is sometimes thought of as meaning the consequences of risk factors, the term *end point* is also used to more clearly indicate the measurement being assessed in a case-control study as well as a cohort study or a randomized controlled trial. Thus, the assessment process may be thought of as the process of measuring the outcome or end point in the study and the control groups.

[1.9] Validity may also be defined as a particular type of accuracy which asks how well the measurement represents the phenomenon of interest. This approach to validity is particularly useful in assessing outcomes in which there is no gold

Appropriate Measure of Outcome

To understand the importance of the appropriateness of a measure of outcome, let us first consider an example of how the use of an inappropriate measure of outcome can invalidate a study's conclusions:

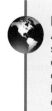

Mini-Study 1.12 ■ An investigator attempted to study whether users of brand A or brand B spermicide had a lower probability of developing tubal infections secondary to chlamydia. The investigator identified 100 women using each brand of spermicide, monitored these women, and performed annual cervical cultures for chlamydia for 5 years. The investigator found that women using brand A spermicide had 1½ times as many positive cervical cultures for chlamydia. The investigator concluded that brand B spermicide is associated with a lower rate of tubal infections.

Chlamydia cultures from the cervix do little to establish the presence or absence of tubal infection. The study may help to establish a higher frequency of chlamydia infection. However, if the intent is to study the relative frequency of tubal infection, the investigator has not chosen an appropriate outcome measurement. Investigators frequently are forced to measure an outcome that is not exactly the outcome they would like to measure. When this occurs, it is important to establish that the phenomenon being measured is appropriate to the question being investigated.

Increasingly, investigations seek to utilize outcomes that represent early evidence of the outcome of interest rather than wait until clear-cut or clinically important outcomes occur months or years later. For instance, when investigating coronary artery disease as an outcome, we would rather detect the disease at the asymptomatic phase using testing rather than wait until there is clinical or electrocardiogram evidence of disease. Despite the desirability of using these early or *surrogate outcomes*, we need to be confident that these outcomes are closely related to the outcome of ultimate interest. As we will see in the chapter on randomized controlled trials, sometimes this is not so easy.

Accurate and Precise Measures of Outcome

Next, we look at what we mean by accurate and precise measures of outcome. It is helpful to think of accuracy and precision as the two criteria for perfect performance. As illustrated in Figure 1.7A–C. We can think of perfect performance as hitting the bull's-eye of a target on every shot. In order to be accurate on average, the bullet does not need to hit the bull's-eye every time. That is, it may be a little high one time and a little low the next time, but if these shots center around the bull's-eye, then the measurement is said to be accurate as displayed in Figure 1.7A.

Precision, however, implies that the bullet always hits nearly the same spot as displayed in Figure 1.7B. Always in the same spot, however, may end up being on one side or other of the

standard such as pain or quality of life. The following types of validity are used in these situations. *Content validity*—asks how well the assessment covers all aspects of the phenomenon under study. For instance, with quality of life questions about intellectual function, vision and hearing, and ability to perform the functions of daily living should all be included. The term *face validity* refers to subjective judgments about whether content validity has been achieved. *Construct validity*—asks about how well an assessment appears to make meaningful distinction consistent with theory. For instance, we would expect that a quality of life scale should produce very different results among a blind population compared to one with full sight. *Criterion validity*—asks about how well an assessment correlates with other well-accepted measurement. *Predictive validity* is a special type of criterion validity in which validity is determined by the ability of a measurement to predict a particular outcome. Researchers are often interested in criterion validity when they use surrogate outcomes. Thus, a study of that uses patients' reports of chest pain as a measurement of coronary artery disease should first establish that chest pain has criterion validity for assessing coronary artery disease. These concepts of validity complement the concepts of validity used in *Studying a Study and Testing a Test*.

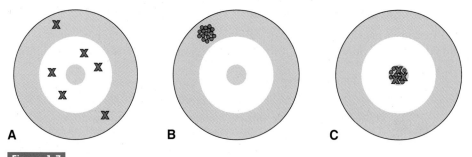

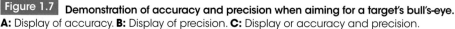

Figure 1.7 **Demonstration of accuracy and precision when aiming for a target's bull's-eye.**
A: Display of accuracy. **B:** Display of precision. **C:** Display or accuracy and precision.

bull's-eye. Thus an ideal measurement is both accurate and precise. An accurate and precise measurement, by definition, hits the bull's-eye every time as displayed in Figure 1.7C.

Measurement of outcome may lack either precision, accuracy, or both. When measurements lack precision and vary widely from measurement to measurement, we say they are not reproducible. Assuming this is due to chance, we call this *random error*. When a measurement is always off target in the same direction, we call this *systematic error* or *assessment bias*.

A large number of reasons for assessment bias have been identified.[1.10] It is helpful to think of these assessment biases as the consequences of obtaining data from different types of sources of information. Thus, together they may be called *information biases*.

Information for measuring outcome may come from three basic sources:

1. The memory of study participants
2. The use of data from their previous records
3. Measurements by the study investigator

Information obtained from the memory of study individuals is subject to two special types of assessment bias—recall bias and reporting bias. *Recall bias* implies defects in memory, specifically defects in which one group is more likely to recall events than other groups. *Reporting bias* occurs when one group is more likely than the other to report what they actually remember. First let us consider the following example of how *recall bias* can occur:

 Mini-Study 1.13 ■ In a case-control study of the cause of spina bifida, 100 mothers of infants born with the disease and 100 mothers of infants born without the disease were studied. Among the mothers of spina bifida infants, 50% reported having had a sore throat during pregnancy versus 5% of the mothers whose infants did not develop spina bifida. The investigators concluded that they had shown an association between sore throats during pregnancy and spina bifida.

Before accepting the conclusions of the study, one must ask whether recall bias could explain its findings. One can argue that mothers who experienced the trauma of having an infant with spina bifida are likely to search their memory more intensively and to remember events not usually recalled by other women.

[1.10] The proliferation of names for biases that occur in specific setting can be avoided by using the structure of M.A.A.R.I.E. to divide bias into two types, bias in assignment and bias in assessment. Selection bias is the fundamental bias of assignment, and assessment bias is the fundamental bias in assessment. The specific types of bias discussed here, such as recall, reporting, and instrument, can be seen as specific types of assessment bias results from different types of problems with obtaining accurate and precise information.

Thus, recall bias is more likely to occur when the subsequent events are traumatic, thereby causing subjectively remembered and frequently occurring events to be recalled that under normal circumstances would be forgotten. We cannot be certain that recall bias affected this study's outcome assessment, but the conditions are present in which recall bias occurs. Therefore, the result of this case-control study may be ascribed, at least in part, to recall bias. The presence of recall bias casts doubts on the alleged association between sore throats and the occurrence of spina bifida.

Reporting bias as well as recall bias may operate to impair the accuracy of the outcome measurement, as illustrated in the following example:

Mini-Study 1.14 ■ A case–control study of the relationship between gonorrhea and multiple sexual partners was conducted. One hundred women who were newly diagnosed with gonorrhea were compared with 100 women in the same clinic who were found to be free of gonorrhea. The women who were diagnosed with gonorrhea were informed that the serious consequences of the disease could be prevented only by locating and treating their sexual partners. Both groups of women were asked about the number of sexual partners they had during the preceding 2 months. The group of women with gonorrhea reported an average of four times as many sexual partners as the group of women without gonorrhea. The investigators concluded that on average women with gonorrhea have four times as many sexual partners as women without gonorrhea.

The women with gonorrhea in this study may have felt a greater obligation, hence less hesitation, to report their sexual partners than did the women without the disease. Reporting bias is more likely to occur when the information sought is personal or sensitive and one group is under greater pressure to report.

Thus, it is possible that women with gonorrhea may simply have been more thorough in reporting their sexual partners rather than actually having had more contacts. Reporting bias in addition to recall error may impair the accuracy of assessment in case-control studies because the participants in a case-control study are already aware of the occurrence or absence of the disease being studied.

When measurements are conducted or interpreted by the investigator, human factors can produce inaccuracies in measurement as a result of both assessment bias and chance. These errors can occur when two investigators perform the same measurements (*interobserver error*) or when the same individual performs the measurements more than once (*intraobserver error*).

Assessment bias may also occur as a result of inaccurate measurement by the testing instruments in all types of studies, as illustrated in the following example:

Mini-Study 1.15 ■ The gastrointestinal (GI) side effects of two nonsteroidal anti-inflammatory drugs (NSAIDs) for arthritis were assessed using an upper GI X-ray. The investigator found no evidence that either drug was associated with gastritis.

The investigator did not recognize that an upper GI X-ray is a very poor instrument for measuring gastritis. Even if a drug caused gastritis, upper GI X-ray examination would not be adequate to identify its presence. Thus, any conclusion based on this measurement is likely to be inaccurate even if it reproducibly measures the wrong outcome.[1.11]

[1.11] When gross instrument error occurs, as in this example, the measurement of outcome also can be considered inappropriate.

Whenever there is a subjective assessment of the outcome, the possibility of assessment bias exists. It may be possible, however, to prevent, recognize, or take into account assessment bias. Human beings, including investigators, see what they want to see or expect to see. Preventing bias may be accomplished by keeping the investigator, who makes the measurement of outcome, from knowing an individual's group assignment. Masked assessment can be used in case-control and cohort studies as well as in randomized controlled trials. Failure to use masked assessment can lead to the following type of bias:

Mini-Study 1.16 ■ In a study of the use of NSAIDs, the investigators, who were the patients' attending physicians, questioned all patients to determine whether one of the NSAIDs was associated with more symptoms that could indicate gastritis. After questioning all patients about their symptoms, they determined that there was no difference in the occurrence of gastritis. They reported that the two drugs produced the same frequency of occurrence of gastritis symptoms.

In this study, the investigators making the assessment of outcome were aware of what the patients were receiving; thus, they were not masked. In addition, they were assessing the patients' subjective symptoms such as nausea, stomach pain, or indigestion in deciding whether gastritis was present. This is the setting in which masking is most critical. Even if the patients were unaware of which medication they were taking, the investigators' assessment may be biased. If the assessment conformed to their own hypothesis, their results are especially open to question. This does not imply fraud, only the natural tendency of human beings to see what they expect or want to see. The investigators' conclusions may be true, but their less-than-perfect techniques make it difficult or impossible to accept their conclusion.

Thus, masking in the process of assessment is important to eliminate this source of assessment bias. Even in the absence of bias, chance can affect the outcome as discussed in Learn More 1.4.

LEARN MORE 1.4 ■ **MISCLASSIFICATION ERROR** ■ Measurements of outcome may misclassify patients as having an outcome such as thrombophlebitis when they do not, or as not having thrombophlebitis when they truly do. This type of misclassification when resulting from chance is known as *nondirectional misclassification* as opposed to directional misclassification or bias. When a measurement is made which frequently misclassifies the outcomes, it is important to examine the consequences that occur, as illustrated in the next example:

Mini-Study 1.17 ■ A cohort study tested for diabetes among those with and without a risk factor. The test used was known to have poor reproducibility. The investigators found that the association between the risk factor and the development of diabetes, while consistent with other investigations was not as strong an association as expected.

The investigators may have diagnosed diabetes when it was not present or failed to diagnosis it when it was present. Assuming this applies to both the study group and the control group, we have an example of nondirectional misclassification or misclassification resulting from chance. The consequence of misclassification error caused by chance is to reduce the magnitude of the association below that which would be found in the absence of misclassification caused by chance. Thus, it is not surprising in this investigation that the association was consistent with previous studies, but much weaker than found in other investigations.

Complete and Unaffected by the Process

Whenever follow-up of patients is incomplete, the possibility exists that those not included in the final assessment had a different frequency of the outcome than those included. The following example illustrates an error resulting from incomplete assessment:

> **Mini-Study 1.18** ■ A cohort study of HIV-positive patients compared the natural history of the disease among asymptomatic patients with a CD4 count of 100 to 200 with a group of asymptomatic patients with a CD4 count of 200 to 400. The investigators were able to obtain follow-up with 50% of those with the lower CD4 counts and 60% of those with the higher CD4 counts. The investigators found no difference in outcome between the groups and concluded that the CD4 count is not a risk factor for developing AIDS.

It can be argued that in this investigation, some of the patients who could not be followed-up were not available because they were dead. If this were the case, the results of the study might have been dramatically altered with complete follow-up. Incomplete follow-up can distort the conclusions of an investigation.

Follow-up does not necessarily mean that patients are actually examined or even that they have continued to be a part of an investigation. At times follow-up may be achieved by searching public records such as death certificates or by obtaining information from relatives or friends based on the participant's agreement to this type of follow-up when they entered the investigation. Using this meaning of follow-up, a high-quality investigation today should achieve nearly 100% follow-up.

Incomplete follow-up does not necessarily mean the patients were lost to follow-up as in the previous example. They may have been monitored with unequal intensity, as the next example illustrates:

> **Mini-Study 1.19** ■ A cohort study of the side effects of birth control pills was conducted by comparing 1,000 young women taking the pill with 1,000 young women using other forms of birth control. Data were collected from the records of their private physicians over a 1-year period. Pill-users were scheduled for three follow-up visits during the year; non–pill-users were asked to return if they had problems. Among users of the pill, 75 women reported having headaches, 90 reported fatigue, and 60 reported depression. Among non–pill-users, 25 patients reported having headaches, 30 reported fatigue, and 20 reported depression. The average pill-user made three visits to her physician during the year versus one visit for the non–pill-user. The investigator concluded that use of the pill is associated with increased frequency of headaches, fatigue, and depression.

The problem of unequal intensity of observation of the two groups may have invalidated the results. The fact that pill-users, and not non–pill-users, were scheduled for visits to their physician may account for the more frequent recordings of headaches, fatigue, and depression. With more thorough observation, commonly occurring subjective symptoms are more likely to be recorded.

Even if a study's outcome or end point meets the difficult criteria of appropriate, accurate, precise, and complete assessment, one more area of concern exists. Investigators intend to measure events as they would have occurred had no one been watching. Unfortunately, the very process of conducting a study may involve the introduction of an observer into the events being measured.

Thus, the reviewer must ask whether the process of observation altered the outcome, as illustrated in the following example:

> **Mini-Study 1.20** ■ A cohort study was conducted of the relationship between obesity and menstrual regularity. One thousand obese women with menstrual irregularities who had joined a diet group were compared with 1,000 obese women with the same pattern of menstrual irregularities who were not enrolled in a diet group. The women were compared to evaluate the effects of weight loss on menstrual irregularities. Those in the diet group had exactly the same frequency of return to regular menstrual cycles as the nondiet group controls.

It is possible that the nondiet-group patients lost weight just like the diet-group patients because they were being observed as part of the study. Whenever it is possible for subjects to switch groups or alter their behavior, the effects of observation may affect an investigation. This is most likely to occur when the individuals in the control group are aware of the adverse consequences of their current behavior and feel pressured to change because they are being observed. This can occur only in a concurrent or prospective cohort study or in a randomized controlled trial because these types of investigation are begun before any of the participants have developed the outcome.

We have now examined the criteria that need to be fulfilled for an ideal measurement of outcome. That is an assessment should be appropriate, accurate and precise, as well as complete and unaffected by the process. We have examined the meaning of each of these criteria and have looked at problems that prevent a measurement from fulfilling these criteria. Now we are ready to use the fourth component of the M.A.A.R.I.E. framework, the results component, to compare the measurements obtained in the study group and in the control group.

REFERENCES

1. Gordis L. *Epidemiology*. 4th ed. Philadelphia, PA: Saunders; 2009.

2. Hulley SB, Cummings SR, Browner WS, et al. *Designing Clinical Research*. 3rd ed. Philadelphia, PA: Lippincott Williams & Wilkins; 2007.

3. Fletcher R, Fletcher S. *Clinical Epidemiology: The Essentials*. 4th ed. Baltimore, MD: Lippincott Williams & Wilkins; 2005.

4. Gehlbach SH. *Interpreting the Medical Literature*. 5th ed. New York, NY: McGraw-Hill; 2006.

5. Greenhalgh T. *How To Read a Paper: The Basics of Evidence-based Medicine*. 3rd ed. Malden, MA: Blackwell Publishing; 2001.

6. Hennekens CH, Buring JE. *Epidemiology in Medicine*. Boston, MA: Little Brown and Company; 1987.

thePoint ✳ Visit http://thePoint.lww.com for interactive Q&A, flaw-catching exercises, searchable eBook, and more!

2 | Studying a Study: M.A.A.R.I.E. Framework—Results

The fourth component of the M.A.A.R.I.E. framework is the results or analysis section. Like the previous components, results require us to address three key questions (1):

- **Estimation:** What is the magnitude or strength of the association or relationship observed in the investigation?
- **Inference:** What statistical technique(s) are used to perform statistical significance testing?
- **Adjustment:** What statistical technique(s) are used to take into account or control for difference between the study and control groups that may affect the results?

ESTIMATION

Strength of Relationship (1–3)

When measuring the strength of a relationship using data from samples, we are attempting to use that information to estimate the strength of the relationship within a larger group called a population. Thus, biostatisticians often refer to any measurement of the strength of a relationship as an *estimate* or *point estimate*. The data from the samples are said to estimate the population's *effect size,* which is the magnitude of the association or the difference in the larger population.[2.1]

When we measure the strength of a relationship, we usually need to define what we mean by the *independent variable(s)* and the *dependent variable*. In general, a dependent variable is the one primary outcome or end point that we wish to estimate based on one or more independent variables. Let us take a look at how we can measure the strength of the relationship between birth control pills, an independent variable, and thrombophlebitis, a dependent variable.[2.2] First, we will look at the basic measure of the strength of an association that is most frequently used in cohort studies. Then we turn to the basic measure used in case–control studies.

Let us assume that we are studying the association between birth control pills and thrombophlebitis. We want to measure the strength of the association to determine how strongly the use of birth control pills affects the risk of thrombophlebitis. Before we do this we must first clarify the concept of *risk*.

When used quantitatively, risk implies the probability of developing a condition over a specified period. Risk equals the number of individuals who develop the condition divided by the

---

[2.1] The measures that we use in this chapter are measures of the strength of an association. *Associations* measure the strength of a relationship in one sample (or population) compared with another. That is, associations are expressed as ratios. *Differences* in contrast subtract a measurement taken in one sample (or population) from those in another sample (or population). Also note that the term effect size does not imply that a cause and effect relationship is present. When describing the data obtained in an investigation, measures of the central tendency such as the *mean* or *average* or alternatively the *median* are used. Measures of the spread or dispersion of the data such as the *standard deviation* are also needed to describe the distribution of continuous data.
[2.2] At times, there will be only a dependent variable and no independent variables. This type of statistical analysis is called *univariable* analysis. Univariable analysis is used primarily in descriptive studies. In contrast, *bivariable* and *multivariable* statistical methods are used primarily in analytical studies. Bivariable analysis implies one dependent and one independent variable. Multivariable analysis implies one dependent and more than one independent variable. In addition to the estimation measures discussed in this chapter, you will also see an estimate of the strength of the relationship for the association between two continuous variables such as blood pressure (BP) and salt intake or body mass index and blood sugar. The basic measurement of the strength of the relationship is known as the *correlation coefficient* (R). The correlation coefficient can vary from +1 to −1. Zero indicates no association or correlation. A correlation coefficient of +1 indicates that as the value of one variable increases the value of the other variable increases. A negative correlation coefficient indicates that as the value of one variable increases the other decreases. In addition, the square of R, or R^2, that is called the *coefficient of determination* provides an estimate of the percentage of the variation that is explained.

total number of individuals who were possible candidates to develop the condition at the beginning of the period. In assessing the 10-year risk of developing thrombophlebitis, we would divide the number of women taking birth control pills who developed thrombophlebitis over a 10-year period by the total number of women in the study group who were taking birth control pills.[2.3]

A further calculation is necessary to measure the relative degree of association between thrombophlebitis for women who are on birth control pills compared with women who are not on birth control pills. One such measure is known as *relative risk*. Relative risk is the probability of thrombophlebitis if birth control pills are used divided by the probability if birth control pills are not used. It is defined as follows:

$$\text{Relative risk} = \frac{\text{Probability of developing thrombophlebitis if birth control pills are used}}{\text{Probability of developing thrombophlebitis if birth control pills are not used}}$$

Generally,

$$\text{Relative risk} = \frac{\text{Probability of the outcome if the risk factor is present}}{\text{Probability of the outcome if the risk factor is absent}}$$

Let us illustrate how the risk and relative risk are calculated using a hypothetical example:

Mini-Study 2.1 ■ For 10 years, an investigator monitored 1,000 young women taking birth control pills and 1,000 young women who were nonusers. He found that 30 of the women on birth control pills developed thrombophlebitis over the 10-year period, whereas only 3 of the nonusers developed thrombophlebitis over the same period. He presented his data using what is called a 2 × 2 table:

	Thrombophlebitis	No Thrombophlebitis	
Birth control pills	$a = 30$	$b = 970$	$a + b = 1,000$
No birth control pills	$c = 3$	$d = 997$	$c + d = 1,000$

The 10-year risk of developing thrombophlebitis on birth control pills equals the number of women on the pill who develop thrombophlebitis divided by the total number of women on the pill at the beginning of the study. Thus, the risk of developing thrombophlebitis for women on birth control pills is equal to

$$\frac{a}{a+b} = \frac{30}{1,000} = 0.030$$

Likewise, the 10-year risk of developing thrombophlebitis for women not on the pill equals the number of women not on the pill who develop thrombophlebitis divided by the total number of women not on the pill at the beginning of the study. Thus, the risk of developing thrombophlebitis for women not on the pill is equal to

$$\frac{c}{c+d} = \frac{3}{1,000} = 0.0030$$

The relative risk equals the ratio of these two risks. A relative risk of 1 implies that the use of birth control pills does not increase thrombophlebitis.

[2.3] When individuals are followed for different periods of time, the denominator used to calculate risk often includes a measure known as *person-years*. A person-year is equivalent to one person followed for one year. Person-years allow us to include individuals who are followed for differing lengths of time by including their data for each year in which they are followed. Person-years are an example of a broader approach that can include any interval of time such as person months, days, or minutes, etc.

$$\text{Relative risk} = \frac{a/(a+b)}{c/(c+d)} = \frac{0.030}{0.003} = 10$$

This relative risk of 10 implies that, on the average, women on the pill have a risk of thrombophlebitis 10 times that of women not on the pill. (2,4) [2.4]

Now let us look at how we measure the strength of association for case–control studies by looking at a study of the association between birth control pills and thrombophlebitis:

Mini-Study 2.2 ■ An investigator selected 100 young women with thrombophlebitis and 100 young women without thrombophlebitis. She carefully obtained the history of prior use of birth control pills. She found that 90 of the 100 women with thrombophlebitis were using birth control pills compared with 45 of the women without thrombophlebitis. She presented her data using the following 2×2 table:

	Thrombophlebitis	No Thrombophlebitis
Birth control pills	$a = 90$	$b = 45$
No birth control pills	$c = 10$	$d = 55$
	$a + c = 100$	$b + d = 100$

Note that in case–control studies the investigator can choose the total number of patients in each group (those with and without thrombophlebitis). She could have chosen to select 200 patients with thrombophlebitis and 100 patients without thrombophlebitis, or a large number of other combinations.

Thus, the actual numbers in each vertical column, the cases and the controls, can be altered at will by the investigator. In other words, in a case–control study, the number of individuals who have and do not have the disease does not necessarily reflect the relative frequency of those with and without the disease. Whenever the number of cases relative to the number of controls is determined by the investigator, it is improper to add the boxes in the case–control 2×2 table horizontally (as we did in the preceding cohort study) and calculate relative risk.

Thus we need to use a measurement that is not altered by the relative numbers in the study and control groups. This measurement is known as the *odds ratio.*

The size of the odds ratio is often very close to the relative risk. That is, the odds ratio is often a good approximation of the relative risk. When this is the situation, it can be used as a substitute for the relative risk. This is the usual situation when the disease or condition under investigation occurs relatively infrequently.

To understand what we mean by an odds ratio, we first need to appreciate what we mean by odds and how odds differ from risk. Risk is a probability in which the numerator contains the number of times the event, such as thrombophlebitis, occurs over a specified period. The denominator of a risk or probability contains the number of times the event could have occurred. Odds, like probability, contain the number of times the event occurred in the numerator. However, in the denominator odds contain only the number of times the event did not occur.

The difference between odds and probability may be appreciated by thinking of the chance of drawing an ace from a deck of 52 cards. The probability of drawing an ace is the number of times an ace can be drawn divided by the total number of cards: 4 of 52 or 1 of 13. Odds, on the other hand, are the number of times an ace can be drawn divided by the number of times it cannot be drawn: 4 to 48 or 1 to 12. Thus, the odds are slightly larger than the probability, but when the event or the disease under study is relatively rare, the odds are a good approximation of the probability.

[2.4] Relative risks may also be presented with the group at lower risk in the numerator. These two forms of the relative risks are merely the reciprocal of each other. Thus, the risk of thrombophlebitis for those not taking birth control pills divided by the risk for those taking birth control pills would be 0.003/0.030 = 0.1 or 1/10.

The odds ratio is the odds of having the risk factor if the condition is present divided by the odds of having the risk factor if the condition is not present. The odds of being on the pill if thrombophlebitis is present are equal to

$$\frac{a}{c} = \frac{90}{10} = 9$$

Likewise, the odds of being on the pill for women who do not develop thrombophlebitis is measured by dividing the number of women who do not have thrombophlebitis and are using the pill by the number of women who do not have thrombophlebitis and are not using the pill. Thus, the odds of being on the pill if thrombophlebitis is not present are equal to

$$\frac{b}{d} = \frac{45}{55} = 0.82$$

Like the calculation of relative risk, one can develop a measure of the relative odds of being on the pill if thrombophlebitis is present versus being on the pill if thrombophlebitis is not present. This measure of the strength of association is the odds ratio. Thus,

$$\text{Odds ratio} = \frac{\text{Odds of being on the pill if thrombophlebitis is present}}{\text{Odds of being on the pill if thrombophlebitis is not present}}$$

$$= \frac{a/c}{b/d} = \frac{9}{0.82} = 11$$

An odds ratio of 1, parallel with our interpretation of relative risk, implies that the odds are the same for being on the pill if thrombophlebitis is present and for being on the pill if thrombophlebitis is absent. Our odds ratio of 11 means that the odds of being on birth control pills are increased 11-fold for women with thrombophlebitis.

The odds ratio is the basic measure of the degree of association for case–control studies. It is a useful measurement of the strength of the association. In addition, as long as the disease (thrombophlebitis) is rare, the odds ratio is approximately equal to the relative risk. Note, however, that the odds ratio is larger than the relative risk. This is a general principle. You can expect the odds ratio to be larger than the relative risk. As the probability of the disease increases, the difference between the odds ratio and the relative risk will increase.

It is possible to look at the odds ratio in reverse, as one would do in a cohort study, and come up with the same result. For instance,

$$\text{Odds ratio} = \frac{\text{Odds of developing thrombophlebitis if pill is used}}{\text{Odds of developing thrombophlebitis if pill is not used}}$$

The odds ratio then equals

$$\frac{a \,/\, b}{c \,/\, d} = 11$$

Note that this is actually the same formula for the odds ratio as the one shown previously, that is, both can be expressed as *ad* divided by *bc*. This convenient property allows one to calculate an odds ratio from a cohort or randomized controlled trial instead of calculating the relative risk. This makes it easier to compare the results of a case–control study with those of a cohort study or randomized controlled trial. Learn More 2.1 looks at a special form of the odds ratio or relative risk that can be used when pairing is used as part of the investigation.

LEARN MORE 2.1 ■ PAIRING AND ESTIMATING THE STRENGTH OF THE ASSOCIATION ■ The relative risk and odds ratio are the fundamental measures we use to measure the strength of an association between a risk factor and a disease. A special type of odds ratio (or relative risk) is calculated when *pairing* is used to conduct an investigation. Pairing implies that one study group individual is linked to one control group individual and the endpoints in the pair are compared. This type of matching, known as pairing, is used to ensure identical distribution of potential confounding variables between study and control groups. When pairing is used, a special type of odds ratio should be used to take advantage of the increased statistical power when estimating the strength of the association.

Let us look at the following example of this measure of the strength of the relationship:

Mini-Study 2.3 ■ Assume that a case–control study of birth control pills and thrombophlebitis was conducted using 100 pairs of patients with thrombophlebitis and controls without thrombophlebitis. The cases and controls were paired so that each member of the pair was the same age and had the same number of previous pregnancies. The results of a paired case-control study are presented using the following 2×2 table[2.5]:

	Controls Using Birth Control Pills	Controls Not Using Birth Control Pills
Cases using birth control pills	30	50
Cases not using birth control pills	5	15

The odds ratio in a paired case–control study uses only the pairs in which the exposure (e.g., the use of birth control pills) is different between the case and control members of a pair. The pairs in which the cases with thrombophlebitis and the controls without thrombophlebitis differ in their use of birth control pills are known as *discordant pairs.*

The odds ratio is calculated using discordant pairs as follows:

$$\frac{\text{Number of pairs with cases using birth control pills and controls not using birth control pills}}{\text{Number of pairs with controls using birth control pills and cases not using birth control pills}} = \frac{50}{5} = 10$$

This odds ratio is interpreted the same way as an odds ratio calculated from unpaired studies.[2.6]

[2.5] The table for a paired case–control study tells us about what happens to a pair instead of what happens to each person. Thus, the frequencies in this paired 2×2 table add up to 100 (the number of pairs) instead of 200 (the number of persons in the study).

[2.6] Pairing, however, has an advantage of greater statistical power. Everything else being equal, statistical significance can be established using smaller numbers of study and control group patients. Pairing may be used in cohort studies and randomized controlled trials as well as case–control studies.

INFERENCE

Statistical Significance Testing (2,4,5)

Most investigations are conducted on only a subset or what is called a *sample* of a larger group of individuals who could have been included in the study. The process of selecting or drawing a sample from a larger population is discussed in Learn More 2.2.

Once a sample is obtained for investigation, researchers are frequently confronted with the question of whether they would achieve similar results if the entire population were included in the study or whether chance selection of those included in the sample may have produced unusual results in their particular sample.

Unfortunately, there is no direct method for answering this question. Instead, investigators are forced to test their study hypothesis using a circuitous method of proof by elimination. This method is known as *statistical significance testing* or *hypothesis testing*.

> **LEARN MORE 2.2 ■ SAMPLING ■** A sample is a subset of all possible measurements from a population. When we are attempting to draw conclusions or inferences about large populations from observations on a sample, we need to assume that the sample is a randomly chosen subset of a larger population of interest. The simplest and most common method for obtaining a sample is called a *simple random sample*. A *random sample* implies that any one individual in the population has a known probability of being included in the sample. In a simple random sample, all individuals in the population have an equal probability of being included. Chance alone, then, dictates which individuals are actually included.
>
> At times, more complex methods of sampling are used to ensure that small subgroups within a population such as members of minorities are included in the observations with enough frequency to draw reliable conclusions about these subgroups. These methods are called *stratified random sampling*.
>
> Frequently, researchers actually obtain samples based upon the ease of obtaining study participants. These types of samples have been called *convenience samples*. Convenience samples are frequently used in randomized controlled trials. However, in randomized controlled trials, participation is restricted by inclusion and exclusion criteria. When a convenience sample or a convenience sample restricted by inclusion and exclusion criteria are used and statistical inferences are drawn, it is important to recognize that the conclusions apply only to a larger population of individuals similar to the one included in the convenience sample.[2.7]

Statistical significance testing, in its most common form, quantitates the probability of obtaining the observed data (or a more extreme result supporting the study hypothesis) if no differences between groups exist in the larger population from which the sample was drawn or obtained. Statistical significance testing assumes that individuals used in an investigation are representative or randomly selected from a larger group or population. This use of the term *random* is confusing because statistical significance testing is used in studies in which the individuals are not randomly selected. This apparent contradiction can be reconciled if one assumes that the larger population consists of all individuals with the same characteristics as those required for entry into the

---

[2.7] The assumption that sampling is random or representative of a larger population relates to the dependent variable. The independent variable may also be sampled using a method that ensures a *representative or naturalist sample* of the larger population. Alternatively, independent variables may be obtained for particular purposes and are not representative of a larger population. This common method of selecting .the independent variables is called *purposive sampling*. The type of sampling of independent variable that is used determines the type of statistical methods, which can be used for bivariable and multivariable methods. Specifically, representative or naturalistic sampling of both the independent and the dependent variables are required for proper use of correlation methods.

investigation. Thus, statistical significance tests actually address questions about larger populations made up of individuals very similar to those used in the investigation.

Statistical significance testing aims to draw conclusions or inferences about a population by studying samples of that population. Therefore, biostatisticians often refer to statistical significance testing as *inference*.

STATISTICAL SIGNIFICANCE TESTING PROCEDURES (2–4)

Statistical significance testing, which is also called hypothesis testing, assumes that only two types of relationships exist: either differences or associations between groups within the study population exist or they do not exist. When we conduct statistical significance tests on study data, we assume at the beginning that no such differences exist in the larger population. The role of statistical significance testing is to evaluate the results obtained from the samples to determine whether these results would be so unusual—if no difference exists in the larger population—that we can conclude that a difference does exist in the large population. Note that the issue is whether or not a difference or association exists. Statistical significance testing itself says little or nothing about the size or importance of the potential difference or association.

Statistical significance testing begins with one *study hypothesis* stating that a difference or association exists in the larger population. In performing statistical significance tests, it is assumed initially that the study hypothesis is false, and a *null hypothesis* is formulated stating that no difference or association exists in the larger population. Statistical methods are then used to calculate the probability of obtaining the observed results in the study sample, or more extreme results, if no difference or association actually exists in the larger population.

When only a small probability exists that the observed results would occur in the study's sample if the null hypothesis were true, then investigators can reject the null hypothesis. In rejecting the null hypothesis, the investigators accept, by elimination, their only other alternative—the existence of a difference or association between groups in the larger population. Biostatisticians often refer to the study hypothesis as the *alternative hypothesis* because it is the alternative to the null hypothesis.

The specific steps in statistical significance testing are as follows:

1. State study hypothesis
2. Formulate null hypothesis
3. Decide statistical significance cutoff level
4. Collect data
5. Apply statistical significance test
6. Reject or fail to reject the null hypothesis

State Study Hypothesis

Before collecting the data, the investigators state a study hypothesis that a difference or association exists between a factor in the study group and in the control group among those in the larger population.

Formulate Null Hypothesis

The investigators then assume that no true difference or association exists between the factor in the study group and in the control group among those in the larger population.

Decide Statistical Significance Cutoff Level

The investigators determine what level of probability will be considered small enough to reject the null hypothesis. In most of health research studies, a 5% chance or less of occurrence is considered unlikely enough to allow the investigators to reject the null hypothesis. However, we are generally left with some possibility that chance alone has produced an unusual set of data. Thus, a null hypothesis that is in fact true will be rejected in favor of the study hypothesis as much as 5% of the time.[2.8]

Collect Data

The data may be collected using a study design such as case–control, cohort study, or randomized controlled trial.

Apply Statistical Significance Test

If a difference or association is observed in the data from the sample, the investigators determine the probability that this difference or association would occur if no true difference or association exists in the larger population. This probability is known as the P value.

In other words, they calculate the probability that the observed data or more extreme data would occur if the null hypothesis of no difference or association were true. To do so, the investigators must choose from various statistical significance tests. Because each type of test is appropriate to a specific type of data, investigators must take care to choose the proper statistical method as we will discuss shortly.

To understand how a statistical significance test uses P values, let us consider an example that uses small numbers to allow easy calculation:

> **Mini-Study 2.4** ■ Assume that an investigator wants to study the question: "Are there an equal number of males and females born in the United States?" The investigator first hypothesizes that more males than females are born in the United States; a null hypothesis that an equal number of males and females are born in the United States is then formulated. Then, the investigator decides the statistical significance cutoff level, which is usually set at 5%, or $P = 0.05$. Next, the investigator samples four birth certificates, using a chance process, and finds that there are four males and zero females in the sample of births.

Let us now calculate the probability of obtaining four males and zero females if the null hypothesis of equal numbers of males and females is true.

Probability of one male	0.50 or 50%
Probability of two males in a row	0.25 or 25%
Probability of three males in a row	0.125 or 12.5%
Probability of four males in a row	0.0625 or 6.25%

Thus, there is a 6.25% chance of obtaining four males in a row even if an equal number of males and females are born in the United States.[2.9] Thus, the P value equals 0.0625. All P values tell us the same basic information. They tell us the probability of producing the observed data, assuming that the null hypothesis is true. Technically they are said to measure the probability of obtaining the observed data, or more extreme data, if no true difference between groups actually exist in the larger population.

[2.8] Investigators also need to decide whether to use a one-tailed or two-tailed statistical significance test. A *two-tailed* test implies that the investigator is willing to accept data that deviate in either direction from the null hypothesis. A *one-tailed* test implies that the investigator is only willing to accept data that deviate in the direction of the study hypothesis. We will assume a two-tailed test unless otherwise indicated.

[2.9] In this example, for simplicity a one-tailed statistical significance test has been used. The births have been assumed to be independent of each other in calculating probabilities. To simplify the calculations, an example has been chosen in which no more extreme possibility exists.

Reject or Fail to Reject the Null Hypothesis

Having obtained a *P* value, the investigators proceed to reject or fail to reject the null hypothesis. If the *P* value is 0.05 or less, that is, the probability of the results occurring by chance is ≤0.05, then the investigators can reject the null hypothesis.

In this situation, the probability is small that chance alone could produce the differences in outcome if the null hypothesis is true. By elimination, the investigators can then accept the study hypothesis that a true difference exists in the outcome between study and control groups in the larger population.

What if the probability of occurrence by chance is >0.05—that is, the *P* value is >0.05 as in the preceding example? The investigators then are unable to reject the null hypothesis. This does not mean that the null hypothesis, that no true difference exists in the larger population, is true. It merely indicates that the probability of obtaining the observed results is too great to reject the null hypothesis and thereby accept by elimination the study hypothesis. When the *P* value is >0.05, we say that the investigation has failed to reject the null hypothesis. The burden of proof, therefore, is on the investigators to show that the data obtained in the samples are very unlikely before rejecting the null hypothesis in favor of the study hypothesis. The following example shows how the statistical significance testing procedure operates in practice:

> **Mini-Study 2.5** ■ An investigator wanted to test the hypothesis that there is a difference in the frequency of mouth cancer among those who chew tobacco and those who do not chew tobacco in the general population. She formulated a null hypothesis stating that mouth cancer occurs with no greater frequency among those who chew tobacco than among those who do not chew tobacco. She then decided that she would reject the null hypothesis if she obtained data that would occur only 5% or less of the time if the null hypothesis was true. She next collected data from a sample of the general population of those who chew tobacco and those who do not chew tobacco. Using the proper statistical significance test, she found that if no difference existed between those who chew tobacco and those who do not chew tobacco in the general population, then data as extreme or more extreme than her data would be observed by chance only 3% of the time—that is, a *P* value of 0.03. She concluded that because her data were quite unlikely to occur if there were no difference in the general population, she would reject the null hypothesis. The investigator thus accepted by elimination the study hypothesis that a difference in the frequency of mouth cancer exists between those who chew tobacco and those who do not chew tobacco.

When the *P value is 0.05 or less*, we say that the results are statistically significant. Remember that we have defined small as a 5% chance or less that the observed results would have occurred in the sample if no true difference exists in the larger population.

The 5% figure may be too large if important decisions depend on the results. The 5% figure is based on some convenient statistical properties; however, it is not a magic number. It is possible to define small as 1%, 0.1%, or any other probability. Remember, however, that no matter what level is chosen, there will always be some probability of rejecting the null hypothesis when no true difference exists in the larger population. Statistical significance tests can measure this probability, but they cannot eliminate it.

Table 2.1 reviews and summarizes the steps for performing a statistical significance test.

ERRORS IN STATISTICAL SIGNIFICANCE TESTING

Several types of errors commonly occur in using statistical significance tests:

■ Failure to state one hypothesis before conducting the study—the multiple comparison problem

TABLE 2.1	How a Statistical Significance Test Works
State study hypothesis	Develop the study question: a difference or association exists in a population.
Formulate null hypothesis	Reverse the hypothesis: no difference or association exists in the population.
Decide statistical significance cutoff level	Equal to or less than 5% unless otherwise indicated and justified.
Collect data	Collect data from samples of the larger population.
Apply statistical significance test	Determine the probability of obtaining the observed data or more extreme data if the null hypothesis were true (i.e., choose and apply the correct statistical significance test).
Reject or fail to reject the null hypothesis	Reject the null hypothesis and accept by elimination the study hypothesis if the statistical significance cutoff level is reached (P value equal to or less than 0.05); fail to reject the null hypothesis if the observed data or more extreme data have more than a 5% probability of occurring by chance if there is no difference or association in the larger population (P value >0.05).

- Failure to draw correct conclusions from the results of statistical significance tests by not considering the potential for a *Type I error*
- Failure to draw correct conclusions from the results of statistical significance tests by not considering the potential for a *Type II error*

Multiple Comparison Problem

The multiple comparison problem occurs when an investigator attempts to investigate multiple hypotheses in the same investigation or attempts to analyze the data without first creating a hypothesis:

The following example illustrates the consequences of failing to state the hypothesis before conducting the study:

Mini-Study 2.6 ■ An investigator carefully selected 100 individuals known to have long-standing hypertension and 100 individuals of the same age known to be free from hypertension. He compared them using a list of 100 characteristics to determine how the two groups differed. Of the 100 characteristics studied, two were found to be statistically significant at the 0.05 level using standard statistical methods: (1) hypertensives generally have more letters in their last name than nonhypertensives and (2) hypertensives generally are born during the first 3½ days of the week, whereas nonhypertensives are usually born during the last 3½ days of the week. The author concluded that although these differences had not been foreseen, longer names and birth during the first half of the week are different between groups with and without hypertension.

This example illustrates the importance of stating the hypothesis beforehand. Whenever a large number of characteristics are used to make a large number of comparisons, it is likely by chance alone that some of them will be statistically significant. It can be misleading to apply the usual levels of statistical significance unless the hypothesis has been stated before collecting and analyzing the data. If differences are looked for without formulating one study hypothesis or only after collecting and analyzing the data, stricter criteria should be applied than the usual 5% probability.

The multiple comparison problem can also occur when investigators analyze the data two or more times. When multiple hypotheses are being examined or the data are being analyzed multiple times, a suggested rule of thumb for the reader of the health literature is to divide the observed P value by the number of hypotheses or comparisons being examined for statistical significance or the number of times the data are analyzed. The resulting P value can then be used to reject or fail to reject the null hypothesis.[2.10]

For instance, imagine that an investigation examined five hypotheses at the same time. To reach a P value that would have the same meaning as $P = 0.05$ for one hypothesis, the P value must be equal to 0.01. That is:

$$\frac{0.05}{\text{Number of comparison}} = \frac{0.05}{5} = 0.01$$

This P value of 0.01 should be interpreted just like a P value of 0.05 if one study hypothesis was stated before beginning the study.

Type I Errors

Some errors are inherent in the method of statistical significance testing. A fundamental concept of statistical significance testing is the possibility that a null hypothesis will be falsely rejected and a study hypothesis will be falsely accepted by elimination. This is known as a Type I error.

In traditional statistical significance testing, there is as much as a 5% chance of incorrectly accepting by elimination a study hypothesis even when no true difference exists in the larger population from which the study samples were obtained. The level of Type I error that is built into the design of an investigation before it is conducted is known as the *alpha level*. Statistical significance testing does not eliminate uncertainty; it aims to measure the uncertainty that exists. Careful readers of studies are, therefore, able to appreciate the degree of doubt that exists and can decide for themselves whether they are willing to tolerate that degree of uncertainty.

Let us see how failure to appreciate the possibility of a Type I error can lead to misinterpreted study results:

Mini-Study 2.7 ■ The author of a review article evaluated 20 well-conducted studies that examined the relationship between breastfeeding and breast cancer. Nineteen of the studies found no difference in the frequency of breast cancer between breastfeeding and formula-feeding. One study found a difference in which the breastfeeding group had an increase in breast cancer. The results of this one investigation were statistically significant at the 0.05 level. The author of the review article concluded that because the study suggested that breastfeeding is associated with an increased risk of breast cancer, breastfeeding should be discouraged.

When 20 well-conducted studies are performed to test a study hypothesis that is not true in the larger population, a substantial possibility exists that one of the studies may show *a P value* at the 0.05 level simply by chance. Remember the meaning of statistical significance with a P value of 0.05: It implies that the results have a 5% probability, or a chance of 1 in 20, of occurring by chance alone when no difference or association exists in the larger population.

Thus, 1 study in 20 that shows a difference should not be regarded as evidence for a difference in the larger population. It is important to keep in mind the possibility that no difference may exist even when statistically significant results have been demonstrated. If the only study

---

[2.10] This method, called *Bonferroni correction*, is a useful approximation for small numbers of variables. As the number of comparisons increases much above 5, the required P value tends to be too small before statistical significance can be declared. This approach reduces the statistical power of a study to demonstrate statistical significance for any one variable. Also note that when a hypothesis is indicated prior to collecting the data, most, if not all, of the variables used in the investigation are collected for purposes of adjustment for potential confounding variables. Thus when analyzing data in this situation, one is not dealing with multiple comparisons. Other methods are used to correct for multiple analyses of the data. The correction needed for multiple analyses is not as large as the correction needed for multiple hypotheses.

showing a relationship had been accepted without further questioning, breastfeeding might have been discouraged.

Type II Errors

A *Type II* error says that failure to reject the null hypothesis does not necessarily mean that no true difference exists in the larger population. Remember that statistical significance testing directly addresses only the null hypothesis. The process of statistical significance testing allows one to reject or fail to reject that null hypothesis. It does not allow one to prove a null hypothesis. Failure to reject a null hypothesis merely implies that the evidence is not strong enough to reject the assumption that no difference exists in the larger population.

A Type II error occurs when we are prevented from demonstrating a statistically significant difference even when a difference actually exists in the larger population. This happens when chance produces an unusual set of data that fails to show a difference, even though one actually exists in the larger population. Efforts to perform statistical significance testing always carry with them the possibility of error.

Investigators may make the problem far worse by using samples that are smaller than recommended based on careful study design. Thus, the chance of making a Type II error increases as the sample's size decreases.

Statistical techniques are available for estimating the probability that a study of a particular size could demonstrate a statistically significant difference if a difference of a specified size actually exists in the larger population. These techniques measure the *statistical power* of the study. The statistical power of a study is its probability of demonstrating statistical significance. Thus, statistical power equals one minus the Type II error. In studies, the probability is quite large that one will fail to show a statistically significant difference when a true difference actually exists. Well-designed studies usually aim for a Type II error between 10% and 20%, that is, they aim for a statistical power of 80% to 90%. A Type II error of 10% is often the goal, with a 20% Type II error being the maximum tolerated consistent with good study design. Without actually stating it, investigators who use relatively small samples may be accepting a 30%, 40%, or even greater probability that they will fail to demonstrate a statistically significant difference when a true difference exists in the larger population. The size of the Type II error tolerated in the design of an investigation is known as the *beta level*. Table 2.2 summarizes and compares Type I and Type II errors.

The following example shows the effect of sample size on the ability to demonstrate statistically significant differences between groups:

> **Mini-Study 2.8** ■ A study of the adverse effects of cigarettes on health was undertaken by monitoring 100 cigarette smokers and 100 similar nonsmokers for 20 years. During the 20 years, 6 smokers developed lung cancer, whereas none of the nonsmokers were afflicted. During the same time period, 30 smokers and 28 nonsmokers developed myocardial infarction. The results for lung cancer were statistically significant, but the results for myocardial infarction were not. The authors concluded that a difference in lung cancer frequency between smokers and nonsmokers had been demonstrated, and a difference between smokers and nonsmokers for myocardial infarction had been refuted.

When true associations between groups are very large, as they are between cigarette smoking and lung cancer, only a relatively small sample may be required to demonstrate statistical significance. When there are true but smaller associations such as those that exist between cigarettes smoking and coronary artery disease, it requires greater numbers to demonstrate a statistically significant difference.

This study would not refute a difference in the probabilities of myocardial infarction in cigarette smokers and nonsmokers. It is very likely that the number of individuals included were too few to give the study enough statistical power to demonstrate the statistical significance of a

TABLE 2.2	Inherent Errors of Statistical Significance Testing	
	Type I Error	**Type II Error**
Definition	Rejection of null hypothesis when no true difference or association exists in the larger population.	Failure to reject the null hypothesis when a true difference or association exists in the larger population. Statistical power equals one minus the Type II error.
Source	Random error.	Random error and/or sample size that is too small to allow adequate statistical power.
Frequency of occurrence	Alpha level prior to conducting the investigation indicates the probability of a Type I error that will be tolerated. After results are obtained, the *P* value indicates the probability of a Type I error.	Beta level prior to conducting the investigation indicates the probability of a Type II error that will be tolerated. If the sample size is small, the probability of a Type II error can be very large, i.e., 50% or greater.

difference. A study with limited statistical power to demonstrate a difference also has limited power to refute a difference.

When the size of an investigation is very large, just the opposite issue may arise. It may be possible to demonstrate statistical significance even if the size or magnitude of the association is very small. Imagine the following results:

> **Mini-Study 2.9** ■ Investigators monitored 100,000 middle-aged men for 10 years to determine which factors were associated with coronary artery disease. They hypothesized beforehand that uric acid might be a factor in predicting the disease. The investigators found that men who developed coronary artery disease had a uric acid measure of 7.8 mg/dl, whereas men who did not develop the disease had an average uric acid measure of 7.7 mg/dl. The difference was statistically significant with a P value of 0.05. The authors concluded that because a statistically significant difference had been found, the results would be clinically useful.

Because the difference in this investigation is statistically significant, it is most likely real in the larger population. However, it is so small that it probably is not clinically important. The large number of men being observed allowed investigators to obtain a statistically significant result for a very small difference between groups.

However, the small size of the difference makes it unlikely that uric acid measurements could be clinically useful in predicting who will develop coronary artery disease. The small difference does not help the clinician to differentiate those who will develop coronary artery disease from those who will not. In fact, when the test is performed in the clinical laboratory, this small difference is probably less than the size of the laboratory error in measuring uric acid. Table 2.2 summarizes and compares Type I and Type II errors.

We learned earlier that statistical significance testing tells us very little about the size of a difference or the strength of an association; that is, the role of estimation. Thus, it is important to ask not only whether a difference or association is statistically significant, but whether it is large or substantial enough to be clinically useful. The world is full of myriad differences between individuals and between groups. Many of these, however, are not large enough to allow us to usefully separate individuals into groups for the purposes of disease prevention, diagnosis, and therapy. That is, they are not clinically important. Statistically significant and substantial or clinically important are two different questions that must be addressed separately. One way to address both of these separate issues is to use *confidence intervals* (CIs).

CONFIDENCE INTERVALS

Statistical significance testing does not directly provide us with information about the strength of an observed association. It is attractive to use a method that provides a summary measure (often called a *point estimate*) of the strength of an association and that also permits us to take chance into account using a statistical significance test.

The calculation of CIs is such a method. CIs combine information from samples about the strength of an observed association with information about the effects of chance on the likelihood of obtaining the observed results. It is possible to calculate the CI for any percentage confidence. However, the 95% CI is the most commonly used. It allows us to be 95% confident that the larger population's difference or association lies within the CI. (3)

CIs are often calculated for odds ratios and relative risks. The reader of the literature may see an expression for relative risk such as "10 (95% CI 8 to12)" or sometime just "10 (8 to12)," which expresses the observed relative risk (lower confidence limit and upper confidence limit). The term *confidence limit* is used to indicate the upper or lower extent of a CI.

Imagine a study in which the relative risk for birth control pills and thrombophlebitis was 10 (95% CI 8 to12). How would you interpret this CI? The 10 indicates the relative risk observed in the sample. The CI around this relative risk allows us to say with 95% confidence that the relative risk in the larger population is between 8 and 12. Because the lower confidence limit is 8, far >1, this allows us to be quite confident that a substantial relative risk is present not only in our sample, but also in the larger population from which our sample was obtained.[2.11]

These expressions of confidence limits, in addition to providing additional information on the size of the estimates of relative risks or odds ratios, have another advantage for the health literature reader. They allow us to rapidly draw conclusions about the statistical significance of the observed data. When using 95% CIs, we can quickly conclude whether or not the observed data are statistically significant with a *P* value ≤0.05.

This calculation is particularly straightforward for relative risk and odds ratio. For these, 1 represents the point at which the probabilities or odds of disease are the same, whether or not the risk factor or intervention is present. Thus, a relative risk or odds ratio of 1 is actually an expression of the null hypothesis, which says the probability or odds of disease are the same whether the risk factor is present or absent. If the CI does not extend to the opposite side of 1, we can conclude that it is very likely that birth control pills increase the chances of thrombophlebitis. That is, it is statistically significant. This is one way of thinking about the meaning of statistically significance.

Thus, if the 95% CI around the observed relative risk does not extend below 1, we can conclude that the relative risk is statistically significant with a *P* value ≤0.05. The same principles hold for odds ratios. Let us look at a series of relative risks and 95% CIs for studies on birth control pill and thrombophlebitis:

A. 6 (95% CI 5 to 8)
B. 6 (95% CI 1.2 to10)
C. 6 (95% CI 0.9 to 12)

The number to the left of the parenthesis is the relative risk, which is obtained from the data in the investigation. The numbers within the parentheses are the lower and upper limits of the 95% CI.

Figure 2.1 provides a graph that can be used to display these CIs.

Figure 2.2 fills in these observed relative risks and the 95% CI.

[2.11] This interpretation of confidence internals is a Bayesian interpretation. An alternative interpretation is often called a *frequentist* interpretation. A frequentist interpretation asks what range of values would be found 95% of the time if the same investigation was repeated an unlimited number of times. The frequentist approach favors presentation of data as *P* values, whereas the Bayesian approach favors CIs. In recent years, a compromise has been reached and many journals now present both *P* values and CIs. CIs can often be calculated using the same data that are needed to perform statistical significance testing. When this is the situation, the CIs are called *test-based CIs*.

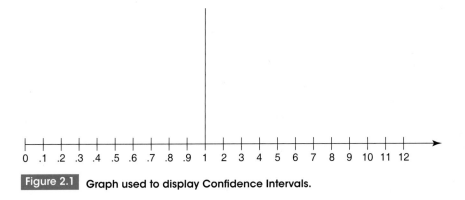

Figure 2.1 | Graph used to display Confidence Intervals.

Examples A and B are both statistically significant because their 95% CIs do not cross to the other side of 1. Note, however, that the CI in example A is much narrower than in example B. Thus, other things being equal, we can be more confident in the results represented by example A than example B. Example C on the other hand is not statistically significant because the 95% CI crosses to the other side of 1.

Now let us look at some observed relative risks and 95% CIs in which the observed relative risk is <1. An observed relative risk of <1 implies that the factor in the numerator reduces the risk or the probability of the outcome. When interventions are investigated, the group receiving the intervention is often placed in the numerator; therefore, relative risk of <1 implies that the study intervention is associated with a better outcome.

Now take a look at the following relative risks and 95% CIs in which the observed relative risk is <1.

D. 0.5 (95% CI 0.3 to 0.65)
E. 0.5 (95% CI 0.2 to 0.9)
F. 0.5 (95% CI 0.1 to 1.5)

Figure 2.3 fills in these observed relative risks and 95% CIs.

In examples D and E, the 95% CIs do not cross 1. Therefore, they are both statistically significant. However, the 95% CI for example D is much narrower than for example E. Thus, other things being equal, we can have more confidence in the results represented by example D. In example F, the 95% CI crosses 1. Therefore, the results are not statistically significant.[2.12]

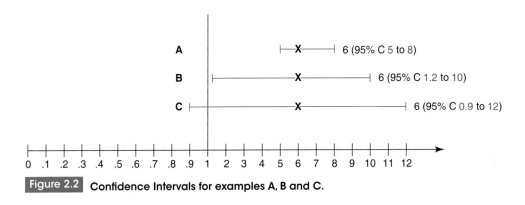

Figure 2.2 | Confidence Intervals for examples A, B and C.

[2.12] By tradition, when the 95% CI reaches but does not extend beyond 1, the results are considered statistically significant. Thus, a P value of 0.05 is considered statistically significant. Often CIs are not symmetrical. CIs around differences can also be calculated. When comparing the CIs of a difference between two groups, however, it is important to recognize that statistical significance is addressed by asking whether the CIs of each group overlap the observed value in the other group. A common misconception holds that the CIs themselves cannot overlap and still have a statistically significant result.

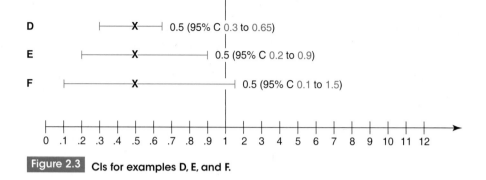

Figure 2.3   CIs for examples D, E, and F.

As a reader of the literature, you will increasingly find the observed value and the confidence limits included in the results section. This is helpful because it allows you to gain a "gestalt," or a feel, for the data. It allows you to draw your own conclusion about the clinical importance of the size or strength of the observed estimate such as the relative risk. Finally, if you want to convert to the traditional statistical significance testing format for hypothesis testing, you can determine whether the results are statistically significant with a *P* value of 0.05 or less.

Thus CIs can help us answer the first two questions of statistics: the estimation of the magnitude of the effect and the inference or statistical significance. Now let us take a look at the third basic question of statistics, adjustment for confounding variables.

ADJUSTMENT

Addressing the Effect of Confounding Variables (2-4)

We have discussed how confounding variables can result from either random error or bias. Chance may produce random error. Unlike bias, the effect of chance is unpredictable. It may either favor or oppose the study hypothesis in a way that cannot be predicted beforehand.

Bias, on the other hand, implies a systematic effect on the data in one particular direction that predictably either favors or opposes the study hypothesis. Bias results from the way the participants were assigned or assessed. Bias and chance may each produce differences between study and control groups, resulting in study and control groups that differ in ways that can affect the outcome of the study.

The investigator is obligated to compare the characteristics of individuals in the study group with those in the control group to determine whether they differ in known ways. If the groups differ substantially, even without being statistically significant, the investigator must consider whether these differences could have affected the results. Characteristics that differ between groups and that may affect the results of the study are potential confounding variables. These potential confounding variables may result either from selection bias or from differences between the study and control groups produced by random error. If a potential confounding variable is detected, the investigator is obligated to consider this in the analysis of results using a process we call *adjustment of data*.[2.13]

[2.13] Many biostatisticians encourage the use of adjustment, even when the differences are small or the importance of differences is not apparent. This has become common, if not routine, with the availability of sophisticated computer software. Also note that multiple variable methods allow for use of data that can include large numbers of potential categories rather than being restricted to data like gender or race that has two or a limited number of potential categories.

In the most straightforward form of adjustment, known as *stratification*, the investigator may separate into groups those who possessed specific levels of the confounding variable. Members of the study group and the control group with the same level of confounding variable are then compared to see whether an association between exposure and disease exists. For instance, if gender is a potential confounding variable, the investigator might subdivide the study group and the control group into men and women and then compare study group versus control group men and study group versus control group women to determine whether the results differ when groups of the same gender are compared. Learn More 2.3 demonstrates the basic process of adjustment for potential confounding variable using a stratification process with an example.

Deciding when to conduct an adjustment procedure may not be as straightforward as is suggested in the male baldness and stroke example. Learn More 2.4 takes a more in-depth look at what we mean by confounding.

Statistical techniques known as multivariable methods are available for adjusting more than one variable at a time.[2.14] Two multivariable methods are often used in the health research literature *logistic regression* and *Cox proportional hazard regression*. Both of these methods allow adjustment for multiple variables when the dependent variable is an either/or variable such as dead/alive or cure/no cure.

Cox proportional hazards regression as opposed to logistic regression allows for multiple measurements for the dependent variables. This is important when the dependent or outcome variable is affected by the length of observations, that is, when the dependent variable is *time-dependent*. Time-dependent dependent or outcome variables are often present in cohort studies as well as randomized controlled trials when groups of individuals are followed over extended periods. Cox proportional hazard regression produces an estimate of the strength of the relationship known as a *hazard ratio*. You can think if a hazard ratio as a relative risk adjusted for multiple potential confounding variables.

When selecting variables for inclusion in any multivariable analysis, it is important to avoid including variables that are themselves associated with other independent variables included in the analysis. Including independent variables that are closely associated with each other produces what is called *collinearity*, which reduces the apparent strength of the relationship for both independent variables. The following scenario illustrates the potential for collinearity:

Mini-Study 2.10 ■ An investigator found an association between high BP and stroke. He then adjusted for multiple potential confounding variables. These included family history of high BP and daily salt intake. After adjustment for these variables, the strength of the association between high BP and stroke was much weaker.

Family history of high BP and daily salt intake are themselves associated with the occurrence of high BP. If the investigator uses these variables as potential confounding variable, they will inevitably weaken the strength of the association between high BP and strokes. This is what we mean by collinearity.

[2.14] Statistical methods that allow for adjustment can incorporate multiple independent variables. They generally cannot address more than one dependent variable. These multivariable methods are often called multivariate methods. Technically multivariate methods refer to special techniques that are able to address multiple dependent variables. When there is more than one dependent variable or more than one hypothesis, the usual approach is to conduct separate analyses, one for each dependent variable. However, when the dependent variable consists of a nominal variable with more than two categories, a chi-square method can be used, which represent true multivariate procedures.

LEARN MORE 2.3 ■ THE PROCESS OF ADJUSTMENT USING STRATIFICATION (5) ■ Let us walk through an example of how adjustment for a confounding variable can be conducted using the process known as *stratification*. Stratification implies that a confounding variable can be taken into account, or controlled for by comparing groups with the same level of a potential confounding variable. If gender is a potential confounding variable, then males can be compared with males and females with females. A similar process can occur for other potential confounding variables such as age, race, or severity of illness:

Mini-Study 2.11 ■ An investigation was conducted of a possible association between male baldness and strokes. The investigators found the following data:

	Stroke		
	Yes	**No**	**Total**
Balding	7,750	92,250	100,000
Not balding	1,900	98,100	100,000
Total	9,650	190,350	200,000

Adopted from Young Epidemiology Scholars Baumgarten M. *Confounding in Epidemiology*. http://yes.collegeboard.org/teaching-units/confounding-epidemiology. Accessed July 21, 2011.

Relative Risk = (7,750/100,000)/(1,900/100,000) = 4.08

These data appear to demonstrate that baldness is associated with stroke. However, if age is a confounding variable related to both balding and coronary artery disease, it would be important to adjust for age. Stratification can be used as a simple method of adjustment by dividing men into two age categories or strata that we will call young and old. Imagine that the stratification by age produced the following results:

Stroke in Older Men

	Stroke		
	Yes	**No**	**Total**
Balding	7,500	67,500	75,000
Not balding	1,000	9,000	10,000
Total	8,500	76,500	85,000

Relative risk for older men = (7,500/75,000)/(1,000/10,000) = 1

Stroke in Younger Men

	Stroke		
	Yes	**No**	**Total**
Balding	250	24,750	25,000
Not balding	900	89,100	90,000
Total	1,150	113,850	115,000

Relative risk for younger men = (250/25,000)/(900/90,000) = 1

Note that in each strata, older men and younger men, the relative risk relating bald to stroke disease is 1. That is, no association exists. Thus taking into account, age has eliminated the impact of male balding.

LEARN MORE 2.4 ■ THE MEANING OF CONFOUNDING ■ Failure to recognize and adjust for a confounding variable can result in serious errors, as illustrated in the following example:

Mini-Study 2.12 ■ An investigator studied the relationship between coffee consumption and lung cancer by monitoring 500 heavy coffee drinkers and 500 coffee abstainers for 10 years. In this cohort study, the risk for lung cancer in heavy coffee drinkers was two times that of coffee abstainers. The author concluded that coffee, along with cigarettes, was established as a risk factor in the development of lung cancer.

Coffee consumption may look like it is related to lung cancer, but this apparent association is most likely the result of the fact that coffee drinking is associated with cigarette smoking. Assume that smoking cigarettes is not only a contributing cause of lung cancer but is also associated with coffee consumption. Thus, when we try to investigate the relationship between coffee consumption and lung cancer, cigarette smoking is a confounding variable. That is, cigarette smoking is associated with both coffee consumption and lung cancer and must be taken into account through the process known as adjustment.

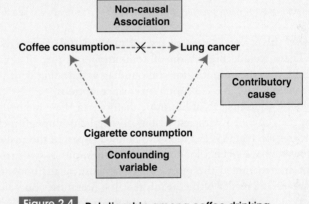

Figure 2.4 **Relationship among coffee drinking, cigarette smoking, and lung cancer.**

Figure 2.4 depicts the relationship among coffee drinking, cigarette smoking, and lung cancer. In adjusting for cigarette smoking, the investigator could divide coffee drinkers into cigarette smokers and nonsmokers and do the same with the coffee abstainers. The investigator would then compare nonsmoking coffee drinkers with nonsmoking coffee abstainers to determine whether the relationship between coffee drinking and lung cancer still holds true. Only after determining that eliminating the impact of cigarette smoking does not eliminate the relationship between coffee drinking and lung cancer can the author conclude that coffee drinking is associated with the development of lung cancer.

The process of conducting adjustments for potential confounding variables has become increasingly easy in recent years as large quantities of data have become available and high-speed computing has made the process much easier to undertake. Increasingly, researchers need to be aware of the potential for *over adjustment.* Let us look at an example of potential over adjustment:

Mini-Study 2.13 ■ Investigators were studying the relationship between obesity and kidney disease. The investigators knew that diabetes is associated with both obesity and strokes. Therefore, they assumed that diabetes was a confounding variable and adjusted for diabetes. They found that after adjustment for diabetes the relationship between obesity and kidney disease nearly disappeared.

(Continued)

Figure 2.5 depicts the relationship among obesity, diabetes, and kidney disease.

Obesity ⟶ Diabetes ⟶ Kidney disease

Figure 2.5 **Relationship among obesity, diabetes, and kidney disease.**

In this example, the investigators have failed to recognize that obesity can lead to diabetes and that diabetes can lead to kidney disease. That is, diabetes is in the chain of causation between obesity and kidney disease. By adjusting for diabetes, they have removed much if not all of the relationship between obesity and kidney disease. We say that they have over adjusted. In general, adjustment should take place when:

- there is an association between a factor and the independent variable and
- there is also an association between the factor and the dependent variable, but
- the factor is not in the chain of causation between the independent and dependent variables.

As we have seen, there are several methods for dealing with potential confounding variables. These include prevention of confounding as part of the design of an investigation and recognition of the potential for confounding and dealing with this possibility as part of the analysis of the results. Table 2.3 summarizes these options.

Often it is possible to utilize more than one of these methods. For instance, matching or pairing can be combined with restrictions on eligibility through inclusion as exclusion criteria. Multiple regression methods can then also be used as part of the analysis of the results.

Now we have taken a look at the basic questions of statistics: estimation, inference, and adjustment and examined the most common statistical methods used to address these questions. However, as a reader of the health research literature, you will encounter a large number of statistical methods whose use depends on the types of data includes in the independent and dependent variables. Thus, let us look at how data can be categorized and how the methods used to address our basic statistical questions is affected by the type of data included in the investigation.

SELECTING STATISTICAL PROCEDURES (1–3)

Statistical procedures can serve several purposes in health research. They are often initially used to summarize the data found in an investigation.[2.15]

[2.15] The data from an investigation can often be summarized using one or two basic summary measurements. When we are dealing with either/or data such as cancer or no cancer, the data can be summarized using one summary measure such as the proportion with the disease, the odds ratio, or the relative risk. When the data have a large number of potential categories, we usually need two measures to summarize the data. One tells us about what is called the *central tendency* and a second measurement that tells us about the spread or *dispersion of the data*. For example, to completely describe a bell shaped or *Gaussian distribution*, two summary measurements are needed—the *mean or average* and the *standard deviation*. The standard deviation measures the dispersion or spread of the sample's data by calculating how far from the sample's mean the individual measurements occur. The standard deviation (σ) is the square root of the variance (σ^2). The variance is equal to the mean square deviation of data (χi) from the mean (μ). The mean is not the only measure of central tendency. Other measures include the *median*, the point at which half the values are greater and half the values are less and the *mode* or location of the greatest number of values. For a Gaussian distribution, but not other types of distributions, the mean, the median, and the mode are equal.

TABLE 2.3	Methods for Dealing with Potential Confounding Variables	
Method	**Meaning**	**Advantages and Disadvantages**
Inclusion and exclusion criteria	Defines criteria for those eligible to be included to ensure a uniform group.	■ Helps assure study and control groups are similar. ■ Narrows range of individuals included, i.e., restricts extrapolation or generalizability of the results.
Group matching	Limits those who are entered into a study to ensure that the study and control groups are similar for key criteria such as age or gender.	■ Ensures similarity of groups but requires excluding some otherwise eligible study participants. ■ Does not take advantage of special statistical techniques for pairing, which have greater statistical power.
Pairing	Linkage of one individual in a study group with one or more similar individuals in a control group to ensure that the study and control groups are similar.	■ Ensures similarity of the study and control individuals and allows use of special statistical techniques with greater statistical power. ■ Need to limit use of pairing to small number of important variables or will not be able to identify pairs. ■ Limits issues that can address if variable of interest is closely associate with variable used for pairing.
Randomization	Assignment of individuals to study and control groups using a chance process.	■ If numbers are large nearly guarantees that the study and control groups will be similar for unknown as well as known confounding variables. ■ Often not ethical or practical at the individual level may not be practical at the community or group level.
Adjustment: stratification	Statistical method for adjustment or taking into account (controlling for) potential confounding variables after collection of the data. Separation of the data into stratum or categories and then comparing of same categories between groups.	■ Makes clear what is being compared and the impact of the adjustment. May be used as initial effort to identify most important variables for subsequent multiple variable adjustment ■ Limited to small number of adjustments especially when sample size is not large.
Adjustment: multiple variable adjustment	Statistical methods for adjustment that permits taking into account multiple confounding variables at the same time.	■ Takes into account multiple variables at the same time and can simultaneously address issues of estimation, inference, and adjustment simultaneously. ■ Need to carefully choose which variables to include avoiding variables that are closely related to each other (collinearity).

When we are dealing with analytical studies, statistical procedures can be used to address the three basic questions of statistics that is estimation, inference, and adjustment.

In order to identify appropriate statistical methods to use to address these basic questions of statistics, we first need to identify the type(s) of data that are represented by each of the independent variable(s) as well as the dependent variable.

Types of Data

To categorize types of data, the first distinction we make is between *continuous* and *discrete* data. Discrete data can in term be subdivided into *ordinal data* and *nominal* or categorical data. Nominal data may have two categories in which case it is also called dichotomous data or more than two categories.

Continuous data are defined as data that provide the possibility of observing any of an infinite number of equally spaced numerical values between any two points in its range of measurement. Examples of continuous data include BP, serum cholesterol, age, and weight. For each of these variables, we can choose any two numerical values and imagine additional intermediate measurements that would be, at least theoretically, possible to observe between those values. We might, for instance, consider the ages of 35 and 36 years. We could think of different ages between 35 and 36 that are distinguished by the number of days since a person's 35th birthday or the number of hours or minutes since that birthday. Theoretically, there is no limit to how finely we can imagine time being measured. Note, however, that continuous data do not need to have an infinite range of possible values but rather an infinite number of possible values within their range. That range may, and usually does, have a lower and an upper boundary. Age is a good example. The lower boundary is zero, and it is difficult to imagine individuals much older than 120 years.

Discrete data, on the other hand, can have only a limited number of values in their range of measurement. Examples of discrete data include number of pregnancies and stage of disease. For each of these variables, we can generally select two values between which it is not possible to imagine other values. For instance, there is no number of pregnancies between two and three pregnancies.

In practice, the distinction between continuous and discrete data can be a bit unclear. For example, the number of hairs on one's scalp is discrete data: We cannot imagine observing a value between 9,999 and 10,000 hairs. Even so, the number of possible numerical values within the entire range of the number of hairs is equally spaced and is very large. Can we consider such a variable to be composed of continuous data? Yes, for most purposes that would be entirely appropriate.

As opposed to continuous data, some types of discrete data measurements are made on *ordinal scales* that are not required to have a uniform interval between consecutive measurements. Data on an ordinal scale have a specific ranking or ordering, as do continuous data, but the interval between consecutive measurements for ordinal data may not be known and may not be constant. A common type of variable measured on an ordinal scale is an ordering of the stage of disease. We know, for instance, that stage 2 is more advanced than stage 1, but we cannot assert that the difference between these two stages is the same as the difference between stage 3 and stage 2.

If we are unable to apply any ordering to discrete data, then we say that the data were measured on a *nominal scale*. Examples of characteristics composed of nominal scale discrete data are gender, race, and eye color. Additional data that we treat as nominal data include dichotomous measurements with two categories even though they might be considered to have an innate order because one is clearly better than the other (e.g., alive vs. dead).

Note that the term "nominal variable" can be confusing. In its common use, a nominal variable is a characteristic, such as gender or race has two or more potential categories. From a statistical point of view, however, one nominal variable is limited to only two categories. Thus, race or eye color should be referred to as nominal data that require more than one nominal variable for inclusion in statistical procedures. The number of nominal variables required is equal to the number of categories of the nominal data minus one. Thus, if we have data on gender with two genders, we require only one nominal variable, but if we have data on race with five races, we require four nominal variables.

Thus, for purposes of selecting a statistical procedure or interpreting the result of such a procedure, it is important to distinguish between three categories of variables:

1. Continuous variables: includes continuous data, such as age, and discrete data that contain a great number of possible values, such as number of hairs.
2. Ordinal variables: includes discrete data that can be ordered one higher than the next and with at least three and at most a limited number of possible values, such as stages of cancer.
3. Nominal variables: includes discrete data that cannot be ordered, such as race, and dichotomous data that can assume only two possible values, such as dead or alive.

The order in which those categories are listed indicates the relative amount of information contained in each type of variable. That is, continuous variables contain more information than ordinal variables, and ordinal variables contain more information than nominal variables. Thus, continuous variables are considered to be at a higher level than ordinal or nominal variables.

Measurements with a particular level of information can be rescaled to a lower level. For example, age (measured in years) can be considered a continuous variable. We could legitimately rescale age to be an ordinal variable by defining persons as being children (0 to 18 years), young adults (19 to 30 years), adults (31 to 45 years), mature adults (46 to 65 years), young elderly (65 to 80 years), and old elderly (80 and older). We could rescale age further to be a nominal variable. For instance, we might simply divide persons into two categories: young and old, or children and adults. We cannot, however, rescale variables to a higher level than the one at which they were actually measured.

When we rescale measurements to a lower level, we lose information. That is, we have less detail about a characteristic if it is measured on a nominal scale than we do if the same characteristic was measured on an ordinal or continuous scale. For example, we know less about a woman when we label her a mature adult than we do when we say that she is 54 years old. If an individual is 54 years old and we measured age on a continuous scale, we could distinguish that person's age from another individual who is 64 years old. However, if age was recorded on the ordinal scale above, we could not recognize a difference in age between those individuals.

Loss of information, when rescaled measurements are used in statistical procedures, has the consistent effect, all else being equal, of increasing the Type II error rate. That is to say, rescaling to a lower level reduces statistical power, making it harder to establish statistical significance and, thus, to reject a false null hypothesis. What we gain by rescaling to a lower level is the ability to circumvent making certain assumptions, such as uniform intervals, about the data that are required to perform certain statistical tests.

We have now reviewed the key steps that must occur in selecting a statistical procedure. These steps are as follows:

1. Identify one dependent variable and all independent variables, if present, on the basis of the study question.
2. Determine for each variable whether it consists of continuous, ordinal, or nominal data.

TABLE 2.4	Selection of Statistical Tests		
Independent variable(s)	Nominal Dependent Variable	Ordinal Dependent Variable	Continuous Dependent Variable
One nominal independent variable	Chi-square	Mann–Whitney test	t-Test
One ordinal independent variable	Convert ordinal variable to nominal variables	Spearman test Convert ordinal independent variable to nominal variables	Convert to nominal dependent variable
One continuous independent variable	Chi-square test for trend	Convert ordinal variable to nominal variables	Pearson correlation or linear regression
More than one nominal independent variable	Mantel–Haenszel (log-rank)	Convert ordinal variable to nominal variables	Analysis of variance
Nominal and continuous independent variables	Logistic regression or Cox proportional hazard regression for time-dependent independent variable	Convert ordinal variable to nominal variables	Analysis of covariance

Table 2.4 organizes many of the commonly used statistical tests based upon the answers to these questions. (1) It provides names of statistical methods that may be appropriate to use in specific circumstances.[2.16]

The results section of the M.A.A.R.I.E. framework addresses the questions of estimation, inference, and adjustment. That is, it asks whether an observed difference or association is substantial (estimation), is likely to be present in the larger population (inference), and is likely due to confounding variables (adjustment). Although the existence of a substantial and statistically significant association that remains after performing adjustment is important, it is only the first criterion for contributory cause or efficacy. To be able to draw conclusions about contributory cause or efficacy, we need to continue on and explore the interpretation component of the M.A.A.R.I.E. framework in Chapter 3.

[2.16] It is important to recognize that many statistical tests require that the data from an investigation fulfill specific assumptions that need to be examined with the assistance of a biostatisticians. At times, statistical tests may be used despite the fact that the data do not completely fulfill these assumptions. In this situation, the statistical tests are said to be *robust*. Many statistical significant tests assume that there is a Gaussian or bell shaped distribution of variables or that a *transformation* can be used to produce a Gaussian distribution. Tests that include a continuous dependent variable may assume an equal variance of the continuous variable for each value of the independent variables. This is known as *homoscedasticity*. A series of exact tests, not included in this table may be used when the expected frequency of the outcome predicted by the null hypothesis is small. For instance, Fisher exact test may be used instead of the chi-square test when any of the expected frequencies of the outcomes under the null hypothesis is <5. Tests designed for paired data such as the McNemar test for one nominal dependent variable and one nominal independent variable are not included in this table.

REFERENCES

1. Sullivan LM. *Essentials of Biostatistics in Public Health*. 2nd ed. Sudbury, MA: Jones and Bartlett Learning; 2011.

2. Hirsch RP, Riegelman RK. *Statistical First Aid: Interpretation of Health Research Data*. Boston, MA: Blackwell Scientific Publications; 1992.

3. Dawson B, Trapp RG. *Basic and Clinical Biostatistics*. 4th ed. New York, NY: McGraw-Hill Companies, Inc; 2004.

4. Motulsky H. *Intuitive Biostatistics*. New York, NY: Oxford University Press; 1995.

5. Young Epidemiology Scholars; Baumgarten M. Confounding in epidemiology. http://yes.collegeboard.org/teaching-units/confounding-epidemiology. Accessed July 21, 2011.

thePoint ✳ Visit http://thePoint.lww.com for interactive Q&A, flaw-catching exercises, searchable eBook, and more!

3 Studying a Study: M.A.A.R.I.E. Framework—Interpretation, Extrapolation

INTERPRETATION

Interpretation asks us to address questions about the meaning of the investigation's results for those who have participated in the investigation. There are three types of questions that can be addressed by interpretation.

- Contributory cause or efficacy: Does the factor being investigated alter the probability that the disease will occur (contributory cause) or work to reduce the probability of an undesirable outcome (efficacy)?
- Harms: Are adverse events that affect the meaning of the results identified?
- Subgroups and interactions: Do the outcomes in subgroups differ and are there interactions between factors that affect outcome?

Questions of contributory cause or efficacy are the first questions that are addressed by interpretation, and at times may be the only questions. Questions of adverse outcomes and questions about subgroups may only be important when there is evidence for contributory cause or efficacy. Therefore, we will take a close look at the issues of contributory cause and efficacy and then outline key concepts for understanding adverse outcomes and subgroups.

Contributory Cause or Efficacy (1,2)

In Chapter 1, we introduced a definition of cause and effect termed *contributory cause*. This same definition is used to establish efficacy. To definitively establish the existence of a contributory cause or efficacy, all three of the following criteria must be fulfilled:

1. **Association:** Does the investigation establish a statistically significant and substantial association that provides convincing evidence that individuals with the "cause" also have an increased probability of experiencing the "effect"?
2. **Prior association:** Does the investigation establish that the "cause" precedes the "effect"?
3. **Altering the cause alters the effect:** Does the investigation establish that altering or modifying the frequency or severity of the "cause" alters the frequency or severity of the disease or other "effect"?

Figure 3.1 again shows the overall framework for using specific types of investigations to establish these criteria.

Association

Establishing the first criterion of contributory cause, association at the individual level requires that we examine the magnitude and the statistical significance of the relationship established in the analysis of results. To establish the existence of an impressive association, we expect a statistically significant and substantial relationship.

Remember, statistical significance testing is designed to help us assess the role of chance when we observe a difference or an association in any of the forms of investigation that we have examined. Thus, the evidence provided in the results section is the basis for determining

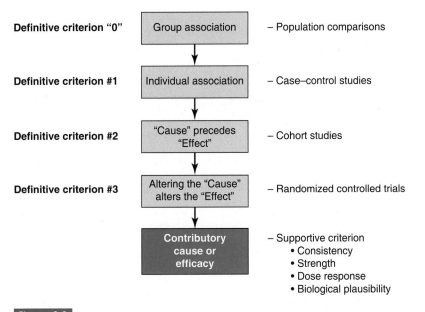

Definitive criterion "0" → Group association — Population comparisons

Definitive criterion #1 → Individual association — Case–control studies

Definitive criterion #2 → "Cause" precedes "Effect" — Cohort studies

Definitive criterion #3 → Altering the "Cause" alters the "Effect" — Randomized controlled trials

Contributory cause or efficacy — Supportive criterion
• Consistency
• Strength
• Dose response
• Biological plausibility

Figure 3.1 Using multiple types of studies to establish criteria for contributory cause and for efficacy.

that an association exists between those with the factor and those with the outcome under investigation.

"Cause" Precedes the "Effect"

To establish the second and third criteria, we must rely on more than statistical analysis. It may appear to be simple to establish that a cause precedes a disease, but let us look at two hypothetical studies in which the authors may have been fooled into believing that they had established that the cause preceding the effect:

Mini-Study 3.1 ■ Two investigators conducted a case–control study to determine whether antacids were taken by patients with myocardial infarction (MI) the week preceding an MI. They were looking for causes of the condition. MI patients were compared with patients admitted for elective surgery. The authors found that the MI patients were 10 times as likely to have taken antacids as the controls were during the week preceding admission. The authors concluded that taking antacids is associated with subsequent MIs.

The authors believed that they established not only the first criterion of causation (an association at the individual level) but also the second criterion (that the cause precedes the effect).

But did they? If individuals have angina before MIs, they may misinterpret the pain and try to alleviate it by self-medicating with antacids. Therefore, the medication is taken to treat the disease and does not truly precede the disease. This study failed to establish that the cause precedes the effect because it did not clarify whether the disease led the patients to take the medication or whether the medication led to the disease. This example illustrates what is called *reverse causality*. It illustrates the potential difficulty encountered in separating cause and effect in case–control studies. At times case–control studies, however, may be capable of providing convincing evidence that the cause precedes the effect. This occurs when there is good documentation of previous characteristics that are not affected by knowledge of occurrence of the disease. Alternatively, we may believe that the characteristic of an individual is not likely to change over time such as the presence of a gene.

Cohort studies often have an advantage in establishing that the possible cause occurs before the effect. The following example, however, illustrates that even in cohort studies we may encounter reverse causality:

> **Mini-Study 3.2** ■ A group of 1,000 patients who had stopped smoking cigarettes within the last month were compared with 1,000 current cigarette smokers matched for total pack-years of smoking. The two groups were monitored for 6 months to determine with what frequency they developed lung cancer. The study showed that 5% of the study group who had stopped smoking cigarettes was diagnosed with lung cancer as opposed to only 0.1% of the currently smoking controls. The authors concluded that stopping cigarette smoking was associated with the subsequent development of lung cancer. Therefore, they advised current smokers to continue smoking.

The cessation of cigarette smoking appears to occur before the development of lung cancer, but what if smokers stop smoking because of symptoms produced by lung cancer? If this was true, then lung cancer stops smoking, and not vice versa. Thus, one must be careful in accepting that the hypothesized cause precedes the effect. The ability of cohort studies to establish that the cause precedes the effect is enhanced when the time lapse between cause and effect relative to the natural history of the disease is longer than in this example. Short time intervals still leave open the possibility that the presumed cause has been influenced by the presumed effect instead of the reverse.

Altering the "Cause" Alters the "Effect"

Even if one has firmly established that the possible cause precedes the effect, to completely fulfill the criteria for contributory cause, it is necessary to establish that altering the cause alters the probability of the effect. This criterion can be established by performing an intervention study in which the investigator alters the cause and determines whether this subsequently contributes to altering the probability of the effect. Ideally, this criterion is fulfilled by performing a randomized controlled trial. As we will discuss in Chapter 5, randomized controlled trials may not be ethical or practical, thus we need to examine other ways to establish the definitive criteria including altering the cause alters the effect.[3.1]

When contributory cause cannot be definitively established, we may need to make our best judgments about the existence of a cause-and-effect relationship. For this situation, a series what have been called *ancillary*, *adjunct*, or *supportive criteria* for contributory cause can be used. These include the following:

1. **Strength of association.** A strong association between the risk factor and the disease as measured, for example, by a large relative risk.
2. **Consistency of association.** Consistency is present when investigations performed in different settings on different types of patients produce similar results.

[3.1] It is important to recognize that contributory cause is an empirical definition. It does not require an understanding of the intermediate mechanism by which the contributory cause triggers the effect. Historically, numerous instances have occurred in which actions based on a demonstration of contributory cause reduced disease despite the absence of a scientific understanding of how the result actually occurred. Puerperal fever was potentially controlled through hand washing before the bacterial agents were recognized. Malaria was controlled by swamp clearance before its mosquito transmission was recognized. Scurvy was prevented by citrus fruit before the British ever heard of vitamin C. Once we understand more about the direct mechanisms that produce disease, we are able to distinguish between indirect and direct contributory causes. What we call a direct cause of disease depends on the current state of knowledge and understanding of disease mechanism. Thus, over time, many direct causes may come to be regarded as indirect causes. In addition, it is important to distinguish these terms from the legal concept of proximal cause. *Proximal cause* refers to the timing of actions that could prevent a particular outcome and should not be confused with the definition of causation used here.

3. **Biological plausibility.** Biological plausibility implies that a known biological mechanism is capable of explaining the relationship between the cause and the effect.[3.2]

4. **A dose-response relationship.** A dose-response relationship implies that changes in levels of exposure to the risk factor are associated with changes in the frequency of disease in a consistent direction.

Data that support each of these four criteria help bolster the argument that a factor is actually a contributory cause. When these criteria are fulfilled, it reduces the likelihood that the observed association is due to chance or bias. These criteria, however, do not definitively establish the existence of a contributory cause.

In addition, none of these four criteria for contributory cause are essential. A risk factor with a modest but real association may in fact be one of a series of contributory causes for a disease. Consistency is not essential because it is possible for a risk factor to operate in one community but not in another. This may occur because of the existence in one community of other prerequisite conditions. Biological plausibility assumes that we understand the relevant biological processes. Finally, demonstrating a dose-hypersensitivity reactions may result from exposure to even a small amount of an agent. Larger exposures may not result in greater reactions. Even when a dose-response relationship is present, it usually exists only over a limited range of values. For cigarettes and lung cancer, one or two cigarettes per day may not measurably increase the probability of lung cancer, and the difference between three and four packs per day may not be detectable. Dose-response relationships may be confusing, as illustrated in the next example:

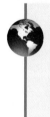

Mini-Study 3.3 ■ An investigator conducted a cohort study of the association between radiation and thyroid cancer. He found that low-dose radiation had a relative risk of five of being associated with thyroid cancer. He found that at moderate levels of radiation, the relative risk was 10, but at high levels, the relative risk was 1. The investigator concluded that radiation could not cause thyroid cancer because no dose–response relationship of more cancer with more radiation was demonstrated.

The relative risk of 10 is an impressive association between radiation and thyroid cancer. This should not be dismissed merely because the relative risk is diminished at higher doses. It is possible that low–dose and moderate–dose radiation contributes to thyroid cancer, whereas large doses of radiation actually kill cells and thus do not contribute to thyroid cancer.

For many biological relationships, a little exposure may have little measurable effect. At higher doses, the effect may increase rapidly with increases in dose. At still higher doses, there may be little increase in effect. Thus, the presence of a dose–response relationship may depend on which part of the curve is being studied.[3.3]

These ancillary, adjunct, or supportive criteria for judging contributory cause are just that: They do not in and of themselves settle the issue. If present, they may help support the argument for contributory cause. These criteria help in understanding issues raised in a controversy and the limitations of the data.

[3.2] The biological plausibility of the relationship is evaluated on the basis of clinical or basic science principles and knowledge. For instance, hypertension is a biologically plausible contributory cause of strokes, coronary artery disease, and renal disease because the mechanism for damage is known and the type of damage is consistent with that mechanism. However, data suggesting a relationship between hypertension and cancer would not be biologically plausible, at least on the basis of current knowledge. Biological plausibility also implies that the timing and magnitude of the cause are compatible with the occurrence of the effect. For instance, we assume that severe, long-standing hypertension is more likely to be a contributory cause of congestive heart failure or renal disease than mild hypertension of short duration.

[3.3] Other ancillary criteria have been developed and used. Although not universally accepted, their presence may increase the probability that a contributory cause is present. These criteria include specificity (i.e., one "cause" produces one "effect") and analogy (i.e., there are other well-established examples of similar relationships). As with the other ancillary criteria, these criteria are not necessary to establish a contributory cause. (1)

Other Concepts of Causation

The approach we have been using for establishing contributory cause has been very useful in studying disease causation especially noncommunicable diseases. The traditional approach to establishing causation for communicable diseases has been quite different. In the 19th century, Robert Koch developed a series of conditions that must be met before a bacterium can be considered the cause of a disease. The series of conditions is known as *Koch's postulates*. Learn More 3.1 takes a look at Koch's postulates and what has been called *Modern Koch's postulates.*

LEARN MORE 3.1 ■ KOCH'S POSTULATES AND MODERN KOCH'S POSTULATES(3,4) ■ Causation in communicable disease has been an issue since the 19th century when the germ theory of communicable disease was first proposed. Critics challenged the theory arguing that bacteria were the result of disease and not its cause. Robert Koch sought to establish definitive criteria for disease causation in communicable disease which then meant bacterial diseases. Koch's postulates first demonstrated for the spread of anthrax in animal populations required the following four criteria be fulfilled:

- The bacteria must be present in every case of the disease.
- The bacteria must be isolated from the host with the disease and grown in pure culture.
- The specific disease must be reproduced when a pure culture of the bacteria is inoculated into a healthy susceptible host.
- The bacteria must be recoverable from the experimentally infected host.

Koch's postulates have been difficult to fulfill for most bacterial diseases and even more difficult for viral diseases in which the causative cannot be grown in pure culture. Koch's postulates can be viewed as the equivalent of necessary and sufficient causation, perhaps an ideal standard but not a practical standard for most clinical and public health efforts.

In recent years, a revised set of criteria for communicable disease causation has been put forth by the National Institutes of Allergy and Infectious disease which parallels the three definitive criteria we have discussed.

- Association: The communicable disease is associated with the pathogen more often than expected by chance, that is, it is associated at an individual level
- Isolation: The pathogen can be isolated from many if not all those with the disease
- Transmission: The pathogen can be transferred to others and produces the same disease

These criteria together parallel the expectations of association at the individual level, the "cause" precedes the "effect" and altering the "cause" alters the effect. They do not require that necessary and/or sufficient cause be established but recognize that not everyone exposed to a disease will develop clinical evidence of the disease and that some clinical syndromes can be produced by more than one organism.

Originally put forth to address the controversy surrounding the etiology of acquired immunodeficiency syndrome (AIDS), the criteria were useful in establishing coronavirus as the cause of severe acute respiratory syndrome (SARS). These criteria help bring together the approaches used in noncommunicable and communicable diseases for establishing causation. The line between these approaches has narrowed considerably or even disappeared in recent years as conditions such as duodenal ulcers have been demonstrated to be caused by *Helicobacter pyroli* and papillomaviruses have been established as a contributory cause of cervical cancer.

Koch's postulates were built on a system of formal logic that requires what is called *necessary and sufficient causation*. Necessary cause goes beyond the requirements we have outlined for establishing contributory cause. Historically, this was very useful in the study of communicable disease when a single agent was responsible for a single disease. However, if the concept of necessary cause is applied to the study of noncommunicable diseases, it is nearly impossible to prove a causal relationship. For instance, even though cigarettes have been well established as a contributory cause of lung cancer, cigarette smoking is not a necessary condition for developing lung cancer; not everyone with lung cancer has smoked cigarettes.

Under the rules of strict logic, causation also requires a second condition known as *sufficient cause*. This condition says that if the cause is present, the disease will also be present. In our cigarette and lung cancer example, sufficient cause would imply that if cigarette smoking is present, lung cancer will always follow.

Even in the area of communicable disease, cause and effect may not be straightforward; for instance, mononucleosis is a well-established clinical illness for which the Epstein-Barr virus has been shown to be a contributory cause. However, other viruses such as cytomegalovirus also have been shown to cause a mononucleosis syndrome. In addition, evidence may show that Epstein-Barr virus has been present in a patient without ever causing mononucleosis or it may manifest itself by being a contributory cause of other diseases, such as Burkitt lymphoma or other cancers. Thus, despite the fact that the Epstein-Barr virus has been established as a contributory cause of mononucleosis, it is neither a necessary nor a sufficient cause of this syndrome. If we require necessary and sufficient cause before concluding that a cause-and-effect relationship exists, we will be able to document very few, if any, cause-and-effect relationships in clinical medicine or public health. The next example illustrates the consequences of strictly applying necessary cause to health studies:

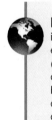

Mini-Study 3.4 ■ In a study of the risk factors for coronary artery disease, investigators identified 100 individuals from a population of 10,000 MI patients who experienced MIs despite normal blood pressure, normal low-density lipoprotein (LDL) and high-density lipoprotein (HDL) cholesterol, regular exercise, no smoking, and no family history of coronary artery disease. The authors concluded that they had demonstrated that hypertension, high LDH and low HDL cholesterol, lack of exercise, smoking, and family history were not the causes of coronary artery disease because not every MI patient possessed a risk factor.

The authors of this study were using the concept of necessary cause as a concept of causation. Instead of necessary cause, however, let us assume that all these factors had been shown to fulfill the criteria for contributory cause of coronary artery disease. Contributory cause, unlike necessary cause, does not require that everyone who is free of the cause will be free of the effect. The failure of known contributory causes to be present in all cases of disease emphasizes the limitations of our current knowledge about all the contributory causes of coronary artery disease and encourages further investigations into additional risk factors. It illustrates the limitations of our current state of knowledge because if all the contributory causes were known, then everyone with disease would possess at least one such factor. Thus, even when a contributory cause has been established, it will not necessarily be present in each and every case.

As we have seen, the concept of contributory cause is very useful because it is directly linked to the use of case–control, cohort and randomized controlled trials. These three basic types of studies may be used together to demonstrate the three definitive criteria for contributory cause. Case–control studies are able to establish individual association; cohort studies can also definitively establish that the "cause" precedes the "effect"; and randomized controlled trials are capable of definitively establishing that altering the "cause" alters the "effect". Contributory cause does not require that all individuals who are free of the contributory cause will be free of the effect. It does not require that all people who possess the contributory cause will develop the effect. In other words, a contributory cause may be neither necessary nor sufficient, but it must be contributory. Its presence must increase the probability of the occurrence of disease, and its reduction must reduce the probability of the disease. There may be more than one contributory cause. Multiple factors may be demonstrated to be contributory causes and multiple interventions may alter the cause and thereby alter the effect.

Harms

Complete interpretation of the results requires us to look beyond contributory cause or efficacy to examine not only the benefits of an intervention but also its potential harms. The approach used for judging the importance of potential harms is different from the approach used for potential benefits or efficacy. As we have seen, investigations are often specifically designed with the aim of demonstrating statistically significant results for the primary end point. Harm or safety is rarely the primary focus of the basic types of investigations. Unless harm or adverse events are themselves the primary end point, most investigations will not have a large statistical power to demonstrate the statistical significance of adverse events observed in an investigation. The importance of under-standing this principle is illustrated in the next example:[3,4]

Mini-Study 3.5 ■ An investigation found that a new treatment for throm-bophlebitis had efficacy in more rapidly resolving clots than the conventional treatment. Life-threatening bleeding, however, occurred in 1% of those receiving the new treatment compared with 0.05% among those receiving conventional treatment. The investigators concluded that this adverse event was not important because the results were not statistically significant.

Despite the small numbers and absence of statistical significance, this finding may be clinically important. We cannot ignore increases in adverse events merely because they are not statistically significant. Most investigations do not have the statistical power to allow us to use statistical signifi-cance testing for adverse events. The investigation of harms is far most complex than the investiga-tion of efficacy or benefits. We will devote a chapter to looking at harms or safety.

Subgroups and Interactions (5)

In addition to drawing conclusions about contributory cause or efficacy and harms, investigators of-ten examine the meaning of the investigation for subgroups of individuals with special characteristics.

Examination of subgroups, or what is called *subgroup analysis*, is an important and error-prone component of interpretation. Ideally, we would like to examine subgroups especially when an intervention has been shown to have efficacy. For instance, we would like to know whether a treatment with efficacy works best for mild versus severe disease, young versus old, males versus females, and so on. Knowing the results for each of these subgroups and many others would assist us in applying the results in practice.

[3,4]The term adverse events is increasingly being used since as opposed to adverse effects or side effects since adverse events does not imply the existence of a cause-and-effect relationship.

Despite the potential usefulness of subgroup analysis, it must be done carefully because there are so many potential subgroups. If all of the potential subgroups are analyzed, we are faced with what we have called the multiple comparison problem—look at enough groups and some of them will inevitably be statistically significant if we use the standard statistical methods.

One approach to subgroup analysis argues that before the investigation begins a limited number of subgroup hypotheses about the outcomes in clinically important subgroups should be identified for later subgroup analysis. These subgroup hypotheses are said to be identified *pre hoc* in contrast to *post hoc* in which no hypotheses are put forward before collecting the data. Pre hoc subgroup hypotheses might include the following: those with more severe disease are expected to have worse than average responses to the treatment or those who receive more intensive treatment are expected to have better than average responses to the treatment. The investigator then could examine these subgroups regardless of the results for the overall investigation.

Another approach argues that subgroup analysis should not be conducted unless the results obtained using the entire study data has demonstrated statistical significance. In this approach, if a statistically significant result based on the primary hypothesis is obtained using the entire study population, a number of large subgroups may be examined. However, in this situation, the investigator needs to limit the number of subgroups examined and take into account the number of subgroups examined.

It is especially important to be careful in drawing conclusions from analyses of subgroups that were conducted in the absence of an overall statistically significant result using post hoc analysis. The consequences of this type of approach are illustrated in the following example:

Mini-Study 3.6 ▪ An investigation of a new treatment for lung cancer found no statistically significant difference between the new treatment and the conventional treatment. However, after examining a large number of subgroups post hoc, the investigators found that those who had left-side primary lesions had a statistically significant improvement in longevity.

As with multiple comparisons in general, when we look at multiple subgroups, we will often eventually find one or more that is statistically significant especially when no hypothesis is put forth before the investigation. Without an overall finding of statistical significance and without an initial hypothesis that left-side primary lesions will respond better, we need to be very cautious in interpreting these results.

Interactions

As part of the investigation of subgroups, we may be able to learn about the interactions between factors that produce better or worse outcomes. Interactions between factors may operate to produce disease or to affect the outcome of disease. Treatment interactions are among the most commonly recognized types of interactions. Interactions between treatments such as drugs are an important part of the evaluation of benefits and harms in clinical practice. Let us extend our previous example to illustrate this point:

Mini-Study 3.7 ▪ The data on patients receiving the new treatment and experiencing more frequent life-threatening bleeding were examined. It was found that these patients had especially rapid dissolution of their clots. The authors concluded that there may be an interaction between the speed of clot breakdown and the probability of life-threatening bleeding. They argued that this relationship makes biological sense, and stressed the potential harm of this new treatment.

The authors correctly focused on the potential interaction. They relate this interaction to what is known about the biology and wisely are cautious about the use of this new treatment.[3.5]

Despite the importance of interactions, statistical methods for identifying and integrating interactions into data analysis are limited. Formal statistical methods usually require statistical significance before labeling the relationship between two factors as interaction. Because of the low statistical power for identifying interaction, the absence of statistical interaction should not be equated with the absence of biological interaction.[3.6]

At times, the impact of interactions is so great that they can be demonstrated to be statistically significant. In these situations, they are added as an additional factor or variable along with the confounding variables. When interactions are found to be statistically significant, it is important to focus on their interpretation, as illustrated in the next example:

> **Mini-Study 3.8** ■ Cigarette smoking is found on average to have a relative risk of 10 for lung cancer. Exposure to environmental factors such as high dose radon is found on average to have a relative risk of 3 for lung cancer. When cigarette exposure and high dose radon exposure were both present, the average relative risk was found to be 30.

This is a type of interaction known as *multiplicative interaction*. Multiplicative interaction implies that the risks multiply rather than add together. That is, if both cigarette smoking and high dose radon exposure are present, the risk for those with both factors compared with those with neither factor is 30 rather than 13. This is an important finding because it suggests that addressing either of the factors will have a much greater than expected impact on the chances of developing lung cancer.

Now we have examined the meaning of the results for those in the investigation. However, our job is not quite done. When reading research, we are interested not only in the meaning for those in the investigation but for those we will encounter in practice. These may be individual patients, at-risk groups, or populations in communities. Thus, the last component of the M.A.A.R.I.E. framework extrapolation asks us to draw conclusion about those who are not included in the investigation.

EXTRAPOLATION

The process of extrapolation requires us to ask what the results of the investigation tell us about individuals not included in the study and for situations not directly addressed by the

---

[3.5] At times, the distinction is made between statistical and biological interaction. This is an example of biological interaction. Despite the biological interaction discussed here, it is unlikely that statistical interaction would be demonstrated. Statistical interaction, even when present, may depend on the scale of measurement used—that is, it may exist for ratios such as relative risk and not exist for differences.

[3.6] It has been argued that use of a P value of 0.05 is not appropriate for statistical significance tests of interaction because of the low power of the tests. In addition, an argument exists that interaction should not be subject to statistical significance testing at all. Note that we do not subject confounding variables to statistical significance tests. However, interactions are very common, and if we introduce a large number of interaction terms into a regression analysis, its statistical power to demonstrate statistical significance for the primary relationship is reduced. Perhaps this is the reason that there is great resistance to raising the acceptable P value for defining interaction or for eliminating the use of statistical significance testing for interaction.

study.[3.7] In conducting extrapolation, the reader must ask how the investigators applied the results to

- Individuals, groups, or populations who are similar to the average participant in the investigation
- Situations that go beyond the range of the study's data
- Populations or settings that differ from those in the investigation

This is not the investigators' job alone. In fact, they are not in the best position to perform extrapolation. The investigators often want their study's conclusions to have the broadest possible implications. But they cannot know the characteristics of the individuals, institutions, or communities to whom the reader wishes to apply the study's evidence. Thus, the reader needs to be the expert on extrapolation.

Let us start by seeing how we can use the data from a study to extrapolate to similar individuals, similar groups at risk, and similar populations or communities. We will then explore extrapolation beyond the data and to different populations and settings.

Extrapolation to Similar Individuals, Groups, or Populations (6,7)

The most cautious form of extrapolation asks the investigator to extend the conclusions to individuals, at-risk groups, and populations that are similar to those included in the investigation. This process can usually proceed using a quantitative approach without the need for additional assumptions on the part of the investigator.

In this form of extrapolation, we may be interested in extrapolating study results to evaluate their overall meaning for an individual who is similar to the average individual included in the investigation. In doing this, we assume that the study's findings are as applicable to other very similar individuals who possess the factor, that is, the risk factor or intervention being studied as it was for the individuals who were actually included in the investigation.

Many case–control and cohort studies estimate the odds ratio or relative risk associated with the development of the disease if a factor is present compared with when it is not present. The odds ratio and relative risk tell us the strength of the relationship between the factor and the disease. A relative risk of 10 means the average individual has 10 times the probability of developing the disease or other outcome over a specified period if the factor is present versus if it is not present.

Relative risk does not, however, tell us the absolute magnitude of the risk of developing the outcome if the factor is present compared with when it is not present. A relative risk of 10 may indicate an increase in probability from 1 per 1,000,000 for those without the factor to 1 per 100,000 for those with the factor. Alternatively, a relative risk of 10 may indicate an increase in probability from 1 per 100 for those without the factor to 1 per 10 among those with the factor. Thus, despite the same relative risk, the *absolute risk* for individuals in these two examples is very different. The absolute risk tells us the probability or rate of occurrence of the event when the risk factor is present and also when it is absence. Knowing these two absolute risks tells us more than knowing their ratio as indicated by the relative risk.

[3.7] Extrapolation is also called *external validity* as well as *generalizability*. Extrapolation is used here because it is the most general term. *Internal validity* as opposed to external validity is a term used to address issues of assessment of the outcome as well as interpretation of the data for those included in the investigation. In the behavioral and social science literature, internal validity often includes content validity: how well the assessment covers all aspects of the phenomenon under study; construct validity: how well the assessment appears to make a meaningful distinction consistent with theory; and criterion validity: how well the assessment correlated with other well accepted measures.

Failure to understand the concept of absolute risk can lead to the following type of extrapolation error:

> **Mini-Study 3.9** ■ A patient has read that the relative risk of death resulting from acute leukemia is increased four times with use of a new chemotherapy for stage III breast cancer. The relative risk of patients dying of stage III breast cancer over the same time period without chemotherapy is 3. She therefore argues that the chemotherapy is not worth the risk of developing acute leukemia.

The absolute risk of dying of stage III breast cancer, however, is far greater than the absolute risk of death from future acute leukemia. The infrequent and later occurrence of acute leukemia means that even in the presence of a risk factor that increases the risk 4-fold, the absolute risk of dying of leukemia is still very small compared with the very high risk of dying of breast cancer. Thus, the absolute risk strongly favors the benefits of treatment despite the small probability of harm. The patient in this example has failed to understand the important difference between relative risk and absolute risk. It is desirable to have information on both the relative risk and absolute risk when extrapolating the results of a study to a particular individual or when comparing one risk to another.[3.8]

Extrapolation to Similar At-Risk Groups

Relative risk and absolute risk are often used to make estimates about the impact on individual patients. Sometimes, however, we are more interested in the average impact that a factor, a risk factor or intervention, may have on groups of individuals with the factor or on a community of individuals with and without the factor.

When assessing the impact of a factor on a group of individuals, we use a concept known as *attributable risk percentage*. Calculation of attributable risk percentage does not require the existence of a cause-and-effect relationship. However, when a contributory cause exists, attributable risk percentage tells us the percentage of a disease that may potentially be eliminated from individuals who have the risk factor if the impacts of that risk factor can be completely and immediately removed.[3.9]

Attributable risk percentage is defined as follows:

$$\frac{\text{Probability of disease if risk factor present} - \text{Probability of disease if risk factor absent}}{\text{Probability of disease if risk factor present}} \times 100\%$$

Attributable risk percentage can be easily calculated from relative risk using the following formula when the relative risk is greater than 1:

$$\text{Attributable risk percentage} = \frac{\text{Relative risk} - 1}{\text{Relative risk}} \times 100\%$$

[3.8] Note that if both absolute risks are known, the relative risk can be calculated as their ratio. When extrapolating to individuals, it is important to appreciate that the data from an investigation addresses issues of averages. Imagine that an intervention is found to have efficacy in an investigation that includes participants with diastolic blood pressure ranging from 90 to 120 mm Hg with an average of 100 mm Hg. The extrapolation to similar individuals should initially address the implications for those similar to the average person in the study, that is, those with a diastolic blood pressure of 100 mm Hg. Those between 90 and 100 mm Hg might be regarded as a subgroup. There are most likely only a small number of participants in the study with a diastolic blood pressure close to 90 mm Hg. Extrapolating results to individuals with a diastolic blood pressure of 90 mm Hg can dramatically increase the number of individuals to whom the results apply, even if there is no evidence that benefit results from treating individuals with a diastolic blood pressure of 90 mm Hg.

[3.9] Attributable risk percentage has also been called attributable fraction (exposed), etiologic fraction (exposed), attributable proportion (exposed), and percentage risk reduction. When efficacy has already been established, attributable risk percentage may be called percent efficacy.

The following table uses this formula to convert relative risk to attributable risk percentage:

Relative Risk	Attributable Risk Percentage (%)
1	0
2	50
4	75
10	90
20	95

Notice that even a relative risk of 2 may produce as much as a 50% reduction in the disease among those with the risk factor.[3.10]

Failure to understand the potential impact of even small increases in relative risk, if the increase in risk is real, may lead to the following extrapolation error:

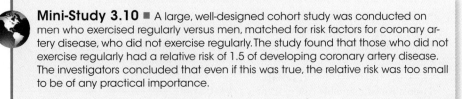

Mini-Study 3.10 ■ A large, well-designed cohort study was conducted on men who exercised regularly versus men, matched for risk factors for coronary artery disease, who did not exercise regularly. The study found that those who did not exercise regularly had a relative risk of 1.5 of developing coronary artery disease. The investigators concluded that even if this was true, the relative risk was too small to be of any practical importance.

Despite the fact that the relative risk is only 1.5, notice that it converts into an attributable risk of >33%

$$\text{Atrributable risk percentage} = \frac{1.5 - 1}{1.5} \times 100\% = 33.3\%$$

This means that among men who do not exercise regularly, one-third of their risk of coronary artery disease could potentially be eliminated if the impact of their lack of exercise could be immediately and completely eliminated. In this example, the lack of exercise may affect a large number of individuals because coronary artery disease is a frequently occurring disease and lack of regular exercise is a frequently occurring risk factor.

An alternative way of expressing the magnitude of the association for a risk group, which is applicable to cohort studies and to randomized controlled trials, is known as the *number needed to treat*. The number needed to treat indicates how many patients similar to the average study participant must be treated, as the average study group patient was, to obtain one less bad outcome or one more good outcome. It is calculated as follows:

$$\text{Number needed to treat} = \frac{1}{\begin{array}{l}\text{Probability of adverse outcome} - \text{Probability of the adverse}\\ \text{in the control group} \qquad \text{outcome in the study group}\end{array}}$$

[3.10] When the relative risk is expressed with the lower risk group in the numerator, the attributable risk percentage can be easily calculated as (1 − relative risk) × 100%. A relative risk <1 implies that the lower risk group is in the numerator. A relative risk <1 can be converted and expressed as a relative risk >1 by using the reciprocal—that is, a relative risk of 0.5 can also be expressed as a relative risk of 2, which implies that the higher risk group in now in the numerator. It can be confusing to compare relative risks >1 with relative risks <1 because relative risks >1 do not have an upper limit, whereas relative risks <1 cannot be <0. Thus, there are advantages of expressing all relative risks as >1. However, it is common to see relative risks expressed as <1 especially when dealing with interventions such as treatment or prevention.

Imagine that an investigation demonstrated a reduction of coronary artery disease over 5 years from 20 per 1,000 in a control group to 10 per 1,000 in the study group. The number needed to treat for 5 years to produce one less case of coronary artery disease would be calculated as follows:

$$\text{Number needed to treat} = \frac{1}{20/1{,}000 - 10/1{,}000} = \frac{1}{10/1{,}000} = 100$$

The number needed to treat of 100 indicates that 100 individuals, like the average participant in the study, need to be treated for 5 years to produce one less case of coronary artery disease.[3.11]

Extrapolation to Similar Populations

When extrapolating the results of a study to a community or population of individuals with and without a risk factor, we need to use another measure of risk known as the *population attributable risk percentage (PAR%)*.[3.12]

If a cause-and-effect relationship is present, the PAR% tells us the percentage of the risk in a population that can potentially be eliminated. To calculate the PAR%, we must know more than the relative risk (expressed as >1). It requires that we know or be able to estimate the proportion of individuals in the population who possess the risk factor (ranging from 0 to 1) that is we need to know the prevalence of the risk factor.[3.13]

If we can estimate the relative risk (expressed as >1) and if we can estimate the proportion of individuals in the population with the risk factor, we can calculate PAR% using the following formula:

$$\text{Population attributable risk percentage (PAR\%)} = \frac{(\text{proportion with risk factor})(\text{relative risk} - 1)}{(\text{proportion with risk factor})(\text{relative risk} - 1) + 1}$$

This formula allows us to relate relative risk, proportion of the population with the risk factor, and PAR% as follows:

Relative Risk	Proportion with the Risk Factor	PAR% (approximate)
2	0.01	1
4	0.01	3
10	0.01	8
20	0.01	16
2	0.10	9
4	0.10	23
10	0.10	46

[3.11] The number needed to treat may be <0. Negative numbers indicate that the control group patients on average had a better result. Thus, a negative number needed to treat indicates how many individuals need to be treated to produce one additional bad outcome. When presented as a positive number, this may also be thought of as the number needed to treat to produce one additional bad outcome or the number needed to harm.

[3.12] PAR% has also been called attributable fraction (population), attributable proportion (population), and etiologic fraction (population).

[3.13] When the odds ratio is a good approximation of relative risk, it may be used to calculate population attributable risk. This interpretation of PAR% like attributable risk percentage requires that a cause-and-effect relationship is present and that the consequences of the cause are immediately and completely reversible. Attributable risk percentages from two or more contributory causes may add to >100%. This is also the situation for PAR%.

Relative Risk	Proportion with the Risk Factor	PAR% (approximate)
20	0.10	65
2	0.50	33
4	0.50	60
10	0.50	82
20	0.50	90
2	1.00	50
4	1.00	75
10	1.00	90
20	1.00	95

Notice that if the risk factor is uncommon in the population (e.g., 1% or proportion with the risk factor = 0.01), the relative risk must be substantial before the PAR% becomes impressive. However, if the risk factor is common (e.g., 50% or proportion with the risk factor = 0.50), even a small relative risk means the potential community impact may be substantial. When the prevalence of the risk factor is 1, or 100% (i.e., when everyone has the risk factor), notice that the PAR% equals the attributable risk percentage. This is expected because attributable risk percentage uses a study group of individuals who all have the risk factor.

Failure to understand the concept of PAR% can lead to the following extrapolation error:

Mini-Study 3.11 ■ Investigators report that a hereditary form of high LDL cholesterol occurs in 1 per 100,000 Americans. They also report that those with this form of hyperlipidemia have a relative risk of 20 for developing coronary artery disease. The authors concluded that a cure for this form of hyperlipidemia would have a substantial impact on the national problem of coronary artery disease.

Using the data and our formula for PAR%, we find that elimination of coronary artery disease secondary to this form of hyperlipidemia produces a PAR% of about 0.02% or one-fiftieth of one percent. Thus, the fact that this type of hyperlipidemia is so rare a risk factor for a common disease means that eliminating its impact cannot be expected to have a substantial impact on the overall occurrence of coronary artery disease.

A final useful measure of the impact of a contributory cause on a population is given by what may be called the *number-prevented-in-the-population (N-P-P)*. The number-prevented-in the population asks about the potential impact of an intervention on a population. It may be expressed as the potential impact on 100,000 people or any sized population. The N-P-P asks how many cases of the disease can potentially be prevented in this population over a specified period such as 1 year. The calculation of the N-P-P requires an estimate of the incidence of the disease as well as the PAR% expressed as a proportion. The formula for N-P-P is as follows:

(Population attributable risk)
  × (incidence of the disease per 100,000 per year) × (100,000 population)

Thus, if the attributable risk percentage is 60% or 0.60 and the incidence per 100,000 is 1,000 per year, then the potential number prevented in the population by eliminating the impact of the factor is

$$(0.60) \times (1,000/100,000 \text{ year}) \times (100,000) = 600 \text{ per year}$$

The N-P-P may be very important to policy makers who are especially interested in the impact of an intervention on large number of people or on the population as a whole. It is important to recognize that the N-P-P like the attributable risk percentage and the PAR% is an estimate of the potential impact of an intervention assuming that there is a cause and effect or contributory cause and that the impact of the factor can be immediately and completely eliminated.

Learn More 3.2 demonstrates how each of these measures can be calculated based on a single set of data that reflect the occurrence of events in a population.

LEARN MORE 3.2 ■ CALCULATION OF MEASURES OF THE STRENGTH OF AN ASSOCIATION ■ When the outcome of an investigation is expressed as either/or data for the dependent and the independent variable, we often present the data using a two-by-two table. The two-by-two table allows us to calculate odds ratios and at times relative risk as we have already discussed. In addition, the data from two-by-two tables can be used to calculate a number of other summary measures of association that can provide useful information about individuals, groups, and/or populations.(5,6)

We have discussed six basic measures that are used to estimate the magnitude of an association when data are expressed as either/or data such as cigarette smoker or nonsmoker and lung cancer or no lung cancer. These measures of the strength of the association are as follows[3.14]:

- Absolute risk: The probability or rate of lung cancer among those who smoke (and among those who do not smoke)
- Relative risk or odds ratio: The probability or odds of lung cancer among those who smoke compared with those who do not smoke
- Attributable risk percentage: The percentage of the risk or probability of lung cancer that can potentially be prevented by elimination of cigarette smoking among current smokers
- Number needed to treat: Number of individuals who need to stop smoking to reduce by one the number of cases of lung cancer
- PAR%: The percentage of the lung cancer in the population that can potentially be prevented by elimination of cigarette smoking among current smokers
- N-P-P: The number of cases of lung cancer that can be prevented in a population of 100,000 by elimination of cigarette smoking among current smokers

Let us look at a hypothetical example of a population of 100,000 to see how we can calculate all of these measures from a two-by-two table. To allow us to do this, we need to assume that the data are representative of the population's prevalence of cigarette smoking and incidence of lung cancer and reflects a defined period of follow-up such as 20 years. In performing these calculations, we use the following hypothetical data:

(Continued)

[3.14]These interpretations of the meaning of these measures assume that a contributory cause has been established and that the impact of the cause (cigarette smoking) can be completely and immediately eliminated. The data reflect a defined period of follow-up that could be 1 year, 20 years or alternatively a lifetime.

LUNG CANCER AND SMOKING OVER 20 YEARS			
	Lung Cancer	No. Lung Cancer	
Regular cigarette smoker	$A = 3,000$	$B = 27,000$	$A + B = 30,000$
Not regular cigarette smoker	$C = 700$	$D = 69,300$	$C + D = 70,000$

The next table shows how to use this data to calculate each of the six measures of the strength of an association.

FORMULAE FOR ESTIMATES OF POTENTIAL IMPACT OF AN INTERVENTION IN A SIMILAR OVER 20 YEARS		
Measurement	Formula	Cigarette and Lung Cancer Example
Absolute risk	With the risk factor = $A/(A + B)$	10%
Relative risk	$\dfrac{A/(A + B)}{C/(C + D)}$	10
Attribute risk percentage	$\dfrac{(A/(A + B)) - (C/(C + D))}{A/(A + B)} \times 100\%$ $\dfrac{\text{Relative risk} - 1}{\text{Relative risk}} \times 100\%$	90%
Number needed to treat	$\dfrac{1}{(A/(A + B)) - (C/(C + D))}$	~11
PAR%	$\dfrac{(\text{Prev. of risk factor})(RR - 1)}{(\text{Prev. of risk factor})(RR - 1) + 1} \times 100\%$ where Prev. of RF = Prevalence of the risk factor or the proportion of the population with the risk factor, i.e., $(A + B)/(A + B + C + D)$	~73%
Number prevented-in-the-population	(No. in population)(incidence rate of the disease)(PAR%)	2,700 in a population of 100,000 over a 20 year period

Extrapolation Beyond the Range of the Data

Extrapolation to new situations or different types of individuals is even more difficult and is often the most challenging step when reading health research. It is difficult because the investigator and the reviewers are usually not able to adequately address the issues of interest to a particular reader. Extrapolation is up to you, the reader. The investigator does not know your community, your institution, or your patients. Despite the difficulty with extrapolating research data, it is impossible to be a health practitioner without extrapolation from the research. Often, we must go beyond the data on the basis of reasonable assumptions. If one is unwilling to do any extrapolation beyond the data, then one is limited to applying research results to individuals who are nearly identical to the average participant in an investigation.

Despite the necessity of extrapolating research data, it is important to recognize the types of errors that can occur if the extrapolation is not carefully performed. When extrapolating to different groups or different situations, two basic types of errors can occur—those due to extrapolations beyond the data, and those resulting from the difference between the study population and the target population, that is the group to which we wish to apply the results.

In research studies, individuals are usually exposed to the factors thought to be associated with the outcome for only a limited amount of time at a limited range of exposure. The investigators may be studying a factor such as hypertension that results in a stroke, or a therapeutic agent such as an antibiotic that has efficacy for treating an infection. In either case, the interpretation must be limited to the range and duration of hypertension experienced by the subjects or the dosage and duration of the antibiotic used in the study. When the investigators draw conclusions that extrapolate beyond the dose or duration of exposure experienced by the study subjects, they frequently are making unwarranted assumptions. They may assume that longer exposure continues to produce the same effect experienced by the study subjects. We will call this type of extrapolation *linear* or *straight line extrapolation*. The following example illustrates a potential error resulting from linear extrapolating beyond the range of the data:

Mini-Study 3.12 ▪ A new antihypertensive agent was tested on 100 patients with hard-to-control hypertension. In 100 patients with hard-to-control hypertension, the agent lowered diastolic blood pressure from 120 to 110 mm Hg at dosages of 1 mg per kg, and from 110 to 100 mm Hg at dosages of 2 mg per kg. The authors concluded that this agent would be able to lower diastolic blood pressure from 100 to 90 mm Hg at doses of 3 mg per kg.

It is possible that clinical evidence would document the new agent's efficacy at 3 mg per kg. Such documentation, however, awaits empirical evidence. Many antihypertensive agents have been shown to reach maximum effectiveness at a certain dosage and do not increase their effectiveness at higher dosages. To conclude that higher dosages produce greater effects without experimental evidence is to make a linear extrapolation beyond the range of the data.

Another type of error associated with extrapolation beyond the range of the data concerns potential adverse events or side effects experienced at increased duration, as illustrated by the following hypothetical example:

Mini-Study 3.13 ▪ A 1-year study of the effects of administering daily estrogen to 100 menopausal women found that the drug relieved hot flashes and reduced the rate of osteoporosis as compared to age-matched women given placebos who experienced no symptom relief. The authors found no adverse effects from the estrogens and concluded that estrogens are safe and effective. Therefore, they recommended that estrogens be administered long term to women, beginning at the onset of menopause.

The authors have extrapolated the data on using estrogens from a 1-year period of follow-up to long-term administration. No evidence is presented to show that if 1 year of administration is free of harms, so is long-term, continuous administration of estrogen. It is not likely that any long-term adverse events would show up in a 1-year study. Thus, the authors have made potentially dangerous extrapolations by going beyond the range of their data.

Linear extrapolation may sometimes be necessary in clinical and public health practice, but we must recognize that linear extrapolation has taken place so we can be on the lookout for new data that may undermine the assumptions and thus challenge the conclusions obtained by linear extrapolation.

Extrapolation to Different Populations or Settings

When extrapolating to a target population, it is important to consider how that group differs from the study's population sample used in the investigation. The following scenario illustrates how differences between countries, for instance, can complicate extrapolation from one country to another:

> **Mini-Study 3.14** ■ In a study involving Japan and the United States, 20% of the Japanese participants were found to have hypertension and 60% smoked cigarettes, both known contributory causes of coronary artery disease in the United States. Among US participants, 10% had hypertension and 30% smoked cigarettes. Studies in Japan did not demonstrate an association between hypertension or cigarettes and coronary artery disease, whereas similar studies in the United States demonstrated a statistically significant and substantial association. The authors concluded that hypertension and cigarette smoking must protect the Japanese from MIs.

The authors have extrapolated from one culture to a very different culture. Other explanations for the observed data are possible. If US participants frequently possess another risk factor, such as high LDL cholesterol, which until recently has been rare in Japan, this factor may override cigarette smoking and hypertension and help to produce the high rate of MIs in the US population.

Extrapolation within countries can also be difficult when differences exist between the group that was investigated and the target population to which one wants to apply the findings, as illustrated in the next example:

> **Mini-Study 3.15** ■ A study of the preventive effect of treating borderline tuberculosis (TB) skin tests (6 to 10 mm) with a year of isoniazid was conducted among Alaskan Native Americans. The population had a frequency of borderline skin tests of 2 per 1,000. The study was conducted by giving isoniazid to 200 Alaskan Native Americans with borderline skin tests and placebos to 200 others with the same borderline condition. Twenty cases of active TB occurred among the placebo patients and only one among the patients was given isoniazid. The results were statistically significant at the 0.01 level. A health official from the state of Virginia, where borderline skin tests occur in 300 per 1,000 skin tests, was impressed with these results. He advocated that all patients in Virginia who had borderline skin tests be treated with isoniazid for 1 year.

In extrapolating to the population of Virginia, the health official assumed that borderline skin tests mean the same thing for Alaskan Native Americans as for Virginians. Other data suggest, however, that many borderline skin tests in Virginia are not caused by TB exposure. They are frequently caused by an atypical mycobacteria that carries a much more benign prognosis and does not reliably respond to isoniazid. By not appreciating the different meaning of a borderline skin test in the residents of Virginia, the health official may be submitting many individuals to useless and potentially harmful therapy.

Extrapolation of study results is always a difficult but extremely important part of reading the health research literature. Extrapolation involves first asking what the results mean for individuals such as the average individual included in the investigation. Thus, one must begin by looking closely at the types of participants and types of settings in which the investigation was conducted. This enables the reader to consider what the results mean for similar individuals and at-risk groups. It also allows the reader to consider the meaning for communities or populations of individuals with and without the characteristics under study.

Often, the reader wants to go one step further and extend the extrapolation to individuals and situations that are different from those in the study. This extrapolation beyond the data must consider the differences between the types of individuals included in the investigation and the target group. Recognizing the assumptions we make in extrapolation forces us to keep our eyes open for new information that challenges these assumptions and potentially invalidates our conclusions.

We have now completed our discussion of the basic approach to reading research using the M.A.A.R.I.E. framework. To better understand how to adapt this approach to different types of investigations, we will now take a look at the application of the M.A.A.R.I.E. framework to specific types of investigations starting with randomized controlled trials in Chapter 4.

Questions To Ask: Studying a Study

The following questions to ask are applicable to the types of investigation we have discussed in the first three chapters. They may be used as a checklist as you read analytical investigations.

Method—The purpose, population, and study sample for the investigation

1. **Study hypothesis:** What is the study question being investigated?
2. **Study population:** What population is being investigated including the inclusion and exclusion criteria for the subjects of the investigation?
3. **Sample size and statistical power:** How many individuals are included in the study and in the control groups? Are the numbers adequate to demonstrate statistical significance if the study hypothesis is true?

Assignment—Allocation of participants to study and control groups

1. **Process:** What method is used to identify and assign individuals or populations to study and control groups?
2. **Confounding variables:** Are there differences between study and control groups, other than the factor being investigated that may affect the outcome of the investigation?
3. **Masking or blinding:** Are the participants and/or the investigators aware of the participants' assignment to a particular study or control group?

Assessment—Measurement of outcomes or end points in the study and control groups

1. **Appropriate:** Does the measurement of outcomes address the study's question?
2. **Accurate and precise:** Is the measurement of outcomes an accurate and precise measure of the phenomenon that the investigators seek to assess?
3. **Complete and unaffected by observation:** Is the outcome measurement nearly 100% complete and is it affected by the participants' or the investigators' knowledge of the study or control group assignment?

Results—Comparison of outcomes in the study and control groups

1. **Estimation:** What is the magnitude or strength of the relationship observed in the investigation?
2. **Inference:** What statistical technique(s) are used to perform statistical significance testing?
3. **Adjustment:** What statistical technique(s) are used to take into account or control for differences between the study group and control group that may affect the results?

Interpretation—Meaning of the results for those included in the investigation

1. **Contributory cause or efficacy:** Does the factor being investigated alter the probability that the disease will occur (contributory cause) or work to reduce the probability of undesirable outcomes (efficacy)?
2. **Harms:** Are adverse events that affect the meaning of the results identified?
3. **Subgroups and interactions:** Do the outcomes in subgroups differ and are there interactions between factors that affect outcome?

Questions To Ask: Studying a Study *(Continued)*

Extrapolation—Meaning of the results for those not included in the investigation

1. **To similar individuals, groups, or populations:** Do the investigators extrapolate or extend the conclusions to individuals, groups, or populations that are similar to those who participated in the investigation?
2. **Beyond the data:** Do the investigators extrapolate by extending the conclusions beyond the dose, duration, or other characteristics of the investigation?
3. **To other populations:** Do the investigators extrapolate to populations or settings that are quite different from those in the investigation?

REFERENCES

1. Bradford-Hill A. The environment and disease: association or causation? *Proc R Soc Med.* 1965;58:295–300.
2. Thagard P. *How Scientists Explain Disease.* Princeton, NJ: Princeton University Press; 1999.
3. Harvard University Library Open Collection Program. Robert Koch 1843–1910. http://ocp.hul.harvard.edu/contagion/koch.html. Accessed July 22, 2011.
4. National Institute of Allergy and Infectious Disease. The evidence that HIV causes AIDS. http://www.niaid.nih.gov/topics/hivaids/understanding/howhivcausesaids/pages/hivcausesaids.aspx. Accessed July 22, 2011.
5. Wang R, Lagakos SW, Ware JH, et al. Statistics in medicine: reporting of subgroup analyses in clinical trials. *N Engl J Med.* 2007;357:2189–2194.
6. Heller R. *Evidence for Population Health.* Oxford, UK: Oxford University Press; 2005.
7. Szklo M, Nieto FJ. *Epidemiology Beyond the Basics.* 2nd ed. Sudbury, MA: Jones and Bartlett Publishers; 2007.

thePoint ✳ Visit http://thePoint.lww.com for interactive Q&A, flaw-catching exercises, searchable eBook, and more!

4 | Randomized Controlled Trials

Randomized controlled trials (RCTs) or randomized clinical trials are now widely considered the gold standard by which we judge efficacy. The U.S. Food and Drug Administration (FDA) requires them for drug approval[4.1]; the National Institutes of Health rewards them with funding; the journals encourage them by publication; and increasingly, practitioners read them and apply their results. When feasible and ethical, RCTs are a standard part of health research. Thus, it is critically important to appreciate what these trials can tell us, what can go wrong, and what questions they cannot address.

RCTs today are usually conducted using an elaborate set of rules and procedures. These apply not only to drugs but increasingly also to a wide range of *interventions* from prevention to palliation. Much of what we discussed in the first three chapters applies to RCTs. In this chapter, we will emphasize the approaches and issues that are unique or especially important for RCTs.

The reporting of RCTs in high-quality journals generally follows the recommendations of what is known as the CONSORT (CONsolidated Standards Of Reporting Trials) Statement.(1) The details for conducting the study need to be defined in what is called the study's *protocol*. Before beginning a RCT, the investigation must be reviewed by an Investigational Review Board (IRB) to evaluate the quality of the study design, the ethics of conducting the study, and the safeguards provided for patients, including a review of the informed consent statement that potential participants will be asked to sign. The IRB is determining whether it is reasonable for a potential participant to be asked to participate. IRBs have taken on increasingly important roles in the conduct of research especially RCTs. Learn More 4.1 reviews roles that IRBs play.

> **LEARN MORE 4.1 ■ INSTITUTIONAL REVIEW BOARDS (2,3) ■** Before beginning an investigation on human beings, a researcher must obtain permission from the Institutional Review Board at each institution in which the research will be conducted. Subsequently, the researcher must obtain the informed consent of all those who are asked to participate. Let us take a look at what is involved in this process.
>
> IRBs are governed by U.S. federal regulations. These regulations derive from the 1978 Belmont Report, which resulted in large part from the Tuskegee study. The Tuskegee study followed approximately 600 poor black males with syphilis beginning in 1932. They were followed without treatment for 40 years despite the fact that effective treatment, penicillin, was available more than two decades earlier.[4.2]
>
> The Belmont report outlined the following principles:
>
> Respect for persons involves recognition of the personal dignity and autonomy of individuals, and special protection of those persons with diminished autonomy.

(Continued)

[4.1] The FDA generally requires convincing results from two independently conducted, well-designed RCTs for approval of a new drug. These investigations may be conducted in the United States or abroad.

[4.2] Note that the Tuskegee study was a cohort study. IRB rules are not limited to RCTs; they cover all studies involving "human subjects research," although exceptions and expedited reviews are available for studies that involve minimal risk to study subjects. *Minimal risk* is defined by the federal guidelines as "… the probability and magnitude of harm or discomfort anticipated in the proposed research are not greater, in and of themselves, than those ordinarily encountered in daily life or during the performance of routine physical or psychological examinations or tests … ." (2) For example, the risk of drawing a small amount of blood from a healthy individual for research purposes is no greater than the risk of doing so as part of routine physical examination.

Beneficence entails an obligation to protect persons from harm by maximizing anticipated benefits and minimizing possible risks of harm.

Justice requires that the benefits and burdens of research be distributed fairly.

The fundamental role of the IRB is to establish that the benefits to the individual and to society are worth the risks. Risk in this context means the potential harm to the individual study participant. To accomplish this goal, the IRB needs to be assured of the quality of the study design since without a well-designed study, little or no benefit can be expected.

An investigator also is expected to establish that there is a need to conduct a RCT. This includes establishing what is called *clinical equipoise*. Clinical equipoise implies that there is sufficient controversy within the expert clinical community about the preferred treatment to justify a RCT. Notice that clinical equipoise does not imply that the investigator is neutral as to the best treatment. Often the investigator will hold a strong opinion as to the best treatment. It is the IRB's responsibility to ensure that safeguards are in place to ensure that the investigator's opinion does not influence the conduct of the investigator.

The federal guidelines outline specific roles for the IRB which include the following:

1. Identify the risks associated with the research, as distinguished from the risks of therapies the subjects would receive even if not participating in research

2. Determine that the risks will be minimized to the extent possible

3. Identify the probable benefits to be derived from the research

4. Determine that the risks are reasonable in relation to the benefits to subjects, if any, and the importance of the knowledge to be gained

5. Ensure that potential subjects will be provided with an accurate and fair description of the risks or discomforts and the anticipated benefits

6. Determine intervals of periodic review, and, where appropriate, determine that adequate provisions are in place for monitoring the data collected

7. Determine the adequacy of the provisions to protect the privacy of subjects and to maintain the confidentiality of the data

If vulnerable populations such as pregnant women, children, or prisoners are included in the research, additional protections are required. Financial compensation is limited to modest compensation for time and effort and is not designed as an incentive to participate. Once the IRB has approved a study, the investigator may seek out individuals who fulfill the inclusion and exclusion criteria and ask for informed consent to participate in the investigation from the individual or their legal representative.

The content and process of informed consent is also governed by federal regulations and guidelines. Informed consent is a process and not just a document. The process of obtaining informed consent must allow potential participants adequate time to ask questions and deliberate on their decision. It must avoid "coercion or undue influence." Situations in which undue influence may occur and special protections are required include those in which potential study participants are in subordinate positions. For instance, undue influence may occur when an investigator is involved in a potential participant's health care or when a faculty requests informed consent from a student or an employer encourages an employee to participate. Informed consent information must be provided clearly and in a language understood by the potential study participant.

(Continued)

Federal guidelines also outline minimum content that needs to be included. The content of informed consent must include the following:

- A statement that the study involves research, an explanation of the purposes of the research and the expected duration of the subject's participation, a description of the procedures to be followed, and identification of any procedures that are experimental.
- A description of any reasonably foreseeable risks or discomforts to the subject.
- A description of any benefits to the subject or to others that may reasonably be expected from the research.
- A disclosure of appropriate alternative procedures or courses of treatment, if any, that might be advantageous to the subject.
- A statement describing the extent, if any, to which confidentiality of records identifying the subject will be maintained.
- For research involving more than minimal risk, an explanation as to whether any compensation is provided for adverse events.
- A statement that participation is voluntary, refusal to participate will involve no penalty or loss of benefits to which the subject is otherwise entitled, and the subject may discontinue participation at any time without penalty or loss of benefits to which the subject is otherwise entitled.

Approval by the IRB and obtaining informed consent from a study participant is a required part of the recruitment process. Once approved by the IRB, those who are asked to participate in the study must be informed and provide their informed consent. An additional review under the Health Insurance Portability and Accountability Act regulations is also now required to ensure the confidentiality of study data.

The CONSORT Statement now expects that a journal article reporting a RCT includes a flow chart that displays the passage of participants through the trial.

Figure 4.1 is the recommended template for reporting the data from RCTs. The terms used are parallel to the first four components of the M.A.A.R.I.E. framework.

- Enrollment = Method
- Allocation = Assignment
- Follow-up = Assessment
- Analysis = Results

Now that we have taken a look at the planning and preparation that is required before beginning a RCT, let us use the M.A.A.R.I.E. framework to examine the unique features of RCTs.

METHOD (4,5)

RCTs generally are used to establish the efficacy of interventions from prevention to cure to palliation. Thus their study hypothesis usually indicates that on average those in the study group will have a better outcome than those in the control group. RCT may include more than two groups allowing comparisons of more than one dosage of a treatment or multiple interventions aimed at

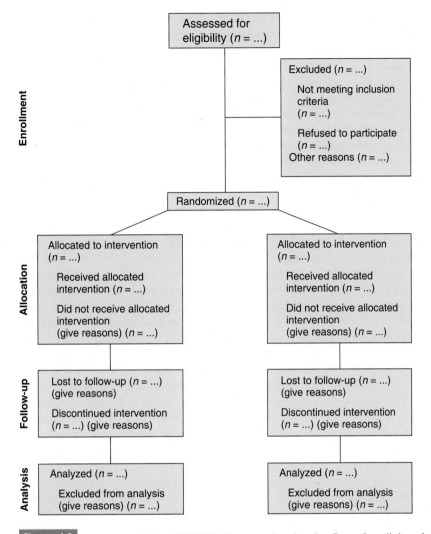

Figure 4.1 Template of the CONSORT diagram showing the flow of participants through each stage of a randomized trial. (Adapted from Consort Statement www.consort-statement.org. Accessed July 20, 2011.)

the same disease. In addition, a type of RCT called a *factorial design* may allow a RCT to address more than one study hypothesis.[4.3]

RCTs are capable of demonstrating all three criteria of contributory cause. When applied to a treatment or other intervention, the term *efficacy* is used instead of *contributory cause*. Efficacy means that in the study group being investigated, the intervention led to an increase in the probability of a desirable outcome. Efficacy, however, needs to be distinguished from effectiveness. *Effectiveness* implies that the therapy works under usual conditions of practice as opposed to the conditions of an investigation.

[4.3] Factorial designs are a method increasingly used in RCTs to examine more than one factor or intervention at a time. Most commonly two treatments or other interventions are investigated each with two levels. The use of two interventions each with two levels requires four different groups. The use of four groups allowed the investigators to study two hypotheses using the same size population that would be required to study one hypothesis. Although factorial design is attractive in terms of the size of studies and their resultant costs, they have a series of potential limitations. If the impacts of the two treatments interact, that is, affect the results of each other, the four groups need to be analyzed separately. The benefits of increased statistical power are then lost and special statistical techniques are required. (4)

RCTs usually have a very specific study hypothesis because they seek to determine whether the intervention works when given according to a defined dosage schedule, by a defined route of administration, and to a defined type of patient.[4.4]

Thus RCTs are expected to have a detailed protocol, including specific inclusion and exclusion criteria. These inclusion and exclusion criteria define the population being investigated. All participants are expected to fulfill these criteria.

A large number of individuals may be evaluated to determine if they meet these inclusion and exclusion criteria. All those who are assessed for eligibility usually do not end up being participants in the investigation. For instance, they may not meet the inclusion or exclusion criteria or they may refuse to participate despite being eligible. Thus the CONSORT Statement's flow chart begins by identifying the number assessed for eligibility and then indicates the number who were excluded and the reasons for their exclusion.

RCTs are not suitable for the initial investigation of a new treatment. When used as part of the drug approval process, RCTs are referred to as *phase 3 trials*. The FDA has traditionally required two independently conducted RCTs conducted for the same indication before reviewing a drug for approval. Ideally, a randomized clinical, or phase 3, trial should be performed before the drug is widely used for the indication being addressed. We will examine the FDA phases of review in greater depth in Chapter 6 when we take a look at harms or safety.

For new drugs that do not have market approval, identifying volunteers may be relatively easy. However, for many procedures and drugs that have been previously marketed and used for other indications, the treatment may have been widely used before RCTs could be implemented. This is a problem because once the treatment has been widely used, physicians and often patients have developed firm ideas about the value of the therapy. In that case, they may not believe it is ethical to enter into a RCT or to continue participation if they discover that the patient has been assigned to the control group.

Once the time is considered right for a RCT, the next question is whether it is feasible to perform one. To answer this, the investigator must define the question being asked in a RCT.

Most RCTs aim to determine whether the new or experimental therapy results in a better outcome, on average, than a placebo or standard therapy. To determine whether a trial is feasible, investigators need to estimate the necessary sample size. They must estimate how many patients are required to have a reasonable chance of demonstrating a statistically significant difference between the new therapy and the placebo or standard therapy. The required sample size as calculated before conducting the investigation depends on the following factors[4.5]:

1. **Size of the Type I error that the investigators will tolerate.** This is the probability of demonstrating a statistically significant difference in samples when no true difference exists between treatments in the larger population. The Type I error is usually set at 5%.

2. **Size of the Type II error that the investigators will tolerate.** This is the probability of failing to demonstrate a statistically significant difference in study samples when a true difference of a selected magnitude actually exists between interventions in the larger population. As we discussed previously, investigators should aim for a Type II error of 10% and accept no more than 20%. A Type II error of 20% indicates an 80% statistical power since the statistical power plus the Type II error add up to 100%. The 80% statistical power implies 80% probability of being able to demonstrate a statistically significant difference between the samples if a true difference of the estimated size actually exists in the larger populations.

3. **Percentage of individuals in the control group who are expected to experience the adverse outcome (death or other undesired outcomes) under study.** Often this can be estimated from previous studies.

[4.4] It is possible to perform a RCT to assess the effectiveness of therapy by using a representative sample of the types of patients to be treated with the therapy and the usual methods that are being used clinically. These types of RCTs will be discussed in Chapter 14.

[4.5] This is all the information that is required for an either/or variable. When calculating sample size for variables with multiple possible outcomes such as continuous data, one must also estimate the standard deviation of the variable.

4. **Improvement in outcome within the study group that the investigators seek to demonstrate as statistically significant.** Despite the desire to demonstrate statistical significance for even small real changes, the investigators need to decide the minimum size of a difference that would be considered clinically important. The smaller this difference between study group and control group therapy that one expects, the larger the sample size required.[4.6]

Let us take a look at the way these factors affect the required sample size. Table 4.1 provides general guidelines for minimum sample size for different levels of these factors.

TABLE 4.1	Sample Size Requirement for Controlled Clinical Trials[a]				
Adverse Outcome in the Control Group	Type II Error (%)	Probability of Adverse Outcome in the Study Group			
		1%	5%	10%	20%
2%	10	3,696			
	20	2,511			
	50	1,327			
10%	10	154	619		
	20	120	473		
	50	69	251		
20%	10	62	112	285	
	20	49	87	218	
	50	29	49	117	
40%	10	25	33	48	117
	20	20	26	37	90
	50	12	16	22	49

[a] All sample sizes obtained from this table assume a 5% Type I error and a two-tailed statistical significance test.

Table 4.1 assumes a Type I error of 5%. Table 4.1 also assumes one study group and one control group of equal size. Finally, it assumes that the investigators are interested in the results whether the results are in the direction of the intervention being investigated or in the opposite direction. Statisticians refer to statistical significance tests that consider data favoring deviations from the null hypothesis in either direction as *two-tailed tests*. Let us look at the meaning of these numbers for different types of studies:

[4.6] The frequency of the outcome under investigation may be estimated from past studies, especially for the control group. It is often more difficult to estimate the expected frequency in the study group, although, as we will discuss, phase 2 trials may assist in making these estimates. Overly optimistic estimates of the results of the new therapy will result in sample size estimates that are too small to demonstrate statistical significance. The treatment used in the control group may influence the estimated frequency of the outcome in the control group. Use of a placebo may have advantages from the perspective of sample size since it may result in a lower rate of desired outcomes in the control group and thus reduce the number of participants needed. As we will discuss later in this chapter, today, the standards for an ethical study require that a placebo not be used if other treatments are available that have greater efficacy than a placebo. One of the consequences of this policy is to increase the sample size needed for RCTs. The terms α-error and β-error are used instead of Type I and Type II errors when estimating sample size before a study because the Type I and Type II errors reflect the results of the investigation.

Mini-Study 4.1 ■ Imagine that an investigator wishes to conduct a RCT on a treatment designed to reduce the 1-year risk of death resulting from adenocarcinoma of the ovary. Assume that the 1-year risk of death using standard therapy is 40%. The investigator expected to be able to reduce the 1-year risk of death to 20% using a new treatment. He believes, however, that the treatment could possibly increase rather than reduce the risk of death. If he is willing to tolerate a 20% probability of failing to obtain statistically significant results, even if a true difference of this magnitude exists in the larger populations, how many patients are required in the study group and in the control group?

To answer this question, we can use Table 4.1 as follows:

Locate the 20% probability of an adverse outcome (death) in the study group on the horizontal axis.

Next, locate the 40% probability of an adverse outcome in the control group on the vertical axis. These intersect at 117, 90, and 49. The correct number is the one that lines up with the 20% Type II error. The answer is at least 90 in each group.

Thus, 90 women with advanced adenocarcinoma in the study group and 90 in the control group are needed to have a 20% probability of failing to demonstrate statistical significance if the true 1-year risk of death is actually 40% using the standard treatment and 20% using the new therapy. Notice that the sample size required for a Type II error of 10% is 117. Thus, a compromise sample size of about 100 in each group would be reasonable for this study.

Also notice that the table includes the numbers required for a 50% Type II error, an error that should not be tolerated. Here 49, that is, about 50 participants, in each group would produce a 50% Type II error.

Thus, a sample size of 100 is an approximate estimate of the number of individuals needed in each group when the probability of an adverse outcome is substantial and the investigators hope to be able to reduce it in half with the new treatment while keeping the size of the Type II error <20%.

Now let us contrast this situation with one in which the probability of an adverse outcome is much lower even without a new intervention:

Mini-Study 4.2 ■ An investigator wishes to study the effect of a new treatment on the probability of neonatal sepsis secondary to premature rupture of the membranes. He assumes that the probability of neonatal sepsis using standard treatment is 10%, and the study group therapy aims to reduce the probability of neonatal sepsis to 5%, although it is possible that the new therapy will increase the risk of neonatal sepsis.

Using the chart as before, we located box that includes 619, 473, and 251. Thus, we see that 619 individuals are needed for the study group and 619 individuals are needed for the control group for a 10% probability of making a Type II, error as is the aim for well-designed studies. If we were willing to tolerate a 20% Type II error, 473 individuals would be required in each group. Thus, approximately 500 individuals each in the study and the control groups is required to be able to demonstrate statistical significance when the true difference between adverse outcomes in the larger population is 10% versus 5%.

The neonatal sepsis example is typical of the problems we study in clinical practice. It demonstrates why relatively large sample sizes are required in most RCTs before they are likely to demonstrate statistical significance. Thus, it is not usually feasible to investigate small improvements in therapy using a RCT.

Let us go one step further and see what happens to the required sample size when a RCT is performed on a preventive intervention in which the adverse outcome is uncommon even in the absence of prevention:

Mini-Study 4.3 ■ Imagine that a new drug for preventing adverse outcomes of pregnancy in women with hypertension before pregnancy is expected to reduce the probability of adverse pregnancy outcomes from 2% to 1%, although the new therapy could possibly increase the risk of adverse outcomes.

From Table 4.1, we can see that at least 2,511 individuals are required in each group even if the investigator is willing to tolerate a 20% Type II error. These large numbers point out the difficulty in performing RCTs when one wishes to apply preventive interventions, especially when the risk of adverse outcomes is already quite low.[4.7]

In summary, the method component of a RCT usually hypothesizes the efficacy of an intervention; it has very specific inclusion and exclusion criteria; and its sample size is calculated to provide at least 80% statistical power to demonstrate statistical significance.

ASSIGNMENT

Participants in a RCT are not usually selected at random from a larger population. Usually, they are volunteers who meet a series of inclusion and exclusion criteria defined by the investigators as we discussed in the methods component.

Individuals entered into RCTs are often a relatively homogeneous group because they share inclusion and exclusion criteria. They are not usually representative of all those with the disease or all those for whom the therapy is intended (i.e., the target population). In addition, they often do not have the type of complicating factors encountered in practice. That is, they usually do not have multiple disease and multiple simultaneous therapies, and they usually do not have compromised ability to metabolize drugs as a result of renal or hepatic disease. Thus, it is important to distinguish between the study population and the target population on whom the intervention will be used when put into practice.

Once an individual has given his or her informed consent to participate in the investigation, he or she may not immediately undergo randomization. Investigators may follow patients before randomizing them to a study or a control group. They may do this to determine whether they are likely to take the treatment, return for follow-up, or in other ways be adherent to the protocol of the investigation. Investigators may use what is called a *run-in period* to exclude patients who do not take prescribed medication, do not return for follow-up, or demonstrate other evidence that they are not likely to follow the study protocol. Because this is an increasingly frequent procedure, it is important to recognize that RCTs often use patients who are especially likely to adhere to treatment and therefore may have an especially good prognosis.

[4.7] These sample sizes are designed for the *primary end point*, which should be an end point expected to occur relatively frequently. However, it may not be the most important end point of interest. For instance, in a study of coronary artery disease, a myocardial infarction may be a primary end point. Other end points that have even more clinical importance but occur less frequently, such as disability or death, are often measured as *secondary end points*. In general, primary but not secondary end points are used for calculating sample size.

Thus before randomization, an investigator often needs to accomplish a series of steps including the following:

1. Obtain IRB approval
2. Identify individuals who meet the inclusion and exclusion criteria
3. Obtain informed consent
4. Complete a run–in period

The randomization of patients to study and control groups is the hallmark of RCTs. An important feature of randomization is called *allocation concealment*. Allocation concealment implies that those assigning participants to groups are not aware of which group the next participant will be assigned to until the moment of assignment. That is, randomization implies unpredictability. The process of allocation concealment is intended to preserve unpredictability. This prevents the person making the assignment from consciously or unconsciously influencing the assignment process. That is, it prevents selection bias.

Randomization implies that any one individual has a predetermined probability of being assigned to each particular study group and control group. This may mean an equal probability of being assigned to one study and one control group or different probabilities of being assigned to each of two or more study and control groups. The proportion of the participants intended for each study and control group is called the *allocation ratio*.

Randomization is a powerful tool for eliminating selection bias in the assignment of individuals to study and control groups. In large studies, it greatly reduces the possibility that the effects of treatment are due to differences in the type of individuals receiving the study and control therapies. It is important to distinguish between randomization, which is an essential part of a RCT, and *random sampling* or random selection, which is not usually a part of a RCT. Random sampling implies that the individuals who are selected for a study are selected by chance from a larger group or population. Thus, random sampling is a method aimed at obtaining a representative sample, one that, on average, reflects the characteristics of a larger group.

Randomization, on the other hand, says nothing about the characteristics of a larger population from which the individuals in the investigation are obtained. It refers to the mechanism by which individuals are assigned to study and control groups once they become participants in the investigation. The following hypothetical study illustrates the difference between random sampling and randomization:

> **Mini-Study 4.4** ■ An investigator wishes to assess the efficacy of a new drug known as Surf-ez. Surf-ez is designed to help improve surfing ability. To assess the value of Surf-ez, the investigator performs a RCT using a group of volunteer championship surfers in Hawaii. After randomizing half the group to Surf-ez and half the group to a placebo, the investigators measure the surfing ability of all surfers using a standard scoring system. The scorers do not know whether a particular surfer used Surf-ez or a placebo. Those taking Surf-ez have a statistically significant and substantial improvement compared with the placebo group. On the basis of the study results, the authors recommend Surf-ez as a learning aid for all surfers.

By using randomization, this RCT has demonstrated the efficacy of Surf-ez among these championship surfers. Because its study and control groups were hardly a random sample of surfers, however, we must be very careful in drawing conclusions or extrapolating about the effects of Surf-ez as a learning aid for all surfers.[4.8]

[4.8] Care must be taken even in extrapolating to championship surfers because we have not randomly sampled all championship surfers. This limitation occurs in most RCTs, which select their patients from a particular hospital or clinical site.

Randomization does not totally eliminate the possibility that study and control groups will differ according to factors that affect prognosis (confounding variables). Known prognostic factors must still be measured and may be found to be different in the study and control groups as a result of chance alone, especially in small studies. If substantial differences between groups exist, these must be taken into account through an adjustment process as part of the analysis.[4.9]

Many characteristics affecting prognosis, however, are not known. In larger studies randomization tends to balance the multitude of characteristics that could possibly affect outcome, even those that are unknown to the investigator. Without randomization, the investigator would need to take into account all known and potential differences between groups. Because it is difficult, if not impossible, to consider everything, randomization helps balance the groups, especially for large studies. The ability to help ensure that unknown factors affecting prognosis are balanced between the groups is the great advantage of randomization.[4.10]

Randomization of individuals to study or control groups is not the only way that randomization is conducted. Learn More 4.2 examines the increasingly common method of group randomization.

LEARN MORE 4.2 ■ GROUP RANDOMIZED TRIALS OR CLUSTER RANDOMIZED TRIALS (5) ■ *Group randomized trials* or *cluster randomized trials* are a special type of RCT in which the unit of randomization is groups such as hospitals, schools, or communities instead of individuals. Group randomized trials have also been called cluster randomized clinical trials and community RCTs because they often investigate questions that can be addressed by groups or populations rather than by individual patients or individual clinicians.

Let us take a look at the types of situations in which group randomized trials are used as illustrated in the next scenario: (7)

Mini-Study 4.5 ■ Researchers were interested in conducting an investigation of the efficacy of a seventh-grade classroom education program for prevention of cigarette smoking. Randomization of individual students was not feasible since it would be so disruptive of classroom routine. In addition, the communications between students outside of class were of concern because it might dilute any effect of the educational program. The investigators decided to randomize pairs of similar schools either to the study group in which the education program was implemented for all seventh-grade students or to the control group in which the educational program was not implemented.

This use of group randomized trials illustrates how randomized by group can address problems associated with interventions designed for groups such as seventh graders. Interventions at the institutional level are increasingly common, ranging from hospital-based programs, such as

(Continued)

[4.9] Many biostatisticians would recommend using a multivariable analysis technique such as logistic regression or Cox proportional hazard regression even when the differences between groups are not substantial. Multivariable analysis then permits adjustment for interaction. Interaction occurs, for instance, when both groups contain an identical age and gender distribution, but one group contains predominantly young women and the other contains predominantly young men. Multivariable analysis then allows one to separate out the interacting effects of age and gender.

[4.10] Randomization as defined by the CONSORT Statement may be divided into simple randomization and restricted randomization. Simple randomization implies that each participant has a known probability of receiving each treatment before one is assigned. Restricted randomization describes any procedure that aims to achieve balance between the groups in terms of either size or characteristics. For instance, *randomization by blocks* implies that randomization is accomplished using blocks of individuals that include a set number of individuals who have given their consent to participate and who are then randomized to study or control groups in a predefined allocation ratio. Randomization by block may be used to ensure that there is balance between those assigned to a study and to a control group in particular study sites in a multisite investigation.

Methicillin-Resistant Staphloccus Aureus (MRSA) control efforts, to restaurant-based programs such as food labeling, to community-based programs such as media campaigns to increase vaccine use. In addition, some interventions require legislation or policy changes that must be applied uniformly to entire governmental jurisdictions, such as restrictions on alcohol use, limitations on cell phone use, or changes in emergency response systems.

It is desirable in all of these types of studies that the unit of randomization be at the group level because that is the level at which implementation will occur if the intervention is found to have efficacy. Despite the fact that the unit of randomization in these types of studies is by institution or geographic unit, the assessment may include changes in the outcomes of individuals. Thus, randomization by group is the cardinal feature of group randomization trials.

Group randomized trials are the gold standard for efficacy of interventions that require group implementation. However, group randomized trials have lower statistical power than studies that conduct randomized trials at the individual level. The considerably smaller number of units being randomized leads to the lower statistical power. Pairing of study and control groups is often an important method for increasing statistical power in group-randomized trials. Statistical methods for adjusting for confounding are also important because the small sample size often means that randomization does not achieve its goal of producing nearly identical study and control groups.

In addition, methods of statistical analysis are available specially designed for group-randomized trials. These methods take into account the fact that the individuals within institutions such as health care facilities and schools and even within communities are not random samples of all possible individuals but rather often share common characteristics unique to their setting. Hospitals may specialize in more severely ill patients; schools may draw from distinct socioeconomic groups; and communities may reflect the culture of a particular ethnic group.

Group randomized trials are an increasingly important type of RCT as researchers focus their interventions not only on one individual at a time but on interventions that can only be implemented at the group or population level. (5)

Randomization is a requirement for a randomized controlled trial. Masking or blinding of study subjects and investigators, however, is a highly desirable feature but not a requirement of a RCT. As we will soon see, the impact of not masking becomes apparent in the third component of the M.A.A.R.I.E. framework, the assessment process.

ASSESSMENT

Assessment in RCTs, as in other types of investigations, requires us to carefully examine the outcome measures being used. Errors in assessing the outcome or end point of a RCT may occur when the patient or the individual making the assessment is aware of which treatment is being administered. This is especially likely when the outcome or end point being measured is subjective or may be influenced by knowledge of the treatment group, as illustrated in the following hypothetical study:

Mini-Study 4.6 ■ A RCT of a new breast cancer surgery compared the degree of arm edema and arm strength among patients receiving the new procedure versus the traditional procedure. The patients were aware of which procedure they underwent. Arm edema and arm strength were the end points assessed by the patients and surgeons. The study found that those receiving the new procedure had less arm edema and more arm strength than those undergoing the traditional mastectomy.

In this study, the fact that the patients and the surgeons who performed the procedure and assessed the outcome knew which patients received which procedure may have affected the objectivity of the way strength and edema were measured and reported. This effect may have been minimized but not totally eliminated if arm strength and edema were assessed using a technology that could not be influenced by the investigators who knew which patients received which therapy. Even a system of masked assessment and objective scoring would not entirely remove the impact of patients and surgeons knowing which surgery was performed. It is still possible that patients receiving the new procedure worked harder and actually increased their strength and reduced their edema. This could occur, for instance, if the surgeon performing the new surgery stressed postoperative exercises or provided more physical therapy for those receiving the new therapy.

In practice, masking is often impractical or unsuccessful. RCTs without masking are called *open* or *open-label trials*. Surgical therapy cannot easily be masked. In addition, the taste or adverse effects of medications are often a giveaway to the patient or clinician. The need to titrate a dose to achieve a desired effect often makes it more difficult to mask the clinician and in some cases the patient. Strict adherence to masking helps to ensure the objectivity of the assessment process. It helps to remove the possibility that differences in adherence, follow-up, and assessment of outcome will be affected by awareness of the treatment received.

Even when objective assessment, excellent adherence, and complete follow-up can be ensured, masking is still desirable because it helps control for the placebo effect. The placebo effect is a powerful biological process that can bring about a wide variety of objective as well as subjective biological effects. The placebo effect extends far beyond pain control and is not limited to situations in which a placebo is used. A substantial percentage of patients who believe they are receiving effective therapy obtain objective therapeutic benefits. When effective masking is not a part of a RCT, it leaves open the possibility that the observed benefit in the study subject is actually the result of the placebo effect.

Thus, when masking is not feasible, doubt about the accuracy of the outcome measures usually persists. This uncertainty can be reduced but not eliminated by using objective measures of end points, careful monitoring of adherence, and complete follow-up of patients.

In addition to attempting masking, the investigators are encouraged by the CONSORT Statement to make an effort to determine whether masking was actually successful. This may be done by asking participants which treatment they believe they received and comparing their response to their actual treatment.

As we have seen, assessment of outcome requires measures of outcome that are appropriate, precise and accurate, complete, and unaffected by the process of observation. The requirements are as important in a RCT as in other types of investigations.

There are some special assessment considerations that apply to RCTs. Investigators often wish to use outcome measures or end points that occur in a short period rather than waiting for more clinically important but longer-term outcomes, such as death or blindness. Increasingly, changes in laboratory tests are substituted for clinically important outcomes. We call these *surrogate outcomes* or surrogate end points. Surrogate outcomes can be very useful if the test is an early indicator of subsequent outcome. If that is not the situation, however, the surrogate outcome can be an inappropriate measure of outcome, as suggested in the following scenario:

Mini-Study 4.7 ■ Researchers note that individuals with severe coronary artery disease often have multiple premature ventricular contractions and experience sudden death, often believed to be caused by arrhythmias. They note that a new drug may be able to reduce premature ventricular contractions. Thus, they conduct a RCT that demonstrates that the new drug has efficacy in reducing the frequency of premature ventricular contractions in patients with severe coronary artery disease. Later evidence indicates that despite the reduction in arrhythmias, those with severe coronary artery disease taking the drug have an increased frequency of death compared with similar untreated patients.

The investigator has assumed that reducing the frequency of premature ventricular contraction in the short run is strongly associated with a better outcome in the longer run. This may not always be the situation, as has been demonstrated with treatment for premature ventricular contractions in this type of setting. The fact that treatment seems like a logical method for reducing deaths caused by arrhythmia may have allowed investigators to accept a surrogate end point. They were assuming without evidence that reduction in arrhythmias would be strongly associated with the end point of interest, which was death in this case.

An additional problem can occur when individuals are lost to follow-up before the study is completed. Even moderate loss to follow-up can be disastrous for a study. Those lost may move to a more pleasant climate because of failing health, drop out because of drug toxicity, or fail to return because of the burdens of complying with one of the treatment protocols.

Well-conducted studies take elaborate precautions to minimize the loss to follow-up. In some cases, follow-up may be completed by a telephone or mail questionnaire. A search of death records should be conducted in an effort to find participants who cannot be located. When outcome data cannot be obtained, resulting in loss to follow-up despite these precautions, it is important to determine, as much as possible, the initial characteristics of patients subsequently lost to follow-up. This is done in an attempt to determine whether those lost are likely to be different from those who remain. If those lost to follow-up have an especially poor prognosis, little may be gained by analyzing the data regarding only those who remain, as suggested by the following hypothetical study:

> **Mini-Study 4.8** ■ In a study of the effects of a new alcohol treatment program, 100 patients were randomized to the new program, and 100 patients were randomized to conventional treatment. The investigators visited the homes of all patients at 9 p.m. on a Saturday and drew blood from all available patients to measure alcohol levels. Of the new treatment group, 30 patients were at home, and one-third of these had alcohol in their blood. Among the conventionally treated patients, 33 were at home, and two-thirds of these had alcohol in their blood. The results were statistically significant, and the investigators concluded that the new treatment reduced alcohol consumption.

Whenever loss to follow-up occurs, it is important to ask what happened to those lost participants. In this study, if those lost to follow-up were out drinking, the results based on those at home would be especially misleading. This is important even if loss to follow-up occurs equally in the study and control groups.[4.11]

One method for dealing with loss to follow-up is to assume the worst regarding the lost participants. For instance, the investigator could assume that the participants not at home were out drinking. It is then possible to redo the analysis and compare the outcome in the study and control groups to determine whether the differences are still statistically significant. When the loss to follow-up is great, this procedure usually indicates no substantial or statistically significant difference between the study and control groups. However, for smaller loss to follow-up, a statistically significant difference may remain. When statistically significant differences between groups remain after assuming the worst case for those lost to follow-up, the reader can be quite confident that loss to follow-up does not explain the observed differences.

[4.11] Loss to follow-up needs to be distinguished from follow-up that occurs despite the participants' withdrawal from the investigation. The term *censored* implies that the event of interest had not occurred at the last time of observation. It implies that no information is available on whether or not the event of interest occurred or would have occurred in the case of death from another cause after the last time of follow-up. Data may be censored because of loss to follow-up, death from another cause, or termination of the investigation.

In an ideal RCT, all individuals would be treated according to the study protocol and monitored over time. Their outcome would be assessed from their time of entry until the end of the study. In reality, assessment is rarely so perfect or complete. Patients often receive treatment that deviates from the predefined protocol. Investigators often label these individuals as *protocol deviants*. Deviating from the protocol, as opposed to loss to follow-up, implies that data on subsequent outcomes were obtained. The occurrence of deviations from the protocol can greatly affect the results of the investigation which is the next component of the M.A.A.R.I.E. framework.

RESULTS (6,7)

In a RCT, it is important to consider what to do with the outcomes from the protocol deviants. To better understand this issue, take a look at the following hypothetical study:

> **Mini-Study 4.9** ■ In a RCT of surgery versus angioplasty for single-vessel coronary artery disease, 100 patients were randomized to surgery and 100 to angioplasty. Before receiving angioplasty, 30 of the patients deviated from the protocol and had surgery. The investigators decided to remove those who deviated from the protocol from the analysis of results.

It is likely that many of the patients who deviated from the protocol and underwent surgery were the ones doing poorly. If that is the situation, then eliminating those who deviated from the protocol from the analysis would leave us with a group of individuals doing especially well.

Because of the potential bias, it is generally recommended that deviants from the study protocol remain in the investigation and be subsequently analyzed as if they had remained in the group to which they were originally randomized. This is known as analysis by *intention-to-treat*. By retaining the protocol deviants, the study question, however, is changed slightly. The study now asks whether prescribing the study therapy produced a better outcome than prescribing the standard therapy recognizing that patients may not actually take the assigned or prescribed treatments. This allows the investigator to better address the effectiveness of the therapy as actually used in clinical practice.

Investigators may perform additional analyses excluding those who deviate from the protocol. These analyses are called *as-treated analysis* or *per-protocol analysis*. Although these analyses may be useful, especially if the intention-to-treat analysis is statistically significant, it is not considered proper methodology to use only an as-treated analysis. Deviations from the protocol are relatively common in RCTs because it is considered unethical to prevent deviations for any reason. Deviation from the protocol may occur when the responsible clinician believes that continued adherence is contraindicated by the patient's condition or when the patient no longer wishes to follow the recommended protocol. Thus, in evaluating a RCT, the reader should understand the degree of protocol adherence and determine how the investigators handled the data from those who deviated from the protocol.

Two other analysis questions face the investigator in a RCT: when to analyze the data and how to analyze the data.

The seemingly simple question of when to analyze the data of a RCT has provoked considerable methodological and ethical controversy. The more times one looks at the data, the more likely one is to find a point when the P-value reaches the 0.05 level of statistical significance using standard statistical techniques.

When to analyze is an ethical problem because one would like to establish that a true difference exists at the earliest possible moment. This is desirable to avoid subjecting patients to therapy that has less benefit. In addition, it is desirable that other patients receive a beneficial therapy at the earliest possible time.

A number of statistical methods called *sequential methods* have been developed to attempt to deal with these problems. When multiple times for analysis of data are planned, these sequential statistical techniques are available to take into account the multiple analyses.

Life Tables and Survival Curves

An important issue that arises in RCTs is the method for presenting data. *Life tables or longitudinal life tables* are the most commonly used method for analyzing data in RCTs. Life-table data are often displayed using what are called *survival plots* or *time-to-event plots*.[4.12]

Let us begin by discussing why life tables are often necessary in RCTs. Then we will discuss the assumptions underlying their use and demonstrate how they should be interpreted.

In most RCTs, individuals are entered into the study and randomized over a period of time as they present for care. In addition, because of late entry or loss to follow-up, individuals are actually monitored for different lengths of time after entry. Therefore, many of the patients included in a study are not followed for the full duration of the study. In addition, the likelihood of an individual experiencing an outcome often depends on the length of follow-up; that is, the probability of the outcome is said to be *time-dependent*. Life tables provide a method for using the data from those individuals who have been included in a study for only a portion of the possible study duration. Thus, life tables allow the investigator to use all the data that they have so painstakingly collected.[4.13]

The life-table method is built on the important assumption that those who were in the investigation for shorter periods would have had the same subsequent experience as those who were actually followed for longer periods. In other words, the "short-termers" would have the same results as the "long-termers" if they were actually followed long term.

This critical assumption may not hold true if the "short-termers" are individuals with a better or worse prognosis than the "long-termers." This can occur if the entry requirements for the investigation are relaxed during the course of a study. Let us see how this might occur by looking at the next hypothetical study:

> **Mini-Study 4.10** ■ A new hormonal treatment designed to treat infertility secondary to severe endometriosis was compared with standard therapy in a RCT. After initial difficulty recruiting patients and initial failures to get pregnant among the study patients, one woman in the study group became pregnant. News of her delivery became front-page news. Subsequent patients recruited for the study were found to have much less severe endometriosis, but the investigators willingly accepted those patients and combined their data with data from their original group of patients.

As this study demonstrates, the same eligibility criteria may not be maintained throughout an investigation. It is tempting to relax the inclusion and exclusion criteria if only severely ill patients are entered into an investigation at the beginning. As the therapy becomes better known in the

---

[4.12] The term *survival analysis* may be used to refer to this overall process. Survival analysis or life-table methods can also be used in cohort studies; thus, they are often called longitudinal life tables. Longitudinal life tables should be distinguished from cross-sectional life tables which are used to calculate life expectancy. In this discussion, the adverse event under study is referred to as death. However, life tables can be used for other effects, such as permanent loss of vision or the occurrence of pregnancy after infertility therapy, and so on.

[4.13] Not all outcomes are time dependent. If there is only one outcome being measured such as a pregnancy outcome, life tables are not needed. Note that this type of life table assumes the end point can occur only once. Thus, it may not be appropriate for studies of diseases such as strep throat, which may recur.

community, at a particular institution, or in the literature, a tendency may occur for clinicians to refer, or patients to self-refer, the less severely ill.

In this case, the short-term study participants are likely to have less severe illness and thus have better outcomes than the "long-termers." This problem can be minimized if the investigators clearly define and carefully adhere to a protocol that defines the type of patients who are eligible for the study on the basis of inclusion and exclusion criteria related to prognosis.

Loss to follow-up may also result in differences between the "short-termers" and the "long-termers." This is likely if loss to follow-up occurs preferentially among those who are not doing well or who have adverse reactions to treatment. We have already discussed the importance of loss to follow-up and stressed the need to assess whether those lost are similar to those who remain.

Life-table data are often presented using a *time-to-event curve*. A time-to-event curve may be referred to as a *survival plot* or *survival curve* even though the outcome may not be death. A time-to-event curve or survival plot is a graph in which the percentage outcome is plotted on the vertical axis, ranging from 100% at the top of the axis to 0% at the bottom. Thus, at the beginning of an investigation, both study and control groups start at the 100% survival mark at the top of the vertical axis. When the outcome represents outcomes other than death, such as blindness or desired outcomes such as pregnancy, the time-to-event curve may start at the 0% point on the bottom of the vertical axis.

The horizontal axis depicts the time of follow-up. Time is counted for each individual beginning with their entry into the study. Thus, time zero is not the time at which the investigation began but the time that each individual was randomized.

Time-to-event curves or survival curves should also include the number of individuals who have been monitored for each time interval. These should be presented separately for the study and the control groups. Thus, a typical life table comparing the 5-year survival data on the study and the control groups might be examined graphically in a survival plot like Figure 4.2. The top row of numbers represents the number of study group participants monitored through the corresponding length of time from their entry into the study, and the bottom row represents the same

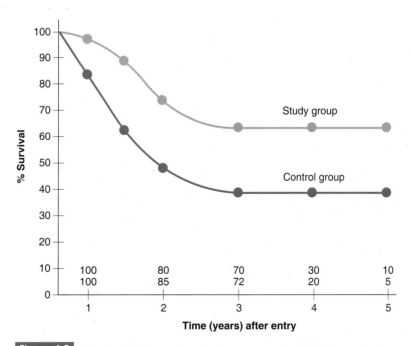

Figure 4.2 A typical study and control group survival plot demonstrating a plateau effect, which typically occurs at the right end of time-to-event plots.

for control group participants. The survival curve can be used directly to estimate the percentage death or survival at, for instance, 5 years; this probability of survival is known as the 5-year *actuarial survival*. For instance, in Figure 4.2, the 5-year actuarial survival read directly from the graph is approximately 60% for the study group and 40% for the control group.

Life-table data are often tested for statistical significance using the log rank or Mantel-Haenszel statistical significance tests. For these tests, the null hypothesis states that no difference exists between the overall life table results for the study and the control groups. Notice that the statistical significance tests do not address the question of which treatment achieves better results at 5 years. In performing these statistical significance tests, one combines data from each follow-up time interval, taking into account the number of individuals being observed during that time interval. Thus, these methods combine data from different time intervals to produce an overall statistical significance test. The combination of data from multiple intervals means that the statistical significance test asks this question: If no true difference exists between the overall effects of the study group and the control group treatments, what is the probability of obtaining the observed or more extreme results?

In other words, if a statistically significant improvement in a study group has been demonstrated on the basis of life-table data, it is very likely that a similar group of individuals receiving the therapy will experience at least some improvement compared with the control group therapy.

As we have seen, life tables can be used directly to obtain estimates of the magnitude of difference in outcome between treatments. Inference can be performed using a statistical significance test that addresses the overall differences. In addition, adjustment for potential confounding variables may be incorporated into the life-table analysis using a technique known as *Cox regression* or *proportional hazards regression*. Thus, life tables can address all three basic questions of statistics: estimation, inference, and adjustment. However, data from life tables are prone to a number of misinterpretations.

When displaying life-table data, it is important to display the number of individuals being monitored at each interval of time in the study group and in the control group. Usually only a small number are monitored for the complete duration of a study. For instance, in Figure 4.2, only 10 individuals in the study group and 5 individuals in the control group are monitored for 5 years. This is not surprising because considerable time is often required to start up a study, and those individuals monitored for the longest time were usually recruited during the first year of the study.

A 5-year probability of survival can be calculated even when only one patient has been observed for 5 years. Thus, one should not rely too greatly on the specific 1-year, 5-year, or any other probability of survival observed unless a substantial number of individuals are actually observed for the full length of the study.

It is important to understand this limitation in the reliability of the estimates obtained from the life table. Failure to recognize this uncertainty can result in the following type of misinterpretation:

Mini-Study 4.11 ■ A clinician looking at the life-table curves in Figure 4.2 concluded that 5-year survival with the study treatment is 60% versus 40% for the control group. After extensive use of the same treatment on similar patients, he was surprised that the study treatment actually produced a 55% survival versus a 50% survival among the control group patients.

If the clinician had recognized that life-table curves do not reliably predict exact 5-year survival, he would not have been surprised about his experience.

Knowledge of the procedures and assumptions underlying life tables also helps in understanding their interpretation. Many time-to-event curves have a flat or plateau phase for long time at the right-hand end of the plot. These may be misinterpreted as indicating a cure once an individual reaches the flat or plateau area of the curve. Actually, this plateau phase usually results because few individuals are monitored for the entire duration of the study. Among those few individuals who are observed for longer periods, the deaths are likely to be fewer and more widely spaced. Because the time-to-event curve moves lower only when an outcome such as death occurs, a plateau is likely when fewer deaths are possible. Thus, an understanding of this *plateau effect* is important in interpreting a life table. We should not interpret the plateau as demonstrating a cure unless large numbers of patients have been observed for long periods.

In addition to the dangers of relying too heavily on the 5-year probability of survival derived from life-table data and of misinterpreting the plateau, it is important to fully appreciate the interpretation of a statistically significant difference between survival plots, as illustrated in the next example:

Mini-Study 4.12 ■ In the study depicted in Figure 4.2, a statistically significant difference in outcome occurred between the study and the control groups on the basis of the 5-year follow-up. The study was subsequently extended for 1 more year, resulting in the survival plot depicted in Figure 4.3, in which the 6-year actuarial survival was identical in the study and the control groups. On the basis of the 6-year data, the authors stated that the 5-year actuarial study was mistaken in drawing the conclusion that the study therapy prolonged survival.

Remember that a statistically significant difference in survival implies that patients receiving one treatment do better than patients receiving another treatment when considering each group's entire experience. Patients in one group may do better only early in the course, midway through, or at the end. Patients who received the better overall treatment may actually do worse early in the treatment because of surgical complications, or at a later point in time as secondary complications develop among those who survive.

Thus, when conducting a study, it is important to know enough about the natural history of a disease and the life expectancy of the individuals in the investigation to choose a meaningful time period for follow-up. Differences in outcomes are unlikely if the time period is too short, such as one that ends before an extended period of therapy is completed.

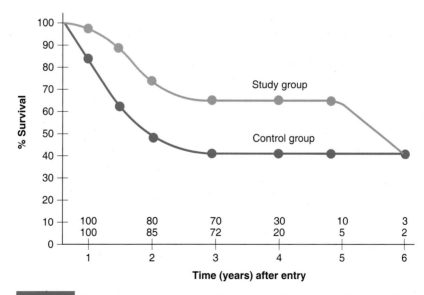

Figure 4.3 Survival plots may meet after extended periods of follow-up. The difference between the overall plots may still be statistically significant.

Similarly, follow-up periods that are too long may not allow the study to demonstrate statistically significant differences if the risks of other diseases overwhelm the shorter-term benefits. For instance, a study that assesses the 20-year outcome among 65-year-olds given a treatment for coronary artery disease might show little difference in survival at 20 years even if differences occur at 5 and 10 years.

INTERPRETATION

RCTs are the gold standard for efficacy. That is, they have the potential to establish all three criteria for efficacy or contributory cause. The following outlines how a RCT can fulfill each of the three criteria:

1. Using randomization, the investigators are able to produce study and control groups that are comparable except for the effects of the intervention. Thus, when substantial and statistically significant differences in outcome occur, the investigator can usually conclude that these differences are associated with the intervention itself.

2. By randomizing individuals to study and control groups at the beginning of the study, the investigators can provide strong evidence that the intervention precedes the effect and is, therefore, a prior association, fulfilling the second criterion of efficacy.

3. Randomization creates similar groups but only the study group receives the intervention designed to alter the outcome, that is, the "effect." By comparing the study and the groups, the investigator can determine whether the intervention alters the outcome, thus fulfilling the third criterion of efficacy.

RCTs, therefore, can establish the existence of an association between an intervention and an outcome, can establish the existence of a prior association, and can demonstrate that altering the "cause" alters the outcome. These are the three criteria necessary for establishing that the new intervention is the cause of the improved outcome.

However, even after establishing that an intervention has efficacy, we need to ask what it is about the intervention that is working. The efficacy may not result from the intervention the investigator intended to study, as suggested in the following study:

Mini-Study 4.13 ■ A RCT of a new postoperative recovery program for posthysterectomy care was performed by randomizing 100 postsurgery women to a standard ward and 100 postsurgery women to a special care ward equipped with experimental beds and postoperative exercise equipment and staffed by extra nurses. Women on the special care ward were discharged with an average length of stay of only 7 days compared with 12 days for women randomized to the regular ward. The results were statistically significant. The investigators concluded that the experimental beds and a postoperative exercise program resulted in a substantially reduced length of stay.

This investigation established that the intervention had efficacy: It worked to produce more rapid recovery and thus to reduce length of stay. However, it is still not clear what actually worked. Before concluding that the experimental beds and the postoperative exercise made the difference, do not forget that extra nurses were also provided. The availability of the extra nurses may have been the cause of the early discharge rather than the beds and the exercise. In an unmasked or open study such as this one, it is possible that the effect of observation itself helped to bring about the observed effect.[4.14]

[4.14] RCTs are increasingly used to compare standard or currently used interventions with new or uninvestigated interventions to try to determine whether the interventions are equivalent. These *equivalence* or *noninferiority* trials are becoming an important component of *comparative effectiveness research*, as we will discuss in Chapter 14.

The interpretation of safety data on adverse events, side effects, or harms is an important, if not definitive, part of RCTs, along with its emphasis on efficacy. We will discuss how RCTs fit into the evaluation of safety in Chapter 6.

With RCTs, as with other types of investigations, questions of subgroups are often of great interest because they help practitioners apply the results of an investigation. The precautions about subgroup analysis that we discussed in Chapter 3 should be kept in mind when interpreting the meaning of the outcomes for subgroups in a RCT.

In RCTs, tests of interaction are often performed that ask whether there is evidence that the effect of treatment differs from one subgroup to another. When interaction is present, close examination of the subgroups can provide important information, as illustrated in the next example:

> **Mini-Study 4.14** ■ A RCT of a new cancer treatment for stage III or IV breast cancer found a modest but statistically significant improvement in outcome. A statistical test for interaction found interaction between the stages and the treatment to be statistically significant. The investigator then examined the data for stage III and stage IV separately and found substantial improvement for those who received the treatment during stage III and slightly poorer average outcome for those who received the treatment during stage IV.

Thus, at times, interaction and the close examination of subgroups can add important clinical information to the interpretation of RCTs.[4.15]

EXTRAPOLATION

An effort to extrapolate the results of an investigation should begin by reexamining the characteristics of the study's population. The strict inclusion and exclusion criteria established in the protocol ensure that study participants in a RCT will be quite similar. This similarity often becomes a limitation when extrapolating to those not included in the investigation.

Individuals included in many RCTs are chosen because they are the type of patients most likely to respond to the treatment. In addition, considerations of time, geography, investigator convenience, and patient compliance are usually of paramount importance in selecting a particular group of patients for an investigation. Pregnant patients, the elderly, the very young, and those with mild disease are usually not included in RCTs unless the intervention is specifically designed for their use. In addition to these inclusion and exclusion criteria that are under the control of the investigator, other factors may lead to a unique group of patients who become participants in a RCT. Every medical center population has its own referral patterns, location, and socioeconomic patterns. A patient population referred to the Mayo Clinic may be quite different from one drawn to a local county hospital. Private practice primary care outpatients may be very different from university hospital subspecialty clinic outpatients. These characteristics, which may be beyond the investigator's control, can affect the types of patients included in a way that may affect the results of the study.

Thus, the patients included in RCTs are often different from the target population; that is, the types of patients whom clinicians are likely to treat with the new therapy in practice. This often creates difficulty in extrapolating the conclusions to patients seen in clinical practice. If the individuals in the investigation are not representative of the target population, extrapolation requires additional assumptions. This does not invalidate the result of a RCT; however, it does mean the clinician must use care and good judgment when adapting the results to clinical practice.

[4.15] Unfortunately, the size of most RCTs provides only low statistical power for demonstrating interactions.

Thus, despite the power and importance of RCTs, the process of extrapolation is still largely speculative. The reader needs to examine the nature of the study institutions and the study patients before applying the study results. Practitioners need to determine whether their own setting and patients are comparable to those in the study. If they are not, the differences may limit the ability to extrapolate from the study.

Patients and study centers involved in an investigation may be different from the usual clinical setting in many ways. For instance,

- Patients in an investigation are likely to be carefully followed up and very adherent to treatment. Adherence and close follow-up may be critical to the success of the therapy.

- Patients in the study may have worse prognoses than the usual patients seen in clinical practice. For this reason, the adverse effects of the therapy may be worth the risk in the study patients, but the same may not be true for patients seen in another clinical setting.

- The study centers may have special skills, equipment, or experience that maximize the success of the new therapy. This may not be true when the therapy is used by clinicians inexperienced with those techniques.

Despite a clear demonstration of a successful therapy using a RCT, clinicians must be careful to account for these types of differences in extrapolating to patients in their own practices. RCTs are capable of establishing the efficacy of treatment performed on a carefully selected group of patients treated under the ideal conditions of an experimental study. They must be used carefully when trying to assess the effectiveness of treatment for clinical care. Thus, well-motivated and conscientious clinicians providing usual care with usual facilities probably cannot always match the results obtained in RCTs.

RCTs, at their best, are capable only of establishing the benefit of treatment under current conditions. Not infrequently, however, the introduction of a new treatment can itself alter current conditions and produce secondary or dynamic effects. RCTs have a limited ability to assess the secondary effects of treatment. This is especially true for those effects that are more likely to occur when the therapy is widely applied in clinical practice. Consider the following hypothetical study:

Mini-Study 4.15 ■ A new drug called Herp-Ex was shown to have efficacy in a RCT. It was shown to reduce the frequency of attacks when used in patients with severe recurrent herpes genitalis. It did not, however, cure the infection. The investigators were impressed with the results of the study and advocated the use of Herp-Ex for all individuals with herpes genitalis.

If Herp-Ex is approved for clinical use, several effects may occur that may not have been expected on the basis of a RCT. First, the drug would most likely be widely used, extending its use beyond the indications in the original trial. Patients with mild attacks or who present with first episodes would most likely also receive the therapy. This often occurs because once a drug is approved, clinicians have a right to prescribe it for other indications. The efficacy shown for recurrent severe attacks of herpes genitalis may not translate into effectiveness for uses that extend beyond the original indications. Second, the widespread use of Herp-Ex may result in strains of herpes that are resistant to the drug. Thus, long-term efficacy may not match the short-term results. Finally, the widespread use of Herp-Ex and short-term success may reduce the sexual precautions taken by those with recurrent herpes genitalis. Thus, over time, the number of cases of herpes genitalis may actually increase despite, or because of, the short-term efficacy of Herp-Ex.

Because of the key role that RCTs play in establishing the efficacy of interventions, considerable attention has been paid to the quality of RCTs. An important component of quality is the ethical rules under which RCTs are conducted. Learn More 4.3 examines many of the current procedures now built into RCTs to address ethical issues.

LEARN MORE 4.3 ■ ETHICAL ISSUES AND RCTs (3,7) ■ Ethical issues are an inherent part of the conduct of RCTs. They are built into the process of IRB approval and informed consent. In addition, specific ethical considerations are part of the design of RCTs and influence each of the components of the M.A.A.R.I. E. process.

Before beginning a RCT, the investigator is expected to register the investigation, which means that the data will be available in the future regardless of the results. Today, registration before beginning a RCT is required for publication in quality journals, and the registration number, often at the end of the abstract, should be looked for as part of the review of methods.

The assignment process in RCTs requires the investigator to consider the type of intervention that should be received by the control group. The use of a placebo is now limited to those situations in which no active treatment is provided as standard or state-of-the-art care. The following example illustrates some of the implications of the current standards for use of placebos:

Mini-Study 4.16 ■ A double-blind RCT was proposed to compare a new treatment to a placebo. The IRB concluded that the use of a placebo was not ethical because an active treatment was part of the current standard of care. The investigation had to be modified to include a larger number of participants in the study and in the control groups.

The use of placebo controls reduces the sample size required for a RCT. This happens because a comparison treatment with some degree of efficacy reduces the anticipated difference between the expected results in the study and the control groups compared with the use of a placebo in the control group. The smaller expected difference means that a larger number of participants are required in each group.

The completeness of the assessment of the outcomes in RCTs may be limited by the ethical principle that participants may leave the investigation at any time for any reason. The investigator often needs to address this issue by seeking permission from the participants, at the beginning of the investigation, to obtain follow-up information using other sources such as contacts with family members.

The fact that participants can and do leave investigations at any time for any reason also influences the analysis process. The intention-to-treat analysis is required in part because individuals who choose to leave the study are often those with a worse outcome or prognosis compared with those who remain.

Today's ethical standards require that an investigation be stopped as soon as efficacy has been established or the harms are believed to outweigh the benefits. In addition, if efficacy is very unlikely to be established based upon the results of what is called an *interim analysis*, a RCT will be stopped. These *stopping rules* are today an important part of RCTs. Stopping rules require the investigator to define the timing and type of interim analyses that will be conducted and the conditions under which an investigation will be stopped.

The interpretation and extrapolation of RCTs may be affected when an investigation is stopped early rather than conducted for the full period envisioned in the original design of the investigation. The following example illustrates how early stopping may influence the interpretation and extrapolation of study results:

Mini-Study 4.17 ■ An investigator conducted an investigation of a new drug for migraine headaches. The investigation was stopped after the second interim data analysis. The independent monitoring board, required by the IRB, found that the drug was associated with an unexpectedly large number of strokes among those in the study group. In addition, the drug's efficacy was no greater than the standard treatment used in the control group, making it very unlikely that efficacy would be established if the investigation were continued.

(Continued)

> Early stopping of an investigation may limit the conclusion that can be drawn about longer-term safety and effectiveness. It is possible that the harms of the drug are limited to a small subgroup, and clinical use could take this into account. Is it possible that with longer-term use, the benefits of the drug would improve? Thus, extrapolation as well as interpretation may be affected by the ethical requirement to stop an investigation at the earliest possible point.
>
> Protections of study participants in RCTs have continued to expand in recent years. The ethical standards that we apply to RCTs can be expected to continue to evolve as new ethical conflicts and new types of interventions develop in the coming years.

RCTs are a fundamental tool for assessing the efficacy of therapy. When carefully used, they serve as a basis for extrapolations about the effectiveness of therapy in clinical practice. New forms of randomized controlled trials are being developed and used that more directly address questions relevant to practice, as we will discuss in Chapter 14. RCTs, however, are not specifically designed to assess the safety of therapy in practice, as we will examine further in Chapter 6.

RCTs represent a major advance. RCTs are central to our current system for evaluating the efficacy of drugs and vaccines and are increasingly being used to evaluate other types of preventive, curative, rehabilitative, and palliative interventions. However, as readers of the health literature, we must understand their strengths and limitations. We must be prepared to draw our own conclusions about the application of the results to our own patients, institution, or community. We must also recognize that RCTs can provide only limited data on effectiveness and safety in practice.

REFERENCES

1. Consort. The Consort statement. http://www.consort-statement.org/consort-statement/overview0/. Accessed July 24, 2011.

2. National Institutes of Health. Information for NIH IRB members. http://ohsr.od.nih.gov/irb/protocol.html. Accessed July 24, 2011.

3. *Institutional Review Board Guidebook*. Chapter III basic IRB review. http://www.hhs.gov/ohrp/archive/irb/irb_chapter3.htm. Accessed July 24, 2011.

4. Hulley SB, Cummings SR, Browner WS, et al. *Designing Clinical Research*. 3rd ed. Philadelphia, PA: Lippincott Williams & Wilkins; 2007.

5. Murry D. *Design and Analysis of Group Randomized Trials*. New York, NY: Oxford University Press; 1998.

6. Szklo M, Nieto FJ. *Epidemiology Beyond the Basics*. 2nd ed. Sudbury, MA: Jones and Bartlett Publishers; 2007.

7. Friedman LM, Furberg CD. *Fundamentals of Clinical Trials*. 4th ed. New York, NY: Springer; 2010.

thePoint ✳ Visit http://thePoint.lww.com for interactive Q&A, flaw-catching exercises, searchable eBook, and more!

5   Observational Studies

Randomized controlled trials are the gold standard for efficacy, but they are not the gold standard for effectiveness or safety. In addition, randomized controlled trials may not be feasible or ethical. They are nearly always very expensive and time consuming. Therefore, there is a great need for other types of analytic studies to complement and prepare for randomized controlled trials. These types of studies are often called *observational studies* because the investigators observe the assignment of study and control groups rather than intervene to create these groups. The importance of observational studies has been emphasized in recent years, and their reporting has become more standardized with the publication of the STROBE statement (STrengthening the Reporting of OBservational studies in Epidemiology), which parallels the Consort Statement for randomized controlled trials (1).

Population comparisons, case-control, and cohort studies are the three basic types of observational studies that are used as part of our efforts to establish contributory cause and efficacy. As we will see, observational studies are also very useful for investigating effectiveness and safety in practice. Let us take a look at each of these types of investigation and examine the relationships between them.

POPULATION COMPARISONS (2,3)

Population comparisons of rates of disease or other outcomes can be used for a number of purposes including the following:

- Studies of etiology often begin with a hypothesis derived from observing a difference or change in rates of disease. For instance,

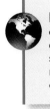

Mini-Study 5.1 ■ An investigator hypothesized that countries with a high consumption of olive oil have a lower rate of death resulting from coronary artery disease compared with countries with a low consumption of olive oil. On the basis of the results of the investigation, he recommended an investigation to determine whether an association at the individual level exists between consumption of olive oil and a lower chance of death resulting from coronary artery disease.

- Screening and diagnostic testing relies on comparing rates to estimate the pretest probability before knowing the patient's symptoms. For instance,

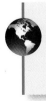

Mini-Study 5.2 ■ An investigator found that the rate of developing coronary artery disease increases with age among men and women, with the rate among women trailing men by approximately 10 years. He used this as the starting point for estimating the risk of coronary artery disease in a 65-year-old man and a 23-year-old woman.

- Prediction of the future often rests on comparing rates of development of disease and the subsequent rates of death or disability. For instance,

Mini-Study 5.3 ■ Among those with a previous myocardial infarction, the rate of death fell steadily from 50 per 1,000 per year to 20 per 1,000 per year between 1982 and 2012. The investigators predicted that the rate would be approximately 10 per 1,000 per year by 2022.

■ Efficacy may be suggested by looking at rates before and after an intervention when other data establishing efficacy are not available. For instance,

Mini-Study 5.4 ■ The rate of developing Reye syndrome was 1.0 per 100,000 children younger than 12 years per year during the 1960s and 1970s when aspirin was promoted for use by children. The rate fell to 0.1 per 100,000 children younger than 12 years per year after aspirin was widely considered contraindicated for young children.

■ Effectiveness can be evaluated using rates once efficacy has been determined by randomized controlled trials. For instance,

Mini-Study 5.5 ■ A vaccine for a common childhood disease was recently approved in the United States after two well-conducted randomized controlled trials demonstrated its efficacy. Its effectiveness was evaluated by collecting data on the number of cases of the disease before and after approval and widespread use of the vaccine. The investigators reported a dramatic decline in the rates of new cases of the disease.

Common to all these examples is the fact that the investigators are looking at rates of disease or rates of outcomes of disease in one population compared with another. Therefore, to understand the population comparisons, we need to take a look at what we mean by rates and how we use them, as discussed in Learn More 5.1.

Population comparisons compare the rates in two or more populations or in the same population over time. They cannot directly relate the data they collect to individuals. Therefore, we say that they aim to establish group relationships or group associations or differences.

The results of population comparisons are often presented as a ratio of rates or a *rate ratio*. Rate ratios may look like relative risk or odds ratios, but since they are derived from population comparisons, they do not ensure that an association exists at the individual level.

Real versus Artifactual Changes or Differences

Population comparisons may examine changes in the same population over time or differences between populations. Regardless of the uses of population comparisons or whether we are interested in changes or differences, it is important to try to determine whether the observed changes or differences in rates are real or *artifactual*. Artifactual changes or differences may also be referred to as spurious or false changes or differences.

LEARN MORE 5.1 ■ **RATES AND THEIR USES** ■ The term rates is a generic term that incorporates a range of measures of the frequency of occurrence of disease or the outcomes of disease. In classifying rates, an important distinction is between *proportions* and *true rates*. A proportion is a fraction in which the numerator is derived from the denominator. That is, the numerator is a subset of the denominator, as illustrated in the following example:

(Continued)

Mini-Study 5.6 ■ An investigator measured the number of cases of lupus erythematosus in a community of 1,000,000 people and finds 1,000 cases. She calculated the number of cases of lupus per 100,000 people and concludes that there are 100 cases of lupus per 100,000 people.

This proportion is known as *prevalence*. Prevalence measures the probability that a disease is present at a particular point in time. That is, a prevalence of 100 per 100,000 represents a probability of 1 per 1,000, or 0.001, or 0.1%.

Another important proportion that is also a probability is known as *case fatality*. Case fatality is a measure of prognosis or the probability of adverse outcomes once a disease has been diagnosed. Case fatality indicates the probability of dying from the disease once the diagnosis is made. Thus, the numerator contains the number of deaths, whereas the denominator contains the number of cases diagnosed. The case fatality is not relevant to conditions that do not result in mortality. In this situation, other adverse outcomes such as blindness or paralysis may be substituted for mortality and can be used as a measure of prognosis.

Strictly speaking, a rate, or what we will call a *true rate*, not only satisfies the conditions of a proportion but also includes a period of time. That is, in a true rate, the numerator is a subset of the denominator and also measures the occurrence of events over a period of time often over a 1-year period, as illustrated in the next example:

Mini-Study 5.7 ■ The lupus erythematosus investigator now identifies all new cases that develop in the community during 2011. She finds 20 new cases per 100,000 people in 2011 and concludes that the rate is 20 per 100,000 per year.

This measurement is known as an *incidence rate*. It measures the probability of the occurrence of an event such as the diagnosis of lupus over the period of a year. Like prevalence, the incidence rate has a numerator that comes from the denominator. Unlike prevalence that measures the situation at one point in time, incidence rates measure the occurrence of events over time. Another important measure that is a true rate is known as the *mortality rate*. Mortality rate is an important type of incidence rate that measures the incidence of death over a year per 100,000 people alive in population at the start of the year.

Incidence rates, prevalence, and case fatality aim to describe three distinct points in the course of a disease. Together, they provide a description of the clinical course of a disease or other condition as follows:

- *Incidence rate* measures the true rate of development of the disease over a period of 1 year.
- *Prevalence measures the probability of having the disease at one point in time.*
- *Case fatality measures the probability of dying or having another adverse outcome once the disease has developed.*

When using rates to compare two or more populations or a single population over time, it is important to clarify which type of rate is being used.[5.1]

[5.1] Rates may utilize different lengths of follow-up time for different individuals. If individuals are followed for differing lengths of time, a measure known as a *person-year is* often used. A person–year is one individual followed for 1 year. At times, the term rate is used as a generic term to indicate any fraction or *ratio* with a numerator and a denominator. A ratio may consist of a numerator that measures one phenomenon and a denominator that measures a different phenomenon. For example, in perinatal mortality rates, the numerator consists of the number of stillbirths in a population and the denominator is the number of live births during the same time period. This special type of ratio can be confusing because the numerator is unrelated to the denominator. This type of ratio does not have any predefined limits. In other words, theoretically, it can vary from zero to infinity since the numerator and the denominator do not depend on each other.

Changes or differences in rates may be the result of real changes in the incidence, prevalence, or case fatality. Alternatively, changes or differences may reflect changes in the method by which the particular disease is measured. Artifactual changes or differences imply that, despite the fact that a change or difference was observed, it does not reflect changes in the disease but merely in the way the disease is measured, sought, or defined.

Artifactual changes or differences result from the following three basic sources:

1. Changes or differences in the ability to recognize the disease. These represent changes in the measurement of the disease.

2. Changes or differences in the efforts to recognize or report the disease. These may represent efforts to recognize the disease at an earlier stage, changes or differences in reporting requirements, or new incentives to search for the disease.

3. Changes or differences in the definition of the disease. These represent changes or differences in the criteria used to define the disease.

The following example illustrates the first type of artifactual change, the effect of a change or difference in the ability to recognize a disease:

Mini-Study 5.8 ■ Because of an improvement in technology, a study of the prevalence of mitral valve prolapse was performed. A complete survey of the charts at a major university cardiac clinic found that in 1977 only 1 per 1,000 patients had a diagnosis of mitral valve prolapse, whereas in 2012, 60 per 1,000 patients had mitral valve prolapse included in their diagnoses. The authors concluded that the prevalence of the condition was rapidly increasing.

Between 1977 and 2012, the use of echocardiography greatly increased the ability to document mitral valve prolapse. In addition, the growing recognition of the frequency of this condition led to a much better understanding of how to suspect it by physical examination. It is not surprising, then, that a much larger proportion of cardiac clinic patients were known to have mitral valve prolapse in 2012 compared with 1977. It is possible that if equal understanding and equal technology were available in 1977, the prevalence would have been nearly identical. This example demonstrates that artifactual changes may explain large differences in the prevalence of a disease.

Changes in the efforts to recognize a disease may occur when the available treatment improves, as illustrated in the following example:

Mini-Study 5.9 ■ A new treatment for migraine headache is approved for use and is widely advertised in the medical journals and in major newspapers. The number of patients presenting for care with migraine headaches doubles in the year after approval of the new drug. These patients meet all the criteria for a diagnosis of migraine.

This apparent doubling of the prevalence of migraine is most likely due to the increased proportion of individuals with migraine headache who present for care after becoming aware of the new treatment. A high proportion of individuals with many self-limited or nonprogressive diseases do not seek health care. Changes in the types of patients who seek care can produce dramatic but artifactual changes in the rates. It is important to recognize that at times the increased ability to diagnose a disease such as mitral valve prolapse or the increased interest in its diagnosis such as migraine headaches may lead to real changes or improvements in the outcomes of the disease.

Finally, artifactual changes or differences in rates may result merely from changes in the definition used to define the disease. The following example illustrates how the definition of a disease may change over time and thus produce an artifactual difference in the apparent rate:

> **Mini-Study 5.10** ■ The incidence rate of acquired immunodeficiency syndrome (AIDS) increased every year between 1981 and 1990. In 1 year during the early 1990s, there was a sudden, dramatic increase in the reported rate. One investigator interpreted this sudden increase as a sign that the epidemic had suddenly entered a new phase. It was later recognized that no sudden change had occurred.

The dramatic increase may have been due to a change in the Centers for Disease Control and Prevention's definition of AIDS, which meant that more individuals with human immunodeficiency virus infection fell within the definition of AIDS. When sudden changes in the incidence rate of a disease occurs, one must suspect artifactual differences, such as changes in the definition of a disease. In this case, one suspects that an artifactual change was superimposed on long-term changes. Long-term changes in rates are referred to as a *temporal* or *secular* trend.

Even if we conclude that the changes or differences in rates are real, we need to be aware that different populations may have differing demographic characteristics that can affect the outcome being investigated. For populations, the most common demographic characteristics for which data are available is age. Age is a strong predictor of many diseases, so differences in age distribution of the populations being compared are important to recognize and to address. Issue of age distribution in a population may occur even when comparing the same population especially over extended periods. Demographic changes can produce a substantial increase in the average age of a population over a period of a few decades. Let us look at the next scenario, which illustrates the importance of recognizing differences in age distribution of the populations being compared:

> **Mini-Study 5.11** ■ The incidence rate of pancreatic cancer in the United States per 100,000 population was compared with the incidence rate in Mexico. The rate in the United States was found to be three times as high as the rate in Mexico per 100,000 population per year. The authors concluded that U.S. residents have a risk of pancreatic cancer three times as high as the risk among Mexicans.

The risk of pancreatic cancer may or may not be higher in the United States. Pancreatic cancer is a disease that increases with age. Therefore, the higher incidence rate may be due to the fact that the United States has an older age distribution than Mexico. Thus, a comparison of pancreatic cancer in Mexico and the United States requires taking into account the age distribution of the two populations. This can be done by calculating the incidence rate per 100,000 population that would have occurred in Mexico if it had the same age distribution of the population as the United States.[5.2]

[5.2] Or, alternatively, the incidence rate for the United States could have been calculated assuming that it had the same age distribution as Mexico. This is known as the direct method of age standardization. There are two basic forms of age adjustment or age standardization known as *direct* and *indirect age standardization*. Direct age adjustment uses the age-specific rates from one population (population A) and applies it to the number of individuals in the corresponding age group in the comparison population (population B). This allows one to ask the question: How many deaths would have occurred in population B if it has the same age distribution as population A? Direct age standardization allows a comparison of the number of deaths that did occur in population B with the number that would have been expected to occur if population B had the same age distribution as population A.

Indirect standardization, as opposed to direct standardization, does not require knowledge of the death rates in each age group in the population of interest. Indirect standardization uses an external population such as the U.S. population in 2000, where the age-specific death rates are known. The age-specific death rates in the U.S. population in 2000 are then applied to the number of individuals at each age in the population of interest. This allows calculation of an expected number of deaths.

The observed or actual number of deaths in the population of interest can then be compared with this expected number of death in the population of interest. This ratio of observed to expected number of deaths is called the *standardized mortality ratio*. Standardization can be misleading when the rates for one age group are increasing while the rates for another are decreasing. In addition, the choice of standard population can affect the results, especially if the population distribution is changing.

Using Population Data to Generate Hypotheses

When using population or group data, investigators frequently have little information about the individuals who comprise the group. Thus, when comparing rates to develop a hypothesis for further study, investigators must be careful not to imply an association among individuals when only a group association has been established. This type of error, known as an *ecological fallacy* or *population fallacy*,[5.3] is illustrated in the following example:

Mini-Study 5.12 ■ A study demonstrated that the rate of drowning in Florida is four times higher than in Illinois. The study data also demonstrated that in Florida, ice cream is consumed at a rate four times that of Illinois. The authors concluded that individuals who eat ice cream have an increased risk of drowning.

To establish an association at the individual level, the authors must first demonstrate that those who eat ice cream are the same people who are more likely to drown. Relying on group figures alone does not provide any information about the existence of an association at the individual level. It may not be the people who eat ice cream who drown. The greater consumption of ice cream may merely reflect the warmer weather in Florida compared with Illinois, which increases both ice cream consumption and drowning. These authors committed a population fallacy. They have drawn a conclusion before establishing an association between eating ice cream with drowning at the individual level.

When using rates in groups to develop hypotheses, it must be recognized that the use of group rates establishes group association and not individual association. Failure to appreciate the distinction between group association and individual association may lead to a population or ecological fallacy. Although it is usually important to follow up population comparisons by establishing the existence of relationships at the individual level, at times population comparisons will detect important relationships that cannot be identified at the individual level, as discussed in Learn More 5.2.

LEARN MORE 5.2 ■ **ADVANTAGES AND DISADVANTAGES OF POPULATION COMPARISON** ■ Despite the limitations of population comparisons in identifying relationships that exist at the individual level, population comparisons at times can uncover important relationships that cannot be detected at the individual level. This may occur for several reasons.

First, population comparisons may compare two or more quite different populations that exhibit far more variation in their level of a risk factor than exists within groups included in other types of studies, as illustrated in the next example:

Mini-Study 5.13 ■ A study was conducted of blood cadmium levels and neurological defects. When comparing the relatively low levels of blood cadmium in the United States with higher levels in some newly industrialized countries, there was an association between specific types of birth defects and the average level of cadmium among pregnant women. When the level of blood cadmium in the United States was studied among pregnant women with and without subsequent specific birth defect, no relationship was found at the individual level.

(Continued)

[5.3] The term *population fallacy* will be used because the term *ecological* is increasingly being used to indicate interaction between factors. In addition, *ecological* is a term that may not convey clear meaning.

When group associations are found, which cannot be demonstrated at the individual level, one possible reason is the greater range of levels that can be studied when comparing populations. It is possible that the explanation for the population association in the absence of an individual association is the greater range of cadmium blood levels seen among pregnant women in newly industrialized societies compared with the United States.

At times, population comparisons are the only way to investigate a relationship because the characteristic being measured only exists at the population or group level. For instance, imagine the following example:

Mini-Study 5.14 ■ An association was observed between countries with democratically chosen governments and the percentage of gross domestic product (GDP) spent on end-of-life care and countries without democratically chosen governments.

This type of relationship is detected using what has been called *global measures*, which can only be investigated at the population or group level. This is the situation in the above example since both the measure of democracy and the measure of percentage of GDP spent on end-of-life care are measures that can only be made at the population level; they have no corresponding meaning at the individual level.

In addition, population or ecological associations may unveil important interventions that can be achieved only at the population levels. The impact of taxation of cigarettes on levels of cigarette smoking or effects of population-wide environmental pollutants, for instance, may only be detected by population comparisons. Thus, even if an association can only be demonstrated at the population or group level, we need to ask whether it suggests important interventions that can be implemented only at the population level.[5.4]

In addition to population comparisons, case-control and cohort studies are two other important types of observational studies. In recent years, a number of special types of case-control and cohort studies have been developed, and the distinction between the two types of studies has become blurred. Let us take a closer look at case-control studies and then at cohort studies to better understand these issues.

CASE-CONTROL STUDIES (4,5)

Case-control studies are the type of observational study that we often use initially to establish the existence of an association at the individual level because they are more rapid and cheaper than cohort studies, especially prospective cohort studies. When using a case-control study to establish the existence of an association at the individual level, the goal is to avoid the problem of selection bias. Selection bias may occur whenever the cases and the controls are not representative of the same population. That is, selection bias occurs when the cases and controls are different in a way that makes a difference in the outcome being measured.

There are three basic types of case-control studies with varying ability to avoid selection bias, namely, (1) *case-based case-control studies,* (2) *population-based case-control studies,* and (3) *nested*

[5.4] An additional reason that individual associations may not detect associations identified at the individual level is interactions that occur at the individual level and that do not occur at the population level. These are especially common with communicable diseases. For instance, studies of dengue fever in villages in Mexico detected an association between communities with high levels of exposure to mosquito larvae and the level of antibody to dengue fever. This association was not detected when investigated at the individual level in specific communities. The reason may have been that once dengue fever spreads within the community, its occurrence does not depend on the level of larvae exposure for any one individual.

case-control studies. All of these types of case-control studies obtain their cases, those with the disease, as new or incidence cases. In contrast, cross–sectional studies identify cases that are present at one point in time, that is, the prevalent cases. Learn More 5.3 discusses these observational studies known as cross–sectional studies.

LEARN MORE 5.3 ■ CROSS-SECTIONAL STUDIES ■ In a cross-sectional study, the assignment and the assessment is conducted at the same point in time. Thus, it is possible to think of a cross-sectional study as a special type of case-control study or alternatively as a special type of cohort study. In a cross-sectional study, the investigator determines whether each individual currently has the risk factor. That is, the condition and the risk factor are measured at the same point in time. Cross-sectional studies can be very useful for investigating conditions such as a genetic relationship, where we can be quite confident that a gene that is currently present was also present in the past.

Cross-sectional studies are often conducted from survey data that identify individuals with and without a disease and simultaneously determine the presence or absence of potential risk factors. Often the data are obtained from surveys conducted for other purposes.[5.5]

Thus, cross-sectional studies are often considered an inexpensive and rapid way to conduct an observational study comparing those with a disease or other condition with those without the disease or condition. Despite the practical advantage of this easy-to-conduct observational study, it has some important limitations.

In a cross-sectional study, the frequency of those with the disease reflects the prevalence of the disease. That is, the frequency of the disease does not represent the probability of developing the disease but rather the probability of having the disease at one point in time, that is, the point in time that the investigation is conducted. Using prevalence of disease represents a problem for observational studies of etiology. Prevalence reflects the incidence times the average duration of the disease. Therefore, a cross-sectional study tends to detect the cases with the longest duration since cases with shorter duration are less likely to be currently present in the population. The following example indicates why the use of prevalent rather than incident cases of disease can produce misleading results:

Mini-Study 5.15 ■ It is known that cigarette smoking is a contributory cause of emphysema; however, those who develop emphysema have an increased probability of stopping smoking, which increases their longevity. A cross-sectional study of emphysema and smoking found a surprisingly weak association between smoking and emphysema compared with that found in case-control studies that included only newly developed cases of emphysema.

The fact that cigarette smoking not only influences the development of emphysema, but that stopping increases the duration of emphysema is the underlying reason that this cross-sectional study produced misleading results. Those living with emphysema are often those who have stopped smoking. Use of incidence or newly diagnosed cases would not have led to this conclusion. This type of error has been called *incidence–prevalence bias.*

Second, cross-sectional studies are even more limited than case-control studies in their ability to determine which came first since the disease and the risk factor are measured at the same point in time. In a cross-sectional study, no attempt is generally made to determine past behavior or exposure. Cross-sectional studies, however, if they are repeated can be helpful in establishing the change in

(Continued)

[5.5] Surveys represent a method of data collection not a type of investigation. Surveys may be conducted to establish the frequency of factors or diseases. Alternatively, they may be conducted to compare current data with the past or to try to predict the future. Survey data such as the National Health and Nutrition Examination Survey, which is conducted in the United States, have the advantage that they include a representative sample of a larger population. If the survey data are representative of the population, cross-sectional studies may reduce the potential for selection bias and allow comparisons of the same population over time.

> prevalence over time. The incidence rate of new cases can at times be estimated based on the changes in prevalence over a period of time.
>
> Thus, cross-sectional studies need to be distinguished from case-control and cohort study, although their methods of analysis often utilize many of the same statistical techniques.

Let us now take a look at each of the three basic types of case-control studies:

■ Case-based case-control studies

■ Population-based case-control studies

■ Nested case-control studies

Regardless of the type of case-control study, the goal is to include cases and controls that are representative of all those in the population from which they were obtained; that is, to avoid selection bias, cases and controls should be representative of what is called the *source population* or the larger population of which they are ideally a representative sample.

The three basic types of case-control studies obtain their cases and control in three different ways that affect their ability to avoid selection bias. Case-based case-control studies obtain their cases from new or incidence cases that develop, or more accurately are diagnosed, at one or more sites, often hospitals. The controls are then chosen from among other patients admitted to the same hospital. This traditional approach to case-control studies has a number of advantages because the controls are often readily accessible and may have time available to participate, and their medical records may be readily available to provide additional data. Unfortunately, case-based case-control studies often result in selection bias when the selection of controls is related to the factor under investigation, as demonstrated in the next scenario:[5.6]

> **Mini-Study 5.16** ■ Patients with postmenopausal uterine cancer were identified at the time of diagnosis in a large community hospital to investigate the relationship between uterine cancer and the level of estrogens in their blood. Controls are age-matched women admitted to a gynecological service for other surgical conditions. The investigators found no relationship between uterine cancer and blood estrogen level. Reviewers of the article questioned the use of control women on gynecological services because many of them had conditions for which estrogen has been commonly prescribed.

This case-based case-control study suffers from selection bias since the controls are chosen because of their admission to a gynecological service and therefore are not representative of all postmenopausal women from the same source population as those with uterine cancer. To circumvent this problem with case-based case-control studies, investigators increasingly conduct studies in the community from which the cases are obtained in an effort to ensure that the cases and controls come from the same source population. These investigations are called population-based case-control studies. This process requires greater effort and cost, but may, if done well, avoid the problem of selection bias. However, selection bias is still possible if the factor under investigation affects the likelihood of participation in the study or the likelihood of being diagnosed with the condition as illustrated in the next scenario:

[5.6] This type of selection bias resulting from the method for selecting hospital controls has also been called the *Berksonian bias*.

> **Mini-Study 5.17** ■ A population-based case-control study was conducted by identifying newly diagnosed women with postmenopausal uterine cancer and age matched postmenopausal controls. All women lived in the same zip code area. A high percentage of control group women were not at home at the time of the study visit and did not participate in the study. The study found a very strong association between blood estrogen levels and postmenopausal uterine cancer. Later it was recognized that this association was magnified by the fact that control women who were at home were less socially and professionally active and had an especially low probability of using estrogens compared with the general population of postmenopausal women.

Thus, population-based case-control studies are less likely than case-based case-control studies to result in selection bias. However, selection bias may still occur because of differing levels of participation or other factors related to the probability of diagnosis.

Population-based case-control studies have additional advantages. If the cases selected are representative of all cases and the population size is known, the incidence of the disease can be calculated. In addition, if the controls are representative of the entire population, including those with the disease, then the frequency of the risk factor among the controls provides an estimate of the prevalence of the risk factor in the population. Being able to estimate the prevalence of the risk factor allows the investigator to calculate the population attributable risk percentage. Being able to also estimate the incidence of the disease allows the investigator to calculate the number-prevented-in-the-population.

The third basic type of case-control study, known as a nested case-control study, is the least likely to produce selection basis. Nested case-control studies imply that the cases are obtained from a cohort study or a randomized controlled trial with participants who are representative of the population of interest i.e. the source population. When this is the situation, the controls can be obtained by random sampling from the remainder of those in the larger investigation. If all cases found in the larger investigation are used, then we can assume that the cases are representative of all cases in the population of interest. If controls are obtained by random sampling of those without the disease in the investigation, then we can assume that the controls are representative of all those without the disease in the population of interest. Thus, both the cases and the controls will be representative of the same population, that is, their source population. Let us see how a nested case-control study might be conducted in the next scenario:[5.7]

> **Mini-Study 5.18** ■ A cohort study enrolled and stored blood on 10,000 post-menopausal women chosen to be representative of all post menopausal women in a large U.S. state. They were followed for over a decade to determine whether they developed coronary artery disease. During this period, 100 women developed uterine cancer. The investigators identified these women as cases and randomly selected 100 controls from among the other 9,900 women in the investigation. The investigator tested the initial blood sample of the cases and controls for estrogen levels and found a strong association between blood estrogen use and uterine cancer. The relationship, however, was not as strong as the one found in the population-based case-control study.

This type of case-control study requires the conduct of a well-designed cohort study or randomized controlled trial. However, the case-control study only requires testing the blood of those who develop

---

[5.7] A special type of nested case-control study has also been called a *case-cohort study*. A case-cohort study implies that the controls have been obtained as a sample of the entire cohort including those with the disease. Controversy exists as to which method provides a better means of ensuring that both the cases and control come from the same source population.

the disease and a small sample of those who do not. When availability of the blood samples is limited or the tests are expensive, the need for only a small number of tests can be an important advantage.

A nested case-control study is considered the gold standard for avoiding selection bias in obtaining cases and controls that are representative of the source population. A nested case-control study is considered a better design than a case-based or population-based case-control study. All three types of case-control studies are currently in use and can produce accurate results if precautions are undertaken to reduce or eliminate selection bias.

All case-control studies share an advantage over cohort studies in that they require a far smaller sample size than cohort studies. Learn More 5.4 explores the sample size requirements for case-control studies.

LEARN MORE 5.4 ■ CASE-CONTROL STUDIES AND SAMPLE SIZE (6) ■ A major advantage of case-control studies is the ability to address associations using a far smaller number of study and control group individuals than would be required in a randomized controlled trial or a cohort study. To get an idea of the number of cases and controls needed to conduct a case-control study, let us look at our original example of the possible relationship between birth control pills and myocardial infarction in young women. Because the incidence of myocardial infarction in young women is very low, a cohort study or randomized controlled trial would need to enroll many thousands of young women in a study and in a control group to observe a substantial number of young women who experience myocardial infarction. Let us take a look at the number of cases and controls that would be needed to conduct this type of case-control study:

Mini-Study 5.19 ■ Let us imagine that previous studies suggest that high-dose birth control pills result in a relative risk (or odds ratio) of 2 for the relationship between birth control pills and myocardial infarction. Then, to have an 80% chance of demonstrating statistical significance (a 20% Type II error), approximately 200 cases and 200 controls would be needed to conduct a case-control study.

If the true odds ratio was actually 2.5, the same study could be conducted with as few as 100 individuals in each group. On the other hand, if we wanted to be able to demonstrate statistical significance for an odds ratio as small as 1.5, we would need approximately 700 cases and 700 controls.[5.8]

Case-control studies can quickly get large as the investigator attempts to demonstrate statistical significance for smaller and smaller odds ratios. Thus, investigators often use other techniques to increase the statistical power. Often it is far easier to identify and include controls without disease than cases with the disease in an investigation. Increasing the ratio of controls to cases to two, three, or even four can increase the statistical power of an investigation. However, there are rapidly diminishing returns as the investigator increases the ratio of controls to cases. A substantial impact on statistical power is achieved by having two cases per control, and up to four cases per control may be helpful. Increasing the number of controls per case above four is not generally worth the cost.

(Continued)

[5.8] These calculations assume a 10% use of high-dose birth control pills in the general population of women of childbearing age, an 80% power, and a 5% two-sided Type I error. One of the reasons that case-control studies are traditionally small compared with other types of investigations is that biases inherent in case-control studies limit their usefulness for small increases in the odds ratio. Thus, investigators do not generally attempt to use case-control studies to demonstrate statistical significance for small odds ratios such as 1.2. If we were interested in detecting an odds ratio of 1.2 in this situation, we would need nearly 4,000 cases and 4,000 controls.

An additional advantage of increasing the number of controls is the ability to use more than one type of control. The best type of individual to use as controls especially in a case-based case-control study is often not obvious. When this is the situation, use of different types of controls may allow the investigator to compare the cases with each type of control group and determine whether any differences are apparent, as illustrated in the next example:

Mini-Study 5.20 ■ A case-control study of the relationship between heartburn and adenocarcinoma cancer of the esophagus utilized 200 cases of adenocarcinoma of the esophagus as cases. Controls consisted of individuals from the same general population including 200 age-matched individuals without cancer, 200 with squamous cell carcinoma of the esophagus, and 200 with adenocarcinoma of the gastric cardia. The investigators found a strong association with adenocarcinoma of the esophagus, a weaker but statistically significant association with adenocarcinoma of the gastric cardia, and no association with squamous cell carcinoma of the esophagus.

This investigation provides important information that takes advantage of the three different control groups. Thus, case-control studies do require the investigator to include far fewer individuals in the investigation. Nonetheless, the number of individuals required can become relatively large, and investigators often need to identify more controls than cases to provide adequate statistical power to conduct the investigation.

Case-control studies and cohort studies are traditionally thought of as two quite different types of investigations. However, in recent years, the similarities between these two basic types of observational studies have been emphasized. The nested case-control study illustrates the similarity of the two different types of studies. In addition, the traditional prospective cohort or concurrent cohort study, which follows individuals forward over time, is increasingly being replaced by retrospective or nonconcurrent cohort studies, which like case-control studies may be conducted using existing databases.

Let us take a look at the types of cohort studies that are being used and distinguish them from each other and from case-control studies. We will also look at how new types of cohort studies are providing data that complement and at times substitute for controlled clinical trials.

COHORT STUDIES (7,8)

The immense growth in computer capacity and the rapid acceleration of data collection in the health care system in recent years have expanded potential approaches to health research. Long-term databases collected for research or other purposes such as billing are potentially available for research. In addition, it is now possible for investigators to use databases collected for the primary purpose of ongoing clinical care. [5.9]

Data that are collected as long-term research databases or collected in the course of health care can be used to conduct case-control studies. More often they are used to conduct cohort studies. The type of cohort study performed using an existing database is called a *retrospective cohort study* or a *nonconcurrent cohort study*. Sometimes, this type of research is called by the generic term *outcomes research* since it is often used to evaluate the effectiveness as well as the safety of interventions.

Remember that a cohort study is defined by the fact that study and control groups are identified or observed before determining the investigation's outcome. Thus, in a cohort study, at the time the investigators determine the assignment to study and control groups, they are not aware of the individual's end point or outcome. In contrast, in all types of case-control studies, the

[5.9] Health Insurance Portability and Accountability Act (HIPAA) regulations have restricted the use of data that can be traced back to the individual, which may make it more difficult to use data that were not developed for research purposes.

investigator and the patient are aware at the beginning of the investigation of the occurrence or absence of the disease. This is the key difference between a case-control and a cohort study.

In preceding chapters, we discussed cohort studies in which individuals are observed over time to determine their outcomes. We call this a prospective cohort study or a concurrent cohort study because individuals are monitored prospectively or concurrently over time. In prospective or concurrent cohort studies, the treatment an individual received, or their observed assignment, is ideally identified at the time they first receive the treatment. For example, we might observe one group of patients who underwent surgery, the study group, and another group of patients who received medical treatment, the control group, in 2007. Then the study and the control groups would be observed over time to determine their outcomes. The surgical and the medical patients might be monitored to assess their outcome from immediately after they were identified until 2013.

With the availability of computerized databases on patients recorded during the course of their health care, it is increasingly feasible to conduct a second type of cohort study, a retrospective or nonconcurrent cohort study. In this type of cohort study, it is not necessary to identify the treatment individuals received at one point in time and then to monitor them over time to determine their subsequent outcomes. In retrospective cohort studies, the information about which treatment an individual received in 2007 can be obtained from a database in 2013. By the time an investigation is conducted in 2013, the data on outcome is already recorded in the computer database. Figures 5.1 and 5.2 illustrate the basic difference between a prospective or concurrent cohort study and a retrospective or nonconcurrent cohort study.

To conduct a retrospective cohort study, the investigators could proceed as follows:

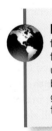

Mini-Study 5.21 ■ In February 2013, investigators begin a study. The investigators first search the database for all patients who underwent surgery and for all patients who received medical treatment for recurrent otitis media in 2007. Those who underwent surgery become the study group, and those who received medication become the control group. After performing this observed assignment, the investigators then search the database to determine the outcomes that occurred from the time of the assignment to study and control groups through January 2013.

A retrospective cohort study is still a cohort study because the study and control groups are assigned before the investigators become aware of the individuals' outcomes. It is not legitimate for the investigators to search the database for the outcomes until they have completed the assignment process, even though these outcomes have already occurred by the time the investigation is begun in February 2013.

Both prospective and retrospective cohort studies may be used to investigate the cause of disease or the benefits and harms of therapy. However, increasingly, retrospective cohort studies are

Study and control groups identified; follow-up begun

Assessment of outcome

2007

2013

Figure 5.1 Time sequence of a concurrent or prospective cohort study.

Study and control groups identified by characteristics in database from 2007; outcome assessed in 2013

2007

2013

Figure 5.2 Time sequence of a nonconcurrent or retrospective cohort study.

being used to study the outcome of therapies, their effectiveness and safety. When the data come from actual clinical practice, it can often complement the information that can be obtained from randomized controlled trials. That is, information from randomized controlled trials and information based on collection of data in the course of clinical practice can be used together to provide a more complete picture than can be obtained from either one alone.

Retrospective cohort studies conducted using ongoing clinical data have several important advantages over randomized controlled trials. First, they may be able to include a large number of individuals with the disease or condition and often an even larger numbers of controls without the condition. Second, there are far fewer ethical constraints since individual patients are not asked to agree to be randomized to a study or control group. Third, when the data come from ongoing clinical care, the patient population often represents the types of individuals on whom the intervention is used in clinical practice. Finally, the low cost and rapid conduct of retrospective cohort studies is an advantage over both prospective cohort studies and randomized controlled trials.

There are various potential uses of retrospective cohort studies that we will explore in this chapter and future chapters, and these include the following:

- Investigating potential improvements in outcomes that are expected to be too small to warrant a randomized controlled trial
- Providing evidence for "altering the cause alters the effect," the third criteria of contributory cause, when randomized controlled trials are not ethical or practical
- Investigating the impact of a therapy in a practice setting to establish effectiveness after efficacy has been established by randomized controlled trials
- Investigating issues of short term and long term safety after a new therapy has been approved for clinical use based on short-term and/or relatively small randomized controlled trials

Now, let us take a look at how retrospective cohort studies differ from randomized controlled trials in terms of each of the components of the M.A.A.R.I.E. framework. We will use the M.A.A.R.I.E. framework to look at how the information retrospective cohort studies provide may complement and at time substitute for the information obtained from controlled trials. We will also examine the limitation of these types of investigations.

METHOD

When investigating an intervention, retrospective cohort studies differ from randomized controlled trials on all three of the methods question. In terms of the study question or study hypothesis, retrospective cohort studies usually address issues of effectiveness and safety. The primary study question for randomized controlled trials, on the other hand, is usually efficacy. Thus, the study question and the hypothesis for these two types of studies will be quite different and often complementary.

The study population used for retrospective cohort studies often includes study and control groups that are representative of those who receive the intervention in clinical practice. In randomized controlled trials, the study population is defined by inclusion and exclusion criteria designed to produce a study population that has a high probability of demonstrating efficacy.[5.10]

In terms of sample size, in retrospective cohort studies, there are a large number of individuals potentially eligible for the study group and an even larger number potentially eligible for the control group. In randomized controlled trials, the size of the study and control groups is often limited to the smallest number compatible with adequate statistical power to demonstrate efficacy.

[5.10] The inclusion and exclusion criteria for a randomized controlled trial are also designed to produce a study population with a low probability of experiencing adverse events.

The next scenario demonstrates the differing approaches of randomized controlled trials and cohort studies:

> **Mini-Study 5.22** ■ A randomized controlled trial using 200 study and 200 control group patients demonstrated the efficacy of nasal polyp surgery for individuals with recurrent sinusitis, aspirin allergy, and asthma. A retrospective cohort study of the effectiveness and safety of the surgery was conducted using a database from ongoing clinical care. Using the database, the investigators identified 20,000 patients who had undergone the same type of nasal polyp surgery and a comparable control group who had not undergone the surgery. The retrospective cohort study did not demonstrate effectiveness. Reviewers of these studies relied on the randomized controlled trial exclusively because of its inherently superior study design.

The randomized controlled trial and the retrospective cohort study address different questions and investigate different populations. Randomized controlled trials are the gold standard for determining efficacy for a specific indication. Efficacy for one clear-cut, narrowly defined indication for treatment such as the patient with recurrent sinusitis, aspirin allergy, and asthma may tell us very little about the outcomes the therapy produces when applied to a broader target population in clinical practice. The outcomes of a therapy when used in clinical practice define its effectiveness. Efficacy, on the other hand, is defined by the results of randomized controlled trials.

Thus, the results of a retrospective cohort study, everything else being equal, may add to or complement the result of a randomized controlled trial by providing information on effectiveness reflecting the way an intervention is actually utilized in clinical practice. Databases from clinical practice can be especially useful for investigating safety issues. We will take a closer look at safety issue in Chapter 6.

In randomized controlled trials, the sample sizes chosen are often designed to be the smallest number that will provide acceptable statistical power (i.e., the largest acceptable Type II error, usually 10% to 20%) in addressing efficacy using what is called the primary end point. As discussed in the chapter on randomized controlled trials, these numbers usually vary from less than 100 in the study group and the control group to several thousand in each group. The sample size in retrospective cohort studies is limited mainly by the availability of patient data in the database. Thousands or even millions of patients may be included. Thus, the potential sample size for retrospective cohort studies may dwarf that of most randomized controlled trials. This difference in sample sizes may have important implications, as illustrated in the next example:

> **Mini-Study 5.23** ■ A randomized controlled trial was conducted comparing removal of colon polyps versus observation. The study and the control groups each included 500 patients. The investigation demonstrated a small but not statistically significant reduction in the subsequent rate of colon cancer. A retrospective cohort study using 10,000 patients who had polyp removal and 10,000 patients who underwent observation also demonstrates a small difference in the subsequent rate of colon cancer, but the *P*-value was 0.00001 and the confidence limits were very narrow.

This type of discrepancy between the results of a randomized controlled trial and those of a retrospective cohort study is expected. If the retrospective cohort study is able to avoid the biases to which it is susceptible, we would expect the retrospective cohort study to have a far greater statistical power. That is, it would have a much greater chance of demonstrating statistical significance if a true difference exists in the population being sampled.

ASSIGNMENT

When discussing retrospective cohort studies and comparing them with randomized controlled trials, we have repeatedly used the phrase "everything else being equal." "Everything else" is not usually equal when we compare these two types of studies because retrospective cohort studies are susceptible to a variety of potential biases. These potential biases are most dramatic in the area of assignment.

Randomized controlled trials, by definition, use randomization for their assignment process. The process of randomization is the hallmark of a randomized controlled trial. Remember that the process of randomization is designed to take into account not only the factors that are known to affect outcome but also those factors that have an effect on outcome we do not anticipate or even understand.

In retrospective cohort studies, assignment of patients to study and control groups is often based on clinicians' treatment of patients. Clinicians try to tailor the treatment to the patient. When clinicians are successful in tailoring treatment to individuals, selection biases are created. Selection bias occurs, for instance, when clinicians assign patients with different prognoses to different treatments. In fact, we can regard the job of clinical care as one of creating biases by tailoring the treatment to the patient. The job of the clinician, then, is to create selection biases, and the job of the researcher is to untangle these selection biases. Selection bias created in database research has been called *case-mix bias*. Let us see how this type of selection bias may influence the results:

Mini-Study 5.24 ■ A randomized controlled trial of a smoking-cessation drug demonstrated a small but statistically significant reduction in smoking among those randomized to the drug. A large, retrospective cohort study identified those prescribed the drug and compared success in quitting among smokers who were prescribed the drug versus smokers who were not prescribed the drug. The investigation demonstrated a much larger reduction in smoking among those prescribed the drug.

The patients prescribed the drug in the retrospective cohort study may have been those who were especially motivated to stop smoking. Clinicians may have tailored their treatment by giving more intensive treatment to the patients they thought would benefit the most. This is a natural and often desirable tendency in clinical care. However, from the researcher's perspective, selecting motivated patients to receive the treatment results in the type of assignment problem we have called selection bias or, specifically in this setting, the case-mix bias. This is the situation, since those who receive the treatment are the same individuals who are especially likely to quit smoking. Recognizing the potential for confounding variables created by the process of clinical care is important so that these confounding variables can be taken into account in the analysis.[5.11]

Randomized controlled trials are often precluded by ethical and practical issues. Once it is suspected that a treatment benefits patients, clinicians and patients will often be unwilling to randomize patients to receive or not to receive the treatment. Thus, a retrospective cohort study may be the best available study design even when a randomized controlled trial would, in theory, be preferable.

In addition to randomized assignment, an ideal randomized controlled trial is also double-masked or double-blinded. That is, neither the patient nor the investigator is aware of the treatment being received. However, as we have seen, in randomized controlled trials double-masked studies are often unethical, impractical, or unsuccessful. Patient masking is not possible in a retrospective

---

[5.11] Unfortunately, databases obtained from clinical care may lack the data needed to measure some important confounding variables that should ideally be taken into account in the analysis.

cohort study of a database from ongoing clinical care. In addition, the clinician who prescribes the treatment is not masked. Thus, for both randomized controlled trials and retrospective cohort studies, we often need to ask what the implications are of a lack of masking. To do this, we usually need to examine how the method of assignment affects the results of the assessment process.

ASSESSMENT

The process of follow-up and assessment in well-conducted randomized controlled trials and retrospective cohort studies is very different. In a randomized controlled trial, patients in the study group and the control group are followed up at predetermined intervals, which are the same for the study and the control groups. The same data are ideally collected on individuals in each group at the predetermined follow-up intervals. The goal of randomized controlled trials is to investigate efficacy. The length of follow-up is usually determined by the minimum length of time needed to establish efficacy. Thus, randomized controlled trials are often short-term trials designed to establish short-term efficacy. Longer-term efficacy may not be well studied in randomized controlled trials. In addition, adverse events that take longer periods to develop may be missed entirely by randomized controlled trials but detected by retrospective cohort studies.

The process of follow-up and assessment in a retrospective cohort study is very different because it occurs as part of the course of health care. Data are collected if and when the patient returns for care. This return visit may be initiated by the clinician or by the patient. Thus, the frequency of data collection, the type of data, and even the accuracy of the data collected are likely to be quite different in randomized controlled trials and retrospective cohort studies. These differences in follow-up may make it more difficult in retrospective cohort studies to detect certain types of adverse events related to treatment, as illustrated in the next example:

> **Mini-Study 5.25** ■ A randomized controlled trial comparing surgery versus medication for benign prostate hypertrophy found that surgery produces far more retrograde ejaculation and impotence than medication. A retrospective cohort study using records from ongoing medical care found no difference in these adverse events, as recorded in the patients' charts.

Unless patients are specifically asked or tested for these adverse events, they may not recognize them or report them to clinicians. Thus, in retrospective cohort studies, the type of outcome measures that can be reliably used may be much more limited than in a randomized controlled trial. In controlled clinical trials potential adverse events can be assessed in the same way for each group at the same time intervals.

RESULTS

In randomized controlled trials, analysis is conducted using the principle of intention-to-treat. Data from individuals are analyzed according to their assignment group even if they deviated from the protocol and never actually received the treatment. Remember that this is done so that individuals with good prognosis are not disproportionately represented among those who are left in the investigation after many participants with a poorer prognosis drop out of the investigation.

In a retrospective cohort study, a process parallel to analysis by intention-to-treat is not feasible because the only patients who appear in the database may be those who actually take the treatment and obtain follow-up, as illustrated in the next example:

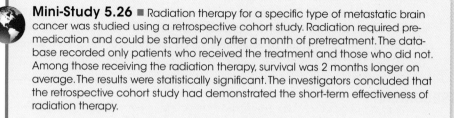

Mini-Study 5.26 ■ Radiation therapy for a specific type of metastatic brain cancer was studied using a retrospective cohort study. Radiation required pre-medication and could be started only after a month of pretreatment. The data-base recorded only patients who received the treatment and those who did not. Among those receiving the radiation therapy, survival was 2 months longer on average. The results were statistically significant. The investigators concluded that the retrospective cohort study had demonstrated the short-term effectiveness of radiation therapy.

The fact that the radiation therapy could not be undertaken for at least a month after it was pre-scribed may mean that those with the worst prognosis had already died or become too ill to receive the radiation therapy. Thus, the retrospective cohort study may have examined a study group with a better prognosis than the control group, indicating the groups may not actually have been analyzed using a method analogous to the intention-to-treat method.

In randomized controlled trials, adjustment is used as a way to account for the known prognostic factors that, despite randomization, differ between the study and control groups. Ran-domization itself usually results in known prognostic factors being similar in the study and control groups. In addition, randomization has the aim to produce similarity even for unknown prognostic factors. Statistical adjustment is still used in a randomized controlled trial; however, its role is only to take into account the differences that occur despite randomization.

In a retrospective cohort study, adjustment has a much larger role. It attempts to recognize and take into account all the known differences between the study and control groups that may affect the outcome being measured. Adequate adjustment in a retrospective cohort study requires the difficult-to-achieve goal of recognizing all potentially important confounding variables and taking them into account in the adjustment process.

INTERPRETATION

As a type of cohort study, retrospective cohort studies are best designed to demonstrate that the treatment is associated with an improved outcome and that the treatment precedes the outcome. Even when this is successful, however, we are often left with some doubt as to the third criterion of contributory cause, or efficacy, of therapy: altering the "cause" alters the "effect."

A special type of retrospective cohort study, however, may help to establish that altering the cause alters the effect. This type of investigation recognizes that a change has occurred in one group over a period of time but not in another comparable group. The probability of a particular outcome before and after the change in each group is then calculated to determine whether the outcome was altered in the group that experienced the change. This type of investigation has been called a *natural experiment* since we are observing changes that occur in the natural course of events, not because of an investigator's intervention. Let us see how a natural experiment may enable us to draw the conclusion that altering the cause alters the effect:

Mini-Study 5.27 ■ Cigarettes were smoked with nearly equal frequency by male physicians and attorneys in the 1960s, and they had a similar probability of developing lung cancer. During the 1970s, a large proportion of male physicians quit smoking cigarettes, whereas a smaller proportion of male attorneys quit smok-ing cigarettes. The investigators observed that both male physicians and male attorneys who stopped smoking had a reduction in their probability of developing lung cancer and that the probability of developing lung cancer among male physicians in subsequent years was far lower than among male attorneys.

A randomized controlled trial of cigarette smoking would have been the ideal method for establishing that altering the cause alters the effect. This type of natural experiment is the next best method. It is often, as in this situation, the only ethical and feasible method for establishing contributory cause.

After analysis of the results and interpretation are completed using all the individuals included in either a randomized controlled trial or a retrospective cohort study, the investigators are often interested in examining the meaning of the results for subgroups included in the investigation. The large numbers of participants included in a retrospective cohort study may allow the investigators to subdivide the study group and control group into subgroups and examine the therapy's effectiveness for each of these groups. Because of the larger numbers, the data from the retrospective cohort studies' subgroups may be more reliable than those from subgroups derived from smaller randomized controlled trials. This may have important implications, as illustrated in the next hypothetical example:

> **Mini-Study 5.28** ■ A randomized controlled trial of one-vessel coronary artery disease demonstrated that angiography had greater efficacy, on average, than drug treatment. Subgroup analysis performed by creating groups that differed in their extent of myocardium served by the vessel, age of the patients, and gender of the patient was not able to demonstrate statistically significant differences between these groups. A large retrospective cohort study demonstrated overall effectiveness of angiography, but it also demonstrated that this effectiveness was limited to younger men and to patients with a lesion supplying a large area of myocardium.

This type of result illustrates the principle that the larger number of patients who may be included in a retrospective cohort study may enable this type of study to better address issues among subgroups than even the most well-designed, randomized controlled trial. This use of randomized controlled trials and retrospective cohort studies demonstrates the potential to use the results of one type of study to supplement the results of the other.

EXTRAPOLATION

Extrapolation of the results of a randomized controlled trial requires making assumptions about the population that will receive the treatment (i.e., the target population). Remember that randomized controlled trials are usually conducted using homogeneous patients. That is, they often exclude patients who are on multiple treatments, who have liver or kidney disease complicating their management, and who have other diseases. In addition, special precautions may be used in randomized controlled trials to exclude patients who have special characteristics, such as those who are not likely to follow up or who are likely to become pregnant. Thus, the patients included in randomized controlled trials are often quite different from those included in retrospective cohort studies. Therefore, the results of a randomized controlled trial and those of a retrospective cohort study may look very different, even when the new therapy is administered using the same implementation procedures, as illustrated in the next example:

> **Mini-Study 5.29** ■ A randomized controlled trial of a new method of home dialysis for newly diagnosed renal failure patients demonstrated substantial improvement in outcome compared with outpatient hemodialysis. The new dialysis method was then made available on a voluntary basis to all dialysis patients throughout the country. All those using the new technique were compared with all those using standard outpatient hemodialysis in a retrospective cohort study. The investigators found no difference in outcome between the new home dialysis method and standard outpatient hemodialysis.

A randomized controlled trial on a small homogeneous group of new dialysis patients may show very different results compared with a retrospective cohort study involving a larger number of more heterogeneous patients. For instance, patients who are accustomed to outpatient hemodialysis may have difficulty switching to the new treatment. Patients with more complications or long-standing outpatient hemodialysis may not do as well on the new therapy.

Thus, we cannot necessarily expect that the results of a randomized controlled trial and those of a retrospective cohort study will be the same even when both are well designed and the therapy is administered using the same implementation procedures. It is still likely that for carefully selected patients, like those in the randomized controlled trial, the new method of home dialysis is better than the standard therapy.

As we discussed, randomized controlled trials are limited to assessing outcomes or end points over a relatively short period. After they are introduced into practice, dynamic effects may occur that may alter the longer-term effectiveness of the therapy. Resistance may occur; the treatment may be used for new indications, producing more or less effectiveness; or patient behavior may change, altering the effectiveness of treatment.

Retrospective cohort studies may be more successful in detecting these changes in effectiveness that occur over time. The large number of patients in a database may allow the investigator to compare the outcomes that occurred when the treatment was prescribed in different years. Alternatively, the degree of effectiveness can be assessed over extended periods to determine whether any benefit observed in the short run persists over a longer period. This advantage of retrospective cohort studies is illustrated in the next example:

> **Mini-Study 5.30** ■ A new high-energy treatment for kidney stones has been demonstrated in a randomized controlled trial to have efficacy in the treatment of obstruction of a ureter compared with surgery when patients are observed for 1 year. A retrospective cohort study was performed on obstruction of a ureter caused by kidney stones treated with the new technique and followed for up to 10 years. The results of the retrospective cohort study demonstrated less effectiveness for the new treatment compared with surgery. Those undergoing surgery actually did better after 1 year.

These two results may both be true. They may complement each other. This could be the case if the new treatment increases the rate of recurrence of kidney stones. The relatively short-term follow-up that is usually possible in randomized controlled trials leaves an important role for retrospective cohort studies using databases obtained from ongoing clinical care in the longer-term assessment of safety and effectiveness.

Remember that randomized controlled trials are the gold standard for assessing efficacy, but they have severe limitations when assessing benefits and harms for the target population. When assessing the longer-term outcomes of treatment and the occurrence of rare but serious adverse events, retrospective cohort studies can complement randomized controlled trials and compensate for some, if not all, of their deficiencies. Table 5.1 summarizes the differences between randomized controlled trials and retrospective cohort studies.

TABLE 5.1	Comparison of Randomized Controlled Trials and Retrospective Cohort Studies	
Studies	**Randomization Controlled Trials**	**Retrospective Cohort Studies**
Method	As small as possible—aim to demonstrate statistical significance for a frequent and important outcome—primary end point inclusion and exclusion criteria used to define homogenous groups of patients	May be large limited only by availability of records obtained in course of ongoing medical care Participants selected as part of ongoing provision of services—may be more representative of the target population for the treatment
Assignment	Randomization Ideally double blinded Potential ethical limitations	No randomization—patients selected in the course of ongoing provision of services with follow-up tailored to patients' progress potentially creating selection biases (case-mix problem) Fewer ethical constraints
Assessment	Follow-up of study and control patients at the same intervals aiming for equal intensity of follow-up Concurrent follow-up needed Data collected under investigator's control facilitating accuracy and precision of data collection	Potential for longer-term follow-up Follow-up as part of ongoing provision of services with unequal intervals of follow-up likely Follow-up has already occurred so quicker and cheaper Data collected in the usual course of provision of services subjecting data to potential for low accuracy and precision
Results	By intention-to-treat with end point Ideally obtained from all individuals who were randomized	Inclusion of only those whose follow-up appears in database
Interpretation	Gold standard for efficacy Relatively small numbers limit interpretation regarding safety especially with respect to rare but serious adverse events Subgroup analysis should generally occur only after overall showing that one treatment is better or subgroup's importance is hypothesized before collecting the data	Conclusions about efficacy more difficult because of potential confounding variables such as prognosis. Thus, therapies may appear to work because of clinicians' skills in assigning treatment Potential to use as "natural experiment" to help establish causation when randomized controlled trial not ethical or feasible Greater potential for assessing rare but serious side effects especially when numbers are large Larger numbers hold greater potential for subgroup analysis
Extrapolation	Efficacy found for homogenous group in the investigation must be extrapolated to target population requiring that assumptions be made Limitations when extrapolating from short-term trials to longer-term use require extrapolation beyond the data	Target population often included in the investigation thus allowing more direct evidence of effectiveness in practice Potential for longer-term follow-up data allowing longer-term conclusions without extrapolation beyond the data

REFERENCES

1. Vandenbroucke JP, Van Elm E, Altman DG, et al. Strengthening the reporting of observational studies in epidemiology (STROBE): explanation and elaboration. *Epidemiology*. 2007;18(6):805–835.

2. Aschengrau A, Seage GR. *Essentials of Epidemiology in Public Health*. 2nd ed. Sudbury, MA: Jones and Bartlett Publisher; 2008.

3. Friis RH, Sellers TA. *Epidemiology for Public Health Practice*. 4th ed. Sudbury, MA: Jones and Bartlett Publishers; 2009.

4. Greenberg RS, Daniels SR, Flanders WD, Eley JW, Boring JR. *Medical Epidemiology*. 4th ed. New York, NY: Lange Medical Books; 2005.

5. Szklo M, Nieto FJ. *Epidemiology Beyond the Basics*. 2nd ed. Sudbury, MA: Jones and Bartlett Publishers; 2007.

6. Hennekens CH, Buring JE. *Epidemiology in Medicine*. Boston, MA: Little Brown and Company; 1987.

7. Gehlbach SH. *Interpreting the Medical Literature*. 5th ed. New York, NY: McGraw-Hill; 2006.

8. Gordis L. *Epidemiology*. 4th ed. Philadelphia, PA: Saunders; 2009.

thePoint ✳ Visit http://thePoint.lww.com for interactive Q&A, flaw-catching exercises, searchable eBook, and more!

6   Safety

Randomized controlled trials are the gold standard for efficacy so we might ask the question: What is the gold standard for safety? Unfortunately, the answer is not so easy since there is no one type of study that can provide us with all the evidence we need. We might think of the gold standard for safety as many years of use by millions of people accompanied by systematic monitoring for adverse events. Although this may be the ideal standard, it presents us with a catch-22. Safety cannot be established without first subjecting millions of people to potential harm.

To understand safety, we need to recognize that most interventions produce harms as well as benefits. The goal of measuring safety is to be sure that the harms are minimized and that the benefits are clearly greater than the harms. The generic term "acceptable harm" is increasingly being used instead of "safe" since the term safe may provide a false sense of security that no undesirable outcomes will occur. Safety also may imply that we understand the relationship between our interventions and any harms that occur after an intervention. The term *adverse events* is increasingly being used instead of side effects or adverse effects to avoid the implication of a clear-cut cause-and-effect relationship since cause-and-effect relationships are especially difficult to establish for harms.

Because of the complexity of the investigation of harm, we need to take a different approach than that used to understand the benefits of interventions. The investigation of harms requires the use of multiple types of studies. The emphasis is not on one type of investigation but on how a range of investigations fit together to provide evidence about potential harms. Thus, we need a multipart systematic approach to evaluating safety recognizing that it will not be perfect.

The U.S. Food and Drug Administration (FDA) has developed and recently expanded its approach to assessing adverse events associated with drugs. This framework is useful in understanding the process and in integrating the various types of research studies that contribute to our understanding of harms. Although developed and used for drug approval and monitoring, it has been extended to use for vaccines and increasingly for other types of interventions. The FDA has begun to utilize what is called a *systems approach* to drug safety. Learn More 6.1 introduces the concept of systems approaches and illustrates its successful use in airline safety.

> **LEARN MORE 6.1 ■ SYSTEMS APPROACHES—AIRLINE SAFETY AND DRUG SAFETY** ■ When examining the role of the FDA in preventing harm, it can be helpful to think about the harms from health interventions as parallel to the safety issues faced by the airline industry. What is known as a *systems approach* to commercial airline safety has been credited with reducing deaths despite the rapidly increasing number of passenger miles flown each year. A systems approach examines the multiple influences on a problem and the interactions of these influences, identifies bottlenecks and leverage points, and looks for changes over time.
>
> Despite the potential harms of airline travel, a complex system of prevention, protection, and response is now in place. The government and the airline industry have developed a complex systematic approach to equipment testing, routine maintenance, training of personnel, protective equipment, and thorough investigation of not only crashes but near misses as well. This has been achieved by examining all the known influences on safety, looking for bottlenecks and leverage points in the process, and performing continuing monitoring to detect new risks and the return of previously known hazards.
>
> Systems thinking or system approaches are based on an *integrative approach* to evidence. An integrative approach implies that evidence from a

(Continued)

variety of sources is brought together to address decision-making and problem-solving issues. In an integrative approach, the interaction between factors is a major focus. This approach contrasts with *reductionist approach* more frequently used in health research. In a reductionist approach, the investigator focuses on one factor at a time. Data are collected on other factors in large part to take these potential confounding factors into account, to control, or to adjust for them. Thus, most of the specific types of investigations that we have discussed take a reductionist approach. However, once we step back and attempt to put together the evidence, we often need to take an integrative or systems approach.

No comprehensive systems approach to safety is in place in health care. As we proceed to think through the issues raised by safety, the airline industry's systems approach provides an illustrative model for what is possible.[6.1]

Our look at harms will focus on drugs and vaccines, but adverse events are possible with all interventions whether they are called surgery, medical devices, or dietary supplements. Surgery, medical devices, and, especially, dietary supplement generally undergo less investigation before their use in clinical practice than drugs and vaccines.

Herbals, vitamins, minerals, and other substances that are classified as dietary supplements do not require demonstrations of efficacy or acceptable harm before being marketed and sold. In fact, marketing and use of dietary supplements do not require FDA approval. Dietary supplements may not be advertised for the treatment or prevention of disease, but they can be and are advertised for use to alter anatomy and physiology from weight to blood pressure to energy to mood. In monitoring for adverse events associated with dietary supplements, the burden is on the FDA to demonstrate that important adverse events occur.

The system for evaluating drugs and vaccines, as we will see, is generally more tightly regulated than surgery, medical devices, or dietary supplements. However, the surveillance system for medical devices is the only one that requires institutions to report the occurrence of all potentially life-threatening failures. Expect to see changes in the regulation of medical devices in coming years.

The system for drug and vaccine monitoring for harms has evolved over the last 100 years reflecting the history of the FDA. Changes have often been instituted after highly publicized tragedies and epidemics caused by drugs or vaccines and therapeutic devices. Learn More 6.2 reviews key elements of this history.

LEARN MORE 6.2 ■ SAFETY AND THE FDA (1) ■ The FDA was established in 1906. Its authority over drugs was initially very limited. It had no authority to require testing for efficacy, and it had very limited authority over safety mostly confined to requiring disclosure of the ingredients. The authority of the FDA over drugs, vaccines, and medical devices has grown enormously since 1906. The following important events led to changes in the FDA law:

- In 1937, an outbreak of kidney failure in children occurred after exposed to a dangerous preparation of the first antibiotics, sulfa. The FDA law was amended to require premarket testing for safety.
- In the mid-1950, distribution of early live polio vaccine produced polio-like illness. The FDA law was amended to establish standards for vaccines.
- The early 1960s thalidomide case in which thousands of children were born especially in Europe with dramatically shortened limbs. Despite the fact that the United States was spared the tragedy

(Continued)

[6.1] Systems approaches are being used to address food safety. The 2010 U.S. federal food safety legislation is built on principles of systems thinking. Motor vehicle injuries have also been addressed using a systems approach.

of thalidomide, the FDA law was amended to greatly strengthen the standards for efficacy testing for the first time integrating randomized controlled trials into the process.

■ The 1970s widespread use of the Dalcon Shield IUD produced an epidemic of tubal infection, infertility, and ectopic pregnancies. The FDA law was amended to provide authority for medical device regulation.

■ In the first decade of the 21st century, the cardiac risks of Cox-II inhibitors were acknowledged only after they were used for years by many millions of people.

In response to this latest tragedy, Congress gave the FDA extensive new authority to take a systems approach, including a wide range of new tools for postmarket monitoring, researching, labeling, and controlling the use of drugs.

FDA PHASES (2)

The FDA's regulation of prescription drugs is organized into the following phases:

■ *Prehuman animal and laboratory testing*
■ *Preapproval-Phase 1*
■ *Preapproval-Phase 2*
■ *Preapproval-Phase 3*
■ *Postapproval-Phase 4*

Let us take a look at the process and limitation of what takes place in each of these phases. Table 6.1 summarizes the key information related to each phase.[6.2]

TABLE 6.1	FDA Phase of Evaluation of Prescription Drugs		
	Definition	**Implementation Issues**	**Limitations**
Prehuman animal and laboratory testing	Evaluation for harms on at least two species at high doses before initial use on humans New approaches being developed	Assess carcinogenic, teratogenic, and fertility effects	High dose effects may not correlate with effects on humans Species differences may result in missing effects that later appear in human testing or after widespread clinical use
Phase 1	Initial testing of drug on humans may include healthy volunteers or terminally ill patients but not generally those on whom drug will be used in clinical practice Small studies, often several studies including 5–10 persons each	Designed to assess pharmacology including metabolism and excretion in effort to establish dose, timing, and route of administration Evaluation for adverse events especially on vulnerable organs including liver, kidney, and bone marrow	Small numbers mean many adverse events may be missed When includes patients not representative of those on whom the drug will be used, may not help predict adverse events

(Continued)

[6.2] The conclusions of this process are generally not published in journals, but are summarized in the official FDA product descriptions that are widely available to clinicians through the *Physicians' Desk Reference*.

TABLE 6.1	FDA Phase of Evaluation of Prescription Drugs *(Continued)*		
	Definition	**Implementation Issues**	**Limitations**
Phase 2	Initial small-scale controlled or uncontrolled trials of efficacy with secondary assessment of harms Size designed to estimate efficacy often 20–200	Designed to establish that there is enough evidence of efficacy to warrant phase 3 randomized controlled trials. Focus not primarily on harms	Primary intent is assessment of efficacy. Small numbers and less than comprehensive assessment of harms often limit ability to draw conclusion about potential harms
Phase 3	At least two independently conducted randomized controlled trials required unless not practical or ethical Size designed to demonstrate efficacy usually ranging from 100 in each group to 3,000 in each group	Designed to establish efficacy in the shortest possible time for one indication for a group defined by uniform inclusion and exclusion criteria. Study group compared with conventional treatment Investigate short-term harms relative to conventional treatment	Uniform characteristics of the participants may result in study and control groups with only one disease who are taking only one medication. Randomized controlled trials often too small, too short, and too simple to detect rare but serious adverse events
Phase 4	Postmarket surveillance A system to monitor interventions such as drugs and vaccines after approval Potentially uses multiple types of data and multiple types of follow-up investigations including surveillance systems, meta-analysis, retrospective cohort studies, and case–control studies May also include limitations on authority to prescribe and/or required testing or monitoring before prescribing or refilling prescription	Once a drug is used in practice, adverse events may be more frequent than seen before approval because of the use on patients with multiple or more severe disease and/or the use of multiple treatments Spontaneous reports to FDA from clinicians and patients form the basis of current postmarket surveillance. There is currently no required reporting of even serious adverse events or universal required follow-up of patients previously treated as part of a randomized controlled trial Meta-analysis, case–control studies, and retrospective cohort studies from clinical practice are increasingly being used to evaluate potential harms	Spontaneous reporting system results may not detect adverse events especially if they are not dramatic, do not occur soon after the intervention, require special testing to detect their presence, are clinically unexpected, and/or are similar to the effects of the disease being treated.

It is useful to categorize these phases as a preapproval or *premarket* process followed by a *postmarket* process that occurs after FDA approval. The first four components through phase 3 can be viewed as premarket; that is, they occur before FDA approval to market the drug. Phase 4 is often called postmarket since it collects data on adverse events after the approval of the drug. Let us walk through these phases to better understand what is involved, how they relate to each other, and why there are still holes in this "safety net." The process we will describe is a general or generic process that may be modified for specific new drugs or categories of drugs or vaccines.[6.3]

Prehuman animal and laboratory testing

Before studying a drug on humans, the FDA requires that animal and laboratory studies be performed. Animal testing is usually administered to two different species at levels well above the weight equivalent dosage expected to be used in humans. Studies are done primarily to detect cancer, birth defects, and effects on fertility. However, toxicity to drug-sensitive organs such as the liver, kidneys, and bone marrow is also investigated. Unfortunately, the effects on animals may fail to either detect subsequent effects in humans or demonstrate high dose effects that are difficult to interpret as illustrated in the following hypothetical example:

 Mini-Study 6.1 ■ A new drug is studied in two animal species. In one species, there was a slightly greater frequency of thyroid cancer seen at doses several times higher than those expected to be used in humans; otherwise, the animal testing did not suggest the potential for harm. When the drug was studied in humans, tests revealed rare but dramatic birth defects but no evidence of cancer.

Humans may absorb, metabolize, and excrete drugs differently than animal species. High dose effects on one animal species alert us to the possibility of similar effects in humans but by no means guarantees their occurrence. In addition, as we will see repeatedly, humans have an enormous range of reactions to drugs even when given by the same route with the dosage adjusted for body weight. Thus, it should not be surprising that animal testing can easily miss the rare but serious adverse events experienced by humans.[6.4]

This phase of drug testing is undergoing revision and hopefully improvement. Advances in our understanding of the mechanism of drug action on a molecular basis may in the future allow us to do a better job of understanding what, where, and how a drug is acting, allowing researchers to focus in on the impacts on a molecular and cellular level. This may require a reexamination of the role of animal testing.

Phase 1—Initial human testing

The initial administration of a drug to human beings is called a phase 1 trial. A phase 1 trial focuses on the pharmacology of the drug including its absorption, metabolism, and excretion. It aims to

---

[6.3] The FDA treats prescription drugs and nonprescription or over-the-counter drugs as two different categories with different requirements and procedures for approval. The FDA's expectations for approval of a drug for over-the-counter use go beyond the requirements discussed here for approval of a prescription drug. The FDA outlines the following five criteria for the approval of a drug for nonprescription use: (1) their benefits outweigh their risks, (2) the potential for misuse and abuse is low, (3) consumer can use them for self-diagnosed conditions, (4) they can be adequately labeled, and (5) health practitioners are not needed for the safe and effective use of the product.

[6.4] Human testing generally awaits the results of initial animal testing, although long-term animal test may continue while initial human testing is underway. Animal testing may also include a measure known as LD50 or the dose that is required to kill 50% of the animals tested at that dose. This data provide information on the potential toxicity of overdoses of the medication.

establish the dose range and route of administration that should be used in subsequent studies. It also looks at issues of harm.

Phase 1 often focuses special attention on effects on organs that are known to be especially sensitive to the actions of drugs. These include the liver, kidney, bone marrow, and testicles. The liver may be especially prone to drug effects because the liver often concentrates drugs as it participates in their metabolism and excretion. The kidneys likewise may be exposed to high doses as part of the excretion process. The rapid rate of cell division in the bone marrow and testicles may make them especially vulnerable to the effects of drugs.

Phase 1 may also focus on effects that might be expected based on the known actions of a particular class of drugs or a particular drug perhaps based on animal studies. A new antidepressant may be subjected to electrophysiological examination of the heart since antidepressants are known to alter the electrical system of the heart. Diuretics may be thoroughly examined for a range of electrolyte and metabolic effects since this class of medication is known to have a range of electrolyte and metabolic effects.

The duration of the exposure to the drug in phase 1 may be quite short, usually days to weeks. The length of exposure may be governed by the length of time needed to determine issues of absorption, metabolism, and excretion. Thus, phase 1 testing cannot be expected to detect longer term or chronic effects.

A phase 1 study is usually quite small, perhaps including only a few dozen individuals. Phase 1 trials do not generally include the types of patients who are expected to receive the drug in clinical practice that is the target population. The type of patients who are asked to participate in phase 1 trials is quite variable. Depending on the intended use of the drug, the patients may be severely ill with little or no chance of benefiting from the drug. Alternatively, they may be healthy volunteers who do not have a need for the drug. As a rule, patients at highest risk such as pregnant women and young children will not be part of a phase 1 trial.

Let us take a look at the some of the limitations of a phase 1 trial as illustrated in the following example:

> **Mini-Study 6.2** ■ A phase 1 trial of a new drug was conducted on 30 healthy, nonpregnant adults who were administered the drug at three different doses over a 1-week period. The investigation monitored the absorption, metabolism, and excretion of the drug, as well as monitoring drug-sensitive organs and clinically observed adverse events. This phase 1 study did not find any clinically important adverse events and did not detect any damage to drug-sensitive organs. When the drug was used for longer periods in later studies, it was found that its effects on the kidneys were frequent and severe enough to preclude its approval for clinical use.

As we have seen, phase 1 trials are designed primarily to understand the pharmacology of the drug. Phase 1 trials also are intended to detect adverse events that occur in the short term and produce undesirable and unintended laboratory or clinical changes. It is expected that additional attention to the detection of adverse events will be needed.

One of the major limitations of phase 1 in particular and assessment of harms in general is the wide range of special sensitivities to drug actions that occur among a small number of people. These sensitivities may occur for a variety of reasons. These individuals may be different in how they metabolize drugs, how other drugs interact with the new treatment, or the way the presence of other diseases complicates the reaction to a new drug. The next hypothetical example illustrates the types of challenges posed by the wide range of reactions that may occur with drugs:

Mini-Study 6.3 ■ A new drug completed phase 1 trials without evidence of important adverse events using healthy volunteers who reflect the age and ethnic distribution of outpatients in a major metropolitan area. When subsequently more widely used, it was found that patients on antidepressants had reduced effectiveness of their medication, that Vietnamese often had dangerously high blood levels, and that those on drugs for Alzheimer often reacted with rapid deterioration of their condition.

These and a range of other adverse events and interactions are difficult to anticipate, identify, and prevent since there are an almost unlimited number of possible interactions. Some of these special sensitivities may be more easily recognized in the future as we better understand how genetically defined groups vary in the way they absorb, distribute, metabolize, and excrete drugs. Although the process of detecting these uniquely vulnerable groups may improve over time, it is unlikely to be completely solved. The challenge of detecting these types of adverse events will require more than phase 1 testing; they will require a comprehensive system of drug monitoring.

Phase 2

Phase 2 is primarily designed to provide suggestive evidence of efficacy of a drug for a particular indication in the shortest possible time. Phase 2 consists of small, sometimes uncontrolled trials designed to determine whether there is a suggestions of efficacy. Phase 2 trials are important since they serve as a precondition for moving ahead with the expense, time, and potential harm of conducting large, randomized controlled trials, which are at the heart of phase 3.

Phase 2 studies can be very useful in helping design phase 3 trials. A phase 2 study can provide an estimate of the magnitude of the effect that can be expected from the drug. Thus, a phase 2 trial can serve as the basis for estimating the sample size needed for phase 3. In addition, a phase 2 trial may suggest specific groups that respond particularly well or poorly to the drug. These may help determine the inclusion and exclusion criteria for a randomized controlled trial. Phase 2 studies may also help estimate the extent of adherence to treatment, the potential costs, and other key information needed to plan a phase 3 randomized controlled trials.

Phase 3

Phase 3 trials focus on randomized controlled trials. As we have seen, randomized controlled trials are the gold standard for establishing efficacy for one particular indication. Their key role in establishing efficacy often means that they are designed around the specific requirements for determining efficacy for a particular disease on a particular type of patient. Randomized controlled trials, even those that are well designed for establishing efficacy for a particular indication, have limitations in establishing effectiveness. They are limited in their ability to determine whether the intervention works on those it will be used on in practice. These same limitations often affect their ability to assess harms. These limitations include the following:

- Randomized controlled trials often focus on one particular group of individuals, who are expected to be particularly responsive to the treatment.
- Randomized controlled trials often include individuals who have only one disease, are not on a spectrum of other treatments, and may not include especially vulnerable groups such as children, pregnant women, etc.
- Randomized controlled trials are designed to be conducted only as long as needed to establish efficacy.
- Randomized controlled trials are designed to establish efficacy for one particular indication.

These general limitations of randomized controlled trials translate into a series of implications for evaluating potential harms.

■ The sample size for randomized controlled trials is determined by the requirements of establishing efficacy. Thus, the number of patients actually receiving the intervention under investigation is generally in the several hundred to several thousand range. These sample sizes are often far too small to fully assess harms.

■ The duration of randomized controlled trials are geared to the length of time necessary to establish efficacy for the particular indication that is being investigated. Thus, an antibiotic for acute infections might be tested for 10 to 14 days, whereas a new drug for acute depression might be tested for 1 to 2 months. Long-term follow-up to assess harms is not an inherent part of randomized controlled trials.

■ The individuals included in the study are carefully defined by inclusion and exclusion criteria. These criteria make it easier to establish efficacy. Thus, we rarely see patients with other complicating disease or those on a variety of other drugs that make them especially susceptible to adverse effects of treatment.

Thus, the shortcomings of randomized controlled trials for assessing harms can be summarized as follows: they are often too small, too short, and too simple. Let us look at some hypothetical scenarios that illustrate the implications of these limitations.

To understand the need for a large sample size to measure harm, let us take a look at the next example:

Mini-Study 6.4 ■ It is known that anaphylaxis occurs on average in approximately 1 in 10,000 intravenous (IV) or intramuscular (IM) administrations of penicillin. An investigator obtained data on the use of IV or IM penicillin on 10,000 individuals and did not find any cases of anaphylaxis. He could not explain this finding.

To appreciate why this can occur, we need to appreciate an important statistical principle known as the *rule-of-three*. The rule-of-three tells us that in order to be 95% certain that we will observe at least one case of a rare but serious adverse event, for example, one with a true probability of once per 10,000 uses, we will require to observe 30,000 individuals. That is, the number of observations that is required is three times the denominator of the true incidence of the adverse event, that is, for penicillin and anaphylaxis 3 × 10,000. A sample size of this magnitude is only feasible once the treatment is used in clinical practice. Thus, we should not be surprised to find that adverse events not observed in randomized controlled trials will be observed in practice.

As a guide to what we can conclude from the absence of adverse events in a randomized controlled trial, we can use the rule-of-three in reverse. The rule-of-three in reverse tells us: If we observe 1,000 individuals who have received the study treatment and no one experiences a severe adverse event, then we can be 95% certain that the true frequency of the adverse event is no greater than 3/1,000 or 1 per 333 uses. Let us see how we can use the rule-of-three in reverse in the following example:

Mini-Study 6.5 ■ A large randomized controlled trial assigned 1,000 patients to a study group and 1,000 to a control group. The investigation did not find any cases of severe adverse events in the trial. When used in practice, the investigators found that the treatment had a frequency of life-threatening adverse events of 1 per 500 uses even among patients similar to those included in the randomized controlled trial.

In this situation, the finding that the true frequency of a life-threatening adverse event was 1 per 500 uses should not surprise us; it is totally consistent with what we would expect from the rule-of-three in reverse. We should not be surprised to find that the incidence of severe adverse events is 1 per 500 uses, which is lower than 1 per 333 uses.

Rare but serious adverse events, by definition, cannot be expected to occur frequently. Thus, randomized controlled trials cannot generally be expected to identify these adverse events. We can say that randomized controlled trials have low statistical power for investigating rare but serious adverse events.

Even when the incidence of adverse events is considerably greater, we should not expect randomized controlled trials to demonstrate statistically significant differences between adverse events in the study and control groups. For instance, take a look at the next scenario:

> **Mini-Study 6.6** ■ A new treatment for heart failure was compared with a conventional treatment in a randomized controlled trial. There were 200 patients assigned to each group. Adverse events reported in the new treatment group included six cases of elevated liver enzymes compared with four in the conventional treatment group. There was one case of aplastic anemia in the new treatment group versus none in the control group. Neither of these differences in adverse events was statistically significant. The authors concluded that no clinically important difference in harms was found between the treatment and the control groups.

When adverse events are observed but are relatively uncommon as is usually the case in randomized controlled trials, we cannot expect the differences in the frequency of harms to be statistically significant since the statistical power to demonstrate statistical significance is low. In fact, the question we should focus on is not statistical significance. We should be asking the following question: if the observed difference in adverse events is real, would it be a clinically important difference? In addition, we should be asking questions such as: Is the timing of administration consistent with a cause-and-effect relationship? Is a cause-and-effect relationship biologically plausible?

As we have discussed, randomized controlled trials have traditionally been conducted for a time period limited to the time needed to adequately establish efficacy for the proposed indication. The relatively short-term nature of phase 3 trials can severely limit what can be learned about longer-term harms as illustrated in the next example:

> **Mini-Study 6.7** ■ The new diabetic medication was tested for 6 months to determine whether it could reduce and maintain a reduction in hyperglycemia. The drug was found to establish efficacy and to satisfy the safety requirements for approval. When used in practice, however, it was found that despite its effectiveness after 6 months, it was associated with a frequency of severe liver disease far above that expected on the basis of the 6-month study.

Short-term studies may or may not produce hints of potential harms that can be monitored in practice. For adverse events that require longer-term exposure to manifest themselves, the short-term nature of efficacy studies is extremely limiting.

Drawing conclusions about what will happen in practice is always a limitation of randomized controlled trials. When we are dealing with the benefits of treatment, we make the distinction between efficacy or how well the intervention works under the conditions of a randomized controlled trial and effectiveness or how well the intervention works under the conditions of practice. Unfortunately, this same distinction is not formally made when we are addressing harms. However, we can think of "safety in practice" as having the same relationship to "safety under research conditions" as effectiveness has to efficacy.

In addition to the relatively small size of randomized controlled trials and the relatively short duration, the uniform characteristics of the eligible patients often make the patient population too simple to draw meaningful conclusions about the harms of the treatment in clinical practice. The inclusion of participants who fulfill specific inclusion and exclusion criteria can severely limit the ability of even large randomized controlled trials to provide useful information on harms as illustrated in the next example:

Mini-Study 6.8 ■ A randomized controlled trial of a new medication for treatment of Type 2 diabetes was used on newly diagnosed Type 2 diabetics without other diseases and who were not taking other medication. The treatment was very successful and no severe adverse events were found. When approved and used in practice, the treatment was quickly found to worsen kidney function among those being treated for hypertension with several antihypertensive medications.

The uniformity of patients in a randomized controlled trial can be an advantage in terms of the ease and cost of establishing efficacy. This advantage for studying efficacy can also be a severe limitation when studying rare but serious adverse events. This is the situation since it is the complicated patient and the complicated treatment where we can expect to observe the greatest frequency of adverse events. The interaction illustrated in this scenario between diabetic and hypertensive medications is impossible to detect in randomized controlled trials when patients are only taking one medication for one disease. Thus, measurement of harms in randomized controlled trials cannot be expected to predict the occurrence of adverse effects among complicated patients in clinical practice.[6.5]

POSTMARKET EVALUATION OF HARM (3)

Understanding the postmarket process of evaluating harms requires that we first understand what the FDA is doing when it approves a drug. In general, FDA approval implies the following[6.6]:

- The drug may be advertised and marketed for a particular indication, the one for which it was studied and approved.
- Once the drug is approved, it may be used by prescribing clinicians for any patient. That is, the prescribing clinician has the authority to use the treatment for indications not specifically approved by the FDA. Use of treatments for indications not approved by the FDA is called *off-label prescribing*.[6.7]

Off-label use of drugs is a very common and at times very useful part of clinical practice as illustrated in the next example:

[6.5] In addition to limitations due to the focus on efficacy, for many years, phase 2 and 3 testing routinely excluded those felt to be at the highest risk of complications, usually pregnant women and children. Recent changes have now made inclusion of children routine if the intention is to include children among those recommended to receive the drug if approved. Pregnant women are still generally omitted from phase 2 and 3 trials except in the unusual circumstance that a treatment is intended for women known to be pregnant.

[6.6] The distinction between pre- and postmarket has become less distinct in recent years as the FDA has attempted to expedite limited noninvestigational clinical use of potentially lifesaving therapies for those with greatest need. Exceptions to FDA procedures such as what is known as *compassionate use* may allow selective clinical use before final FDA approval.

[6.7] Recent changes in FDA procedures have allowed the FDA to restrict the right to prescribe a drug and to require specific tests such as a pregnancy test before filling or refilling a prescription. Currently, these authorities are being used only in very specific circumstances.

Mini-Study 6.9 ■ A new β-blocker was first approved and marketed for treatment of angina. Clinicians observed that it also reduced blood pressure in many patients and began to use it off-label as a treatment for hypertension. The β-blocker was subsequently studied and approved by the FDA for treatment of hypertension. Clinicians continued to use it for off-label indications including migraine headaches and tremors well before the FDA approved it for these indications.

This example illustrated the potential value of allowing clinicians to prescribe drugs for new uses after a drug has been approved for a different indication. This process may allow clinicians to more rapidly incorporate new evidence into their practice and to adopt treatments to individual patients. However, it is important to recognize that drugs prescribed off-label have not undergone review for adverse effects for the new use or been compared with other currently used treatments. Thus, clinicians who utilize drugs for off-label indications should be aware that the potential harms may not outweigh the potential benefits.

Thus once approved, a drug may be prescribed for other conditions, at alternative doses, and for longer durations that those recommended for the particular indication for which the drug is approved.

As we have seen, a full evaluation of harms does not occur until a treatment has been widely used in clinical practice. Its reason(s) for use in clinical practice may be quite different from its use in randomized controlled trials. Even when the treatment is used for the same indication at the same dosage as in the randomized controlled trials, the complexities of patients and treatments in clinical practice may lead to frequent adverse events that may or may not be easily recognized.

Occasionally, an individual clinician treating an individual patient can produce convincing evidence of a cause–and–effect relationship between a drug and an adverse effect as discussed in Learn More 6.3.

LEARN MORE 6.3 ■ **N-OF-1 STUDIES MAY ESTABLISH CAUSE-AND-EFFECT BASED ON A SINGLE PATIENT (4)** ■ Demonstrating cause-and-effect relationships for adverse events is often very difficult. One approach that can sometime produce convincing results that are widely applicable relies on the consequences of starting and stopping treatment in a single individual. This type of investigation has been called an *n-of-1* study. In an n-of-1 study, each patient serves as his or her own control. The treatment is administered to one individual who has developed an adverse outcome such as a rash, and then the therapy is discontinued and the patient is observed to see whether and when the presumed side effect resolves. The final step is to readminister the treatment to see whether the adverse outcome occurs again.

Let us see how an n-of-1 trial may be used to strongly suggest a cause-and-effect relationship that has wide applicability as illustrated in the next example:

Mini-Study 6.10 ■ A patient reported that he developed wheezing after he used a new nasal spray that included a new form of aerosol not previously reported to have adverse effects. The prescribing clinician asked the patient to record the frequency, severity, and timing of the wheezing. The clinician then asked the patient to stop the new nasal spray and substituted another commonly used nasal spray. Follow-up monitoring indicated that the wheezing disappeared. Since the original wheezing did not pose a potential for major harm to the patient, the patient agreed to again use the new nasal spray. The wheezing now returned with a similar pattern. It was soon found that on close questioning of other patients, mild degrees of wheezing were very common with the new nasal spray.

(Continued)

> This approach incorporates the concepts of association, prior associa-
> tion, and altering the cause alters the effect to help establish a cause-and-
> effect relationship for an adverse event. This n-of-1 study has helped establish
> a cause-and-effect relationship and suggest that the cause-and-effect rela-
> tionship might be applicable to a large number of other patients.

MONITORING OF ADVERSE EVENTS

How are adverse events monitored after a drug is approved? The system for monitoring drugs is undergoing extensive review and modification because of the recent appreciation of just how common and serious adverse events associated with of drugs can be.

For many years, the system for detection of adverse events associated with drugs was largely limited to what is known as a *spontaneous reporting system*. In this system, those who prescribe the drug, and increasingly, patients themselves are encouraged to report adverse events to the FDA. However, they are not required to do so.

When a drug is associated with unusual or dramatic adverse events, spontaneous report-ing systems may be useful in detecting their occurrence. These types of adverse events are often called *sentinel events*. The role of the clinician in looking for and reporting sentinel events is essen-tial for the early detection of serious adverse events. For instance, imagine the following scenario:

Mini-Study 6.11 ■ A new vaccine to prevent a respiratory infection and gas-troenteritis in young children resulting from rotavirus was approved for use after successful completion of the required randomized controlled trials. In practice, clinicians reported a small number of dramatic cases of intussusception with small bowel obstruction within a few weeks of receiving the vaccine. The dramatic nature of this condition, its unusual occurrence, and its proximity in time to the vac-cination resulted in the FDA withdrawal of the vaccination.

This is the type of situation where we can expect a spontaneous reporting system to work well. The adverse event was dramatic, it is an unusual condition seldom seen by the average clinician, and it had a close relationship in time to the vaccination. However, spontaneous reporting systems often do not work this well since they have a number of limitations including

- Even with serious adverse events, only a small percentage may be reported especially when the event is not dramatic or closely linked in time to the treatment.
- Unsuspected and even severe adverse events may escape detection or not be attributed to the treatment.
- Adverse events that can occur as a result of other potential causes or are similar to the consequences of the disease being treated may be difficult to recognize and attribute to the treatment.

Let us look at how these limitations of spontaneous reporting may affect the ability of a spontane-ous reporting system to recognize adverse events. First, spontaneous reporting systems may not receive reports of the occurrence of adverse events especially those that are not dramatic or closely linked in time to the treatment as illustrated in the next example:

Mini-Study 6.12 ■ A new treatment for asthma resulted in slowly progressive asymptomatic liver disease after 6 or more months of treatment. Few clinicians and fewer patients recognized this delayed and subtle adverse event and there-fore did not report it through the spontaneous reporting system.

The type of adverse event that occurs may have a large impact on whether or not it is reported or detected in some other way. Adverse events that are not dramatic or closely linked in time with the administration of the drug often are missed by the spontaneous reporting system.[6.8]

With severe unsuspected adverse events, even one case may be of great importance, yet it may escape detection or not be attributed to the treatment as illustrated in the next example:

Mini-Study 6.13 ■ A new diet drug was approved by the FDA. During the first year after approval, only expected adverse outcomes were reported to the FDA. A clinician then found and reported that one of her patients taking the new diet drug from the time it was first approved had fibrosis of a heart valve on echocardiography. The clinician sent other patients on the drug who were doing well for echocardiography and found additional cases of mild fibrosis. It was later appreciated that this unsuspected complication was actually quite common and had not been attributed to the drug when seen on an echocardiogram.

This example illustrates the importance of the alert clinician in detecting not just the clear-cut sentinel events but the unsuspected and subtle relationships that may otherwise be missed.[6.9]

Finally, when an adverse event mimics the complications of the disease itself, it can easily go unrecognized. These types of adverse events are illustrated in the next example:

Mini-Study 6.14 ■ Patients taking a new drug for diabetes developed neuropathy in association with use of the drug approximately once in 20 long-term uses. Because neuropathy is so common among those with diabetes, the adverse event was not attributed to the new drug.

Neuropathy can be produced by a large number of other conditions of which diabetes is among the most common. When an adverse event due to a drug mimics the adverse consequences of the disease itself, it may be especially difficult to recognize.

The spontaneous reporting system cannot be expected to rapidly or completely detect adverse events or accurately reflect their frequency. Patients who receive a new treatment over the first few months to the first few years after initial marketing approval need to be regarded as part of the experiment or what has been called *phase 4*.

POSTMARKET STUDIES AND OTHER METHODS TO MEASURE HARMS (5)

We may conclude that the spontaneous reporting of adverse events, although important, does not in-and-of-itself provide a comprehensive system for evaluating harms associated with drugs. There

---

[6.8] In recent years, the spontaneous reporting system has been available on the Web and has allowed patients as well as clinicians to report adverse events. The large number of reports makes it more likely that rare but serious adverse event will be reported. Unfortunately, the large number of reports also makes it far more difficult to distinguish which adverse events are actually caused by the treatment.

[6.9] This case illustrates the potential to use what the airlines call a near-miss procedure. When even one incident can be attributed to a defect, the airlines are required to review other similar events even if they were merely near misses. This can be more easily accomplished in the airline industry because near-miss reporting is a routine part of the data system.

are a number of types of studies that can be used to supplement the spontaneous reporting system and to detect and evaluate the adverse events associated with interventions.

As we have discussed, randomized controlled trials have an important but limited role in measuring the adverse events associated with a drug or other intervention. The impact of randomized controlled trials may be enhanced by continuing to follow the patients enrolled in a randomized controlled trial after the completion of the study and the approval of the drug as illustrated in the next scenario:

Mini-Study 6.15 ■ A new drug for depression was approved after two large, well-conducted randomized controlled trials demonstrated its efficacy and acceptable harm during a 6-month period. After the randomized controlled trial was completed, those in the control group were offered the option of taking the new treatment and those in the study group were offered the option of continuing the treatment. The investigation continued to follow both groups for the next 2 years. The follow-up study demonstrated reduced efficacy after 1 year but did not demonstrate any new or unexpected adverse events.

This type of follow-up of a randomized controlled trial is a form of a prospective or concurrent cohort. However, it has the advantage that data are also available from the randomized controlled trial, thus, allowing more extended observation for adverse events, as well as for efficacy among those assigned to the study group. It also provides data on those taking the new drug for the first time.

Other types of investigations are often needed to evaluate adverse events including the following:

■ Premarket studies: previous investigations that used a treatment for different indications and in different settings, may at times be combined using a procedure called meta-analysis that we will discuss in Chapter 7. Combining studies may provide numbers that are adequate to demonstrate the potential for serious adverse events or provide evidence that they are unlikely to occur.[6.10]

■ Large databases derived from clinical care and from pharmacy data may allow performance of retrospective cohort studies identifying adverse events not recognized in randomized controlled trials.

■ Case–control studies focusing on patients with and without specific adverse events may be able to identify associations between adverse events and treatments using relatively small number of patients.

Retrospective cohort studies based upon combining data from large databases obtained from electronic medical records plus clinical pharmacy records are becoming a key strategy for evaluating safety in practice. A national network of institutions in the United States are now collaborating with the FDA to include tens of millions of patients in these investigations. These retrospective cohort studies may detect a large number of associations many of which may be due to chance.

[6.10] Issues of harms and adverse events lend themselves to the use of meta-analysis as we will discuss in Chapter 7 since the number of adverse events in any one particular investigation is often limited. By combining the results of multiple investigations, meta-analyses of safety issues may be able to achieve adequate statistical power to demonstrate the statistical significance of the occurrence of an adverse event in association with an intervention. In addition, a meta-analysis may be able to provide an accurate measure of the probability of occurrence of the adverse event. Finally, meta-analyses, if they are large enough may be able to look at subgroups and provide useful information on the types of patients and the types of uses that are most prone to the development of adverse events.

Let us see, however, how this type of a retrospective cohort study might be used to investigate the association between use of a new antibiotic and pancreatitis:

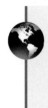

> **Mini-Study 6.16** ■ A large clinical database that combined clinical records and pharmacy records was used to identify more than 10,000 patients who received the new antibiotic and a control group of patients with the same indication for treatment who received an unrelated antibiotic. Follow-up of the clinical records for both groups of patients found a substantial and statistically significant increase in the incidence of pancreatitis in patients receiving the new antibiotic.

The finding that this antibiotic was associated with pancreatitis might lead researchers to investigate whether other drugs in the same pharmacological classification could also be associated with pancreatitis. To conduct this investigation, they might perform the following case–control study:

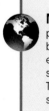

> **Mini-Study 6.17** ■ Two hundred patients with pancreatitis of unknown cause and 200 age- and hospital-matched patients without pancreatitis were included in a case–control study. Drugs taken within the month before diagnosis were obtained. The case–control study found that several drugs from the same chemical class as the suspect antibiotic were also strongly associated with pancreatitis.

This investigation illustrates how case–control studies can provide useful information that builds upon the evidence obtained from retrospective cohort studies. At times, case–control studies are the best and at times the only way to address specific questions of drug safety as suggested in the next scenario:

> **Mini-Study 6.18** ■ The safety of an over-the-counter antinausea drug during pregnancy was investigated using a case-control study. The medication that had been used for many years was none-the-less suspected of causing birth defects especially spina bifida. The investigators identified 500 pregnancies that resulted in spina bifida and paried them with 500 pregnancies that resulted in normal infants. The investigators found a relative risk of three, suggesting that spina bifida was associated with the use of the medication.

Here, even the most extensively developed database connecting pharmacy and clinical records is not likely to include comprehensive data on over-the-counter medication use. Thus, a newly conducted case–control study may be the only way to obtain evidence on the association between the over-the-counter antinausea drug and spina bifida. It is important to recognize, however, that in case-control studies it may be difficult to establish which came first. Here, it is possible that the birth defect produced nausea leading to use of the anti-nausea medication.

Population comparisons, case-control studies, prospective and retrospective cohort studies, randomized controlled trials, and meta-analyses can all contribute evidence to issues of drug safety. Table 6.2 outlines uses of these types of investigations in each of the FDA phases.

TABLE 6.2 | Roles of Study Types in Evaluating Potential Harms

Type of Investigation	Role in Evaluating Potential Harms	Limitations of Role
Prehuman and laboratory testing	Tested on at least two selected animal species to assess teratogenicity, carcinogenicity, and fertility effects, as well as potential impact on vulnerable organs	May not correlate well with human studies
Uncontrolled human studies—phases 1 and 2	Assessment of pharmacological action of drugs including absorption, metabolism, and excretion. Able to identify short-term and relatively common adverse effects on vulnerable organs as well as drug-specific clinical and laboratory impacts that are focused on as part of the investigation	Usually performed on healthy volunteers and cannot assess interactions between interventions, impacts on vulnerable populations, or longer-term adverse events
Randomized controlled trials—phase 3	Provides standardized assessment and relatively complete short-term follow-up to assess adverse events and compare their impact to the observed benefits	Often too small to detect rare but serious adverse events, too short to detect long-term adverse events, too simple to detect interactions with other diseases, or other interventions
Spontaneous reporting system—phase 4	Spontaneous reporting system may allow important information on unusual and dramatic adverse events with close temporal relationship to administration of the intervention	Difficult to attribute adverse events to an intervention especially when adverse events are common and/or there is no clear temporal relationship
Prospective cohort study- open label follow-up of randomized controlled trial—phase 4	Open label follow-up of patients enrolled in randomized controlled trials allows for more extended period of follow-up for adverse events and for effectiveness. This is a type of prospective cohort study	Patients in randomized controlled trials continue to be different from those receiving the drug in practice in ways that may alter benefits as well as harms
Meta-analysis—phase 4	Combining adverse events from multiple investigations with different study designs to obtain adequate numbers of adverse events to achieve adequate statistical power	Reporting of adverse events often based on differing definitions and differing intensity of observation
Retrospective cohort studies—phase 4	Retrospective cohort studies have potential to link pharmacy and clinical records to assess adverse events associated with drugs	When used without prior hypotheses need careful attention to multiple comparison issues and recognition of limitation in drawing cause-and-effect conclusions
Case–control studies—phase 4	Useful for focused investigation of well-defined adverse events as part of postmarketing or phase 4	Requires prior recognition of an adverse event and its potential relationship to an intervention

LEARN MORE 6.4 ■ RECENT AMENDMENT TO THE FDA LAW— NEW AUTHORITY FOR REGULATION OF DRUGS (6) ■ In response to the need for FDA to withdraw a series of previously approved medications from the market including Cox II inhibitors such as Vioxx, in late 2007 the U.S. Congress passed a comprehensive revision of the FDA law providing a series of additional authorities to the FDA. Together, these amendments provide the basis for the development of a systems approach to drug safety. Among the most important provisions are the following:

- The FDA was provided authority to require that more representative patients be included in randomized controlled trials with the aim to have randomized controlled trials more closely reflect the populations on whom the drug will be used.
- The FDA was given authority to require follow-up studies of approved drugs to monitor their performance in clinical practice.
- The FDA was given authority to develop large database systems to link pharmacy record with electronic medical records to assess adverse events on an ongoing basis.
- The FDA was given authority to place increased restrictions on who can prescribe a particular drug and what conditions need to be fulfilled before it can be prescribed including required testing before filling a prescription.
- The FDA was given increased authority to approve and monitor drug advertising to clinicians and directly to patients to ensure that they conform to FDA approved language and accurately communicate risks.
- The FDA was given greater authority to withdraw drugs from the market when serious issues of safety are raised.

Together these amendments provide authority to improve drug safety regulation both premarket and postmarket. They also provide the FDA with authority to respond rapidly to new safety problems and to protect the public against violations of existing drug safety regulations. The implementation of these provisions is an ongoing process, and full implementation is expected to continue for years, if not decades.

The process of putting together the pieces of drug safety into a coherent whole has been a long and difficult challenge. The most recent and ongoing efforts to make this happen resulted from recent amendment to the FDA law. Learn More 6.4 examines these amendments and their potential role in creating a system designed to maximize the benefits and minimize the harms of drugs.

SAFETY OF VACCINES, MEDICAL DEVICES, AND PATIENT SAFETY (7,8)

The focus of this chapter has been on drug safety. Drugs both prescription and nonprescription have been the initial focus of most safety research. Other areas of safety research are now rapidly emerging.

Vaccines safety has been an issue since the 1950s, when the live polio vaccine produced large numbers of clinical cases of polio. However, in recent years, there has been increased attention to vaccine safety stimulated in part by the rapidly expanding number of childhood vaccines and the concern about autism. The studies that refuted the relationship between vaccines and autism used the same basic methods that we have described for postmarket research on drugs.

For vaccines, in parallel with drugs, a national adverse reporting system exists called the vaccine adverse events reporting system. In contrast to drugs, a no-fault system for compensation of vaccine associated adverse events exists called the Vaccine Injury Compensation Program. Thus, more complete and systematic data are becoming available on the adverse effects related to vaccines, and the issues of cause-and-effect are receiving considerable attention. The investigation of adverse events associated with vaccines may form the basis for a better understanding of the biological effects of vaccines and the production of safer vaccines as illustrated in the next example:

> **Mini-Study 6.19** ■ The initial vaccine for rotavirus was removed from the market after reporting of cases of intussusception closely connected in time with the administration of the vaccine. The close connection raised the concern that the vaccine had over stimulated the immune system, leading to localized inflammation resulting in intussusception. Thus, the occurrence of intussusception was biological plausibility. New vaccines were developed to address this issue, and careful monitoring for adverse events was integrated into the pre- and postmarket investigation of the second vaccine. The newer vaccine was associated with far fewer adverse events.

The system for regulation of medical devices is currently based on different principles than drugs and vaccine safety. As part of what is called the 510(k) clearance process, most medical devices need only to demonstrate "substantial equivalence" to devices currently on the market. These existing devices have not generally undergone review either before or after they were marketed. The Institute of Medicine has concluded that the current system does not generally provide assurance of efficacy or safety. Expect to see efforts to create a new structure for medical device regulation, perhaps one that looks at medical devices as part of an overall safety system.

Perhaps the biggest change in recent years has been the emergence of patient safety and quality research. The recognition that nearly 100,000 deaths in the United States each year are associated with adverse events that occur in hospitals has led to a wide range of new types of research. This research often begins using qualitative methods including close examination of individual cases plus in-depth interviews with clinicians, administrators, and at time patients. The potential for patient safety and quality research is illustrated in the following example:

> **Mini-Study 6.20** ■ Children with cancer were found to be at high risk of death from infection while receiving inpatient treatment. Careful postmortem reviews demonstrated that in-dwelling catheters were a likely source of infection. The development of a step-by-step protocol for use and monitoring of in-dwelling catheters were demonstrated to be acceptable as part of an integrated system of care. A multi-institution study then demonstrated its acceptance and ability to reduce the number of systemic infections.

Patient safety and quality research is rapidly emerging as a new approach to research that brings to bear qualitative as well as quantitative methods, relies heavily on demonstration studies, and takes a broad systems approach to understanding the factors that affect the outcome of disease.

A range of types of studies are now used to identify and evaluate potential harms related to our diverse interventions. Expect to see these approaches expand in coming year. Like the old autopsy conference, the new approaches often begin by looking closely at individual cases. Today, however, we have research methods that allow us to study the impact of interventions on groups and to examine the way they fit together as part of a system.

A comprehensive system for preventing harms, parallel to the one in place in the airline industry, does not yet exist in health care. Safety research is now in the take-off phase after a long wait on the runway.

REFERENCES

1. U.S. Food and Drug Administration. History. http://www.fda.gov/AboutFDA/WhatWeDo/History/default.htm. Accessed July 25, 2011.

2. U.S. Food and Drug Administration. Drugs. http://www.fda.gov/Drugs/ResourcesForYou/Industry/default.htm. Accessed July 25, 2011.

3. U.S. Food and Drug Administration. Postmarket drug information for patients and providers. http://www.fda.gov/Drugs/DrugSafety/PostmarketDrugSafetyInformationforPatientsandProviders/default.htm. Accessed July 25, 2011.

4. Guyatt G, Rennie D. *Users' Guides to the Medical Literature: A Manual for Evidence-based Practice*. Chicago, IL: AMA Press; 2002.

5. Weiss NS. *Clinical Epidemiology: The Study of the Outcome of Disease*. 3rd ed. New York, NY: Oxford University Press; 2006.

6. ReedSmith. The FDA Amendments Act of 2007. http://www.reedsmith.com/library/search_library.cfm?FaArea1=CustomWidgets.content_view_1&cit_id=16812. Accessed July 25, 2011.

7. Centers for Disease Control and Prevention. Vaccine safety. http://www.cdc.gov/vaccinesafety/Activities/vaers.html. Accessed August 6, 2011.

8. Institute of Medicine. *Medical Devices and the Public's Health: The FDA 510(k) Clearance Process at 35 Years*. Washington, DC: National Academies Press; 2011.

thePoint ✳ Visit http://thePoint.lww.com for interactive Q&A, flaw-catching exercises, searchable eBook, and more!

7 Meta-analysis

Thus far, we have examined the basic types of investigations in the health research literature that are designed to compare study and control groups. These investigations often provide consistent results. At times, however, studies published in the health research literature seem to conflict with one another, making it difficult to provide definitive answers to important study questions.

It is often desirable to be able to combine data obtained in a variety of investigations and to use all the information to address a study question. *Meta-analysis* is a collection of methods for quantitatively combining information from different investigations to reach conclusions or address questions that were not possible on the basis of a single investigation.

Meta-analysis aims to produce its conclusion by combining data from two or more existing investigations. Traditionally, this process of research synthesis has been the review article's role. In recent years, it has been increasingly recognized that the informal and subjective process of literature review has not always produced accurate conclusions. Meta-analysis of observational studies and randomized controlled trials has now become a standard part of health research as reflected in the publications of standard methods for their reporting with their own acronyms PRISMA (**P**referred **R**eporting **I**tems for **S**ystematic **R**eviews and **M**eta-**A**nalyses) (1) and MOOSE (**M**eta-analysis **o**f **O**bservational **S**tudies in **E**pidemiology) (2).

Meta-analysis can be viewed as one method to be used as part of what is called a *systematic review*. Learn More 7.1 discusses systematic reviews and their relationship to meta-analysis.

LEARN MORE 7.1 ■ SYSTEMATIC REVIEWS ■ Meta-analyses are often a component of a larger research effort known as a *systematic review*. Systematic reviews or overviews aim to comprehensively identify and analyze all the research literature on a given topic ranging from the etiology of a disease, to a diagnostic or screening test, to a potential preventive, curative, or rehabilitative intervention. Systematic reviews are often considered the gold standard for summarizing the literature. They utilize methods of systematic literature review designed to identify all existing studies regardless of the type of study or whether they were published in the peer review literature. Unlike meta-analysis, systematic reviews addresses all previously researched questions related to a defined topic. The distinction between a meta-analysis and a systematic review is illustrated in the following scenario:

Mini-Study 7.1 ■ A systematic review of the impact of exercise on coronary artery disease was conducted using a systematic literature review and examining the physiological, epidemiological, and clinical interventional research related to etiology, prevention, and treatment of coronary artery disease including the use of exercise for rehabilitation. As part of the systematic review, a meta-analysis was conducted to measure the magnitude of the impact of moderate levels of regular exercise on the occurrence of first episode of myocardial infarction.

Notice that a systematic review casts a wide net. Meta-analysis as opposed to a systematic review focuses on a narrower and more clearly defined

(Continued)

questions, often ones that have already been extensively investigated. The process and structure of systematic reviews have been formalized by the Cochrane Collaborative, an international network that produces and updates systematic review on a wide range of subjects (3). The Cochrane Collaborative has developed a standard format for developing and reporting systematic reviews. These Cochrane Reviews are far too extensive to publish in research journals. They are available on the Cochrane Collaboration Web site at http://www2.cochrane.org/reviews/. The structure of the report of a Cochrane Review includes all of the following components:

1. Plain-language summary—A short statement summarizing the review, specifically aimed at lay people.
2. Structured abstract—A structured summary of the review, subdivided into sections similar to the main review. This may be published independently from the review and appears on the medical bibliographic database MEDLINE.
3. Background—An introduction to the question considered, including, for example, details on causes and incidence of a given problem, the possible mechanism of action of a proposed treatment, uncertainties about management options, and so on.
4. Objectives—A short statement of the aim of the review.
5. Selection criteria—A brief description of the main elements of the question under consideration.
6. Search strategy for identification of studies.
7. Methods of the review—A description of how studies eligible for inclusion in the review were selected, how their quality was assessed, how data were extracted from the studies, how data were analyzed, whether any subgroups were studied or any sensitivity analyses were carried out, and so on.
8. Description of studies—A description of how many studies were found, what were their inclusion criteria, how big they were, and so on.
9. Methodological quality of included studies—Were there any reasons to doubt the conclusions of any studies because of concerns about the study quality?
10. Results—What do the data show? The results section may be accompanied by a graph to show a meta-analysis, if this was carried out.
11. Discussion—This includes interpretation and assessment of results.

Systematic reviews are also becoming the starting point for development of clinical guidelines or evidence-based recommendation, as we will see in the Chapter 13.

Let us begin our approach to meta-analysis by illustrating one reason why it is important to combine the results of investigations when addressing a previously researched question. Let us examine one extreme example indicating why the conclusion reached by combining investigations might be different from those reached by examining one investigation at a time:

Mini-Study 7.2 ■ Assume that we are interested in examining a recent innovation in the treatment of coronary artery disease known as transthoracic laser coronaryplasty (TLC). TLC is designed to treat coronary artery disease through the chest wall without using invasive techniques. The first two studies of TLC produced the following results:

Study 1

	Die	Live	Total
TLC	230	50	280
Control	530	210	740

$$\text{Relative risk} = \frac{230/280}{530/740} = \frac{0.821}{0.716} = 1.15$$

$$\text{Odds ratio} = \frac{230/50}{530/210} = \frac{4.60}{2.52} = 1.83$$

Study 2

	Die	Live	Total
TLC	190	405	595
Control	50	210	260

$$\text{Relative risk} = \frac{190/595}{50/260} = \frac{0.319}{0.192} = 1.66$$

$$\text{Odds ratio} = \frac{190/405}{50/210} = \frac{0.469}{0.238} = 1.97$$

The investigators concluded that both studies suggested that TLC produced worse outcomes than the control treatment increasing the chance of dying. Before relegating this technique to history, however, they decided to combine the results of the two studies and see what happened. Combining the data from the two studies produced the results shown below.

Combined Studies 1 and 2

	Die	Live	Total
TLC	420	455	875
Control	580	420	1,000

$$\text{Relative risk} = \frac{420/875}{580/420} = \frac{0.480}{0.580} = 0.827$$

$$\text{Odds ratio} = \frac{420/875}{580/420} = \frac{0.923}{1.381} = 0.668$$

Notice that after combining study 1 and 2 the results have changed and it now looks like TLC produces better outcomes than the control treatment. The odds ratio and relative risk now suggest that TLC reduces the chances of dying. Thus, combining studies may produce some surprising results.[7.1]

This process sets into motion a widespread effort to evaluate the use of TLC in a variety of settings and for a variety of indications worldwide. Most studies focused on single-vessel coronary artery disease as assessed by new noninvasive procedures. Over the next several years, dozens of studies resulted in apparently conflicting results. Thus, it was considered important to conduct

---

[7.1] This is known as *Simpson's Paradox*. It is a very unusual situation illustrated here because of its dramatic impact. Its occurrence requires large differences between the numbers of study group and control group participants in the two studies.

a full-scale meta-analysis evaluating the effects of TLC on single-vessel coronary artery disease. Let us now look at the steps in conducting a meta-analysis using the M.A.A.R.I.E. framework.

METHOD (4)

The process of combining information using meta-analysis can be best understood if we regard each of the studies included in the analysis as parallel to one study site in a multiple-site investigation. In a multiple-site investigation, the investigator combines the data from multiple sites to draw conclusions or interpretations. In meta-analysis, the investigator combines information from multiple studies to draw conclusions or interpretations. This parallel structure allows us to learn about meta-analysis using the M.A.A.R.I.E. framework.

As with our other uses of the M.A.A.R.I.E. framework, we start by defining the study question or study hypothesis. Meta-analysis can be used to accomplish a variety of purposes. It may begin by defining a hypothesis related to the specific purpose for conducting the meta-analysis. Meta-analysis might be used to accomplish any of the following purposes:

- Establish statistical significance when studies are conflicting
- Establish the best possible estimate of the magnitude of the effect
- Evaluate harms when small numbers of adverse events are observed in earlier studies
- Examine subgroups when the numbers in each previous investigation are not large enough to examine subgroups

As with our other types of investigations, the investigators ideally begin with a study hypothesis and proceed to test that hypothesis and draw inferences. When they do this for a therapy, for instance, they may hypothesize that the treatment has been shown to have efficacy.

The studies that should be included in a meta-analysis depend on the purpose of the analysis. Thus, the study hypothesis of the meta-analysis helps to determine the inclusion and exclusion criteria that should be used in identifying relevant studies. The following example shows how the hypothesis can help to determine which studies to include:

> **Mini-Study 7.3** ■ In preparation for a meta-analysis, researchers searched the world's literature and obtained the following 25 studies of TLC for single-vessel coronary artery disease. These investigations had characteristics which allowed them to be grouped into the following types of studies:
>
> 1. Five studies of men with single-vessel disease treated initially with coronary bypass surgery versus medication versus TLC
> 2. Five studies of men and women treated initially with TLC versus bypass surgery
> 3. Five studies of men and women treated initially with TLC versus medication
> 4. Five studies of men treated with TLC versus medication after previous bypass surgery
> 5. Five studies of women treated with repeat TLC versus medication after previous TLC

If the meta-analysis is designed to test a hypothesis, then the studies to be included are chosen because they address issues relevant to the hypothesis. For instance, if the investigator wanted to test the hypothesis that men do better than women when TLC is used to treat single-vessel coronary artery disease, then studies B and C should be used in the meta-analysis. These investigations include comparisons of the outcomes in both men and women.

If the investigators were interested in testing the hypothesis that initial TLC is better than surgery for single-vessel coronary artery disease, then studies A and B should be used in the meta-analysis because these studies compare TLC versus surgery as the initial therapy. Alternatively, if the researcher hypothesized that medication was the best treatment for single-vessel coronary artery disease, then studies A, C, D, and E would be used. In general, the studies that are used are determined by the purpose of the investigation as defined by the study hypothesis of the meta-analysis.

Despite the many similarities between meta-analysis and a multiple-site investigation, there is one important difference. In original research the investigator may define the study question and then identify settings and study participants that are suited to addressing the question and obtaining the needed sample size. In meta-analysis, the questions we may ask are often limited by the availability of previous studies. Thus, the study population and the sample size are largely outside the investigator's control.

To try to circumvent this problem, meta-analysis researchers often define a question or issue broadly and begin by identifying all investigations related to that issue. When this is done, the investigators are conducting an *exploratory meta-analysis* as opposed to a *hypothesis-driven meta-analysis*.

In conducting an exploratory meta-analysis of TLC, for instance, the investigator might initially include all 25 studies just mentioned. Thus, the meta-analysis researcher would define the study group as consisting of those who received TLC, and the control group would consist of all the individuals receiving other therapy.

This process of using all available studies without a specific hypothesis is parallel to the process of conducting a conventional investigation without defining a study hypothesis. This type of exploratory meta-analysis can be useful, but must be conducted carefully and interpreted differently from hypothesis-driven meta-analysis. Despite the potential dangers of combining studies with very different characteristics, the limited number of available studies makes it important for meta-analysis to include techniques for combining very different types of studies.

Meta-analysis attempts to turn the diversity of studies into an advantage. Combining studies with different characteristics may allow us to harness the benefit of diversity. By including apples and oranges, we can ask whether it makes a difference if a fruit is an apple or an orange or whether it is enough that it is a fruit.

The approach for harnessing the benefit of diversity is discussed later. For now, we must recognize that there are actually two types of meta-analysis, hypothesis-based and exploratory.

It is important to remember that the fundamental difference between meta-analysis and other types of investigations is that the data have already been collected and the researcher's choice is limited to including or excluding an existing study from the meta-analysis. Thus, the sample size in meta-analysis is limited by the existence of relevant studies.

Other types of investigations usually start by defining the question to be investigated. This question determines the types of individuals who should be included in the investigation. Similarly, the question to be addressed by a meta-analysis determines the types of studies that should be included in the meta-analysis. Thus, in hypothesis-driven meta-analysis, the first question we need to ask is whether a particular study is relevant to the meta-analysis's study question or hypothesis.

ASSIGNMENT (4,5)

Process of Assignment

Once the study question is defined, the investigators can determine which studies to include in a meta-analysis. This identification of studies to include is the assignment process, requires us to ask the question: Have all the relevant studies been identified?

Identifying all relevant studies is an essential step in the assignment process of a meta-analysis. It is important that the investigator describes the method used to search for research reports, including enough detail to allow subsequent investigators to obtain all the identified literature. This can even include unpublished data. Doctoral dissertations, abstracts, grant reports, and registries of studies are other possible ways to locate previous research.[7.2]

Confounding Variable: Publication Bias

An extensive search for research reports as part of the assignment process in a meta-analysis is important because of the potential for a special type of selection bias known as *publication bias*. Publication bias occurs when there is a systematic tendency to publish studies with positive results and to not publish studies that suggest little or no differences in outcome. Small investigations are frequently not submitted or are rejected for publication which can lead to publication bias. The next example illustrates what we mean by publication bias:

Mini-Study 7.4 ■ After identifying the studies available through a computerized search of published articles, the TLC meta-analysis researchers identified 20 studies of the relationship between TLC and single-vessel coronary artery disease. There was a wide variation in the sample sizes of the studies and in the outcomes, as shown in Table 7.1.

TABLE 7.1	Data from 20 Studies of Transthoracic Laser Coronaryplasty	
Study Number	**Odds Ratio**	**Sample Size (Each Group)**
1	4.0	20
2	3.0	20
3	2.0	20
4	1.0	20
5	0.5	20
6	3.5	40
7	2.5	40
8	1.5	40
9	2.5	60
10	1.5	60
11	1.0	60
12	1.5	80
13	1.0	80
14	1.5	100
15	1.0	100
16	0.5	100
17	1.5	120
18	1.0	120
19	0.5	120
20	1.0	140

[7.2] In performing this search, it is important to avoid double counting. Studies originally presented as abstracts, for instance, will often subsequently appear as original articles. Including the same data two or more times jeopardizes the accuracy of the results of a meta-analysis by violating the assumption that the data obtained in each of the studies are independent of the other studies

One technique that can be used to assess the presence and extent of possible publication bias is known as the *funnel diagram*. A funnel diagram can be drawn using the data in Table 7.1 which produces the funnel diagram displayed in Figure 7.1A.

The funnel diagram is based on the statistical principle that smaller studies, by chance alone, are expected to produce results with greater variation. A funnel diagram that does not suggest the presence of publication bias should look like a funnel, with larger variation in results among smaller studies. Cases in which the lower side of the funnel is incomplete, as shown in Figure 7.1A, suggest that some studies are missing.[7.3]

Now imagine that the TLC meta-analysis researchers searched further and came up with five additional studies. They redrew their funnel diagram plotting the additional studies and obtained Figure 7.1B. From this funnel diagram, which has a more complete funnel appearance, they concluded there was no longer evidence of publication bias and they had likely obtained all or most of the relevant studies.

Even after extensive searching, it is possible that investigations will be missed. This does not preclude proceeding with a meta-analysis. It is possible, as we will see, to take into account this potential publication bias as part of the results component.

Another important part of the assignment process in a meta-analysis is to determine whether there are differences in the quality of studies that justify excluding low-quality studies from the meta-analysis.

There are two potential approaches to this issue. It has been argued that study types with the potential for systematic biases should be excluded from a meta-analysis. For this reason, some meta-analysis researchers have favored the exclusion of all studies except randomized controlled trials, arguing that this type of study is the least likely to produce results that have a systematic bias in one direction or the other.

If randomized controlled trials as well as other types of studies are available, however, an alternative approach is to include all types of studies, at least initially. All investigations are then evaluated to determine their quality. Quality scores ideally can be obtained from two readers of the research report, each using the same standardized scoring system without knowledge of the other reader's score or the authors' identities. Then, it is possible to compare the results of high-quality studies with those of low-quality studies, and randomized controlled trials with observational studies to determine if the results, on average, are similar. Let us examine what might happen when we combine high-quality and low-quality studies in the next example:

Mini-Study 7.5 ■ A meta-analysis of the strength of the relationship between TLC and the outcome of single-vessel coronary artery disease included all known studies, including case–control, cohort, and randomized controlled trials. The investigators had two readers score, each investigation using the same standardized scoring system without knowledge of the other reader's score or the authors' identities. The outcomes on average were the same for randomized controlled trials and for observational studies, but the magnitude of the effect was considerably larger for the low-quality studies compared with the high-quality studies. Thus, the investigators decided to retain in their meta-analysis all high-quality studies whether they were randomized controlled trials or observational studies.

In this meta-analysis it was determined that high quality studies produced different results from the low quality studies. Therefore it was legitimate to include only the high quality studies. If on the other hand the results did not differ between high and low quality studies the investigators would need to include all of the investigations.

[7.3] Note that the scale for the odds ratio is defined so that it is equally spaced above and below 1. Thus, a study with an odds ratio <1 is converted to its reciprocal and then plotted below the horizontal line, for instance study numbers 5, 16, and 19 are converted from 0.5 to their reciprocal 2 and then plotted.

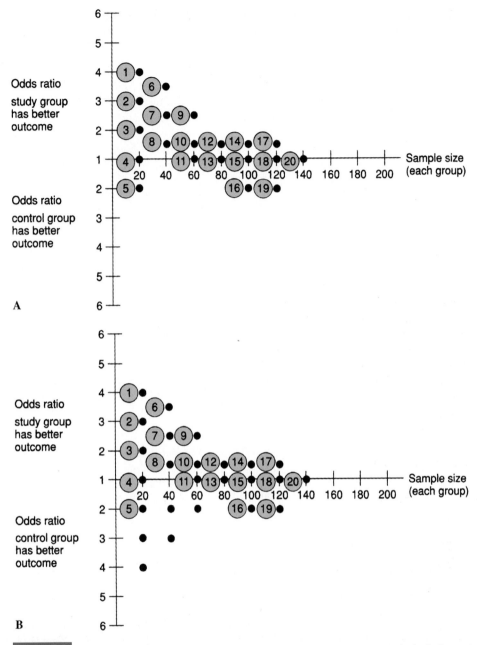

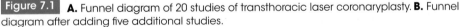

Figure 7.1 **A.** Funnel diagram of 20 studies of transthoracic laser coronaryplasty. **B.** Funnel diagram after adding five additional studies.

A variety of potential confounding variables can affect the outcome of a meta-analysis. As with conventional investigations, it is important that the investigator recognizes these characteristics to take them into account. The usual approach is to recognize the differences as part of the assignment process and take them into account as part of the results component.

For instance, in the TLC studies, we should know whether some studies used only older patients, more severely ill patients, or those with other characteristics or prognostic factors that often result in a poorer outcome in coronary artery disease. In addition, we would want to know whether there were important variations in the treatment given, such as different TLC techniques or different adjunct therapy, such as duration of anticoagulation. Thus, in the assignment process in a meta-analysis, we need data on the degree of uniformity of the patients and of the procedures used among the studies included in the meta-analysis.

Masking

Masking of assignment in meta-analysis has a somewhat different meaning than in other types of investigations. In one sense, the meta-analysis relies on the methods used in the individual studies to mask the participants and investigators. In meta-analysis, masking of assignment can also be achieved by preventing the investigators from being biased by knowledge of the results, the authors, or other characteristics of an investigation when determining whether a particular investigation should be included in the meta-analysis. More than one individual may be asked to judge whether an investigation meets the predefined criteria for inclusion in the meta-analysis.

ASSESSMENT

In conventional investigations, whether they are case–control, cohort, or randomized controlled trials, the investigators define the techniques used to measure the outcome and collect the data to assess the outcome. In meta-analysis, the researcher is usually limited to the techniques used by the primary investigator for assessing the study outcome.

The meta-analysis is also limited by the extent of data presented and the statistical methods used in the original article. However, it is increasingly possible to go back and obtain the original data. Some journals are beginning to ask investigators who submit research articles to make available a complete data set from their study for later review by other investigators or for use in a meta-analysis. In the future, this may allow meta-analysis researchers to reexamine and redefine the various studies' outcomes so that each investigation uses the same or similar measurements.

Precision and Accuracy

Currently, the meta-analysis researcher usually must live with what is available in existing articles. Because of the differences in the definitions and measurements of outcomes in different studies, the researcher performing a meta-analysis is faced with a series of unique issues. First, the meta-analysis researcher must determine which outcome to use in comparing studies. This may pose a serious problem, as illustrated in the next example:

> **Mini-Study 7.6** ■ In the studies of TLC, the following outcome measures were assessed. Ten studies used time until a positive stress test, time until evidence of occlusion on noninvasive angiography, and time until myocardial infarction as the outcomes. Ten other studies used only time until a positive stress test as their measure of outcome. Five studies used time until a positive stress test and evidence of occlusion on noninvasive angiography as their measures of outcome. As a result of the different outcome measurements used, the researcher concluded that a meta-analysis could not be performed.

The need to use precise and accurate measures of outcomes does pose major issues in meta-analysis.

The researcher may be interested in an accurate and early measure of outcome, which, in this case, may be a positive noninvasive angiography indicating closure of the treated vessel. Despite the desirability of using this outcome measure, if it is used to assess outcome, 10 of the 25 studies would need to be excluded. Thus, the researcher performing this meta-analysis may be forced to use time until a positive stress test as the measure of outcome if he or she wishes to include all the studies.

Even after determining that the measure of outcome will be time until a positive stress test, the meta-analysis researcher's problems are not solved, as shown in the following example:

Mini-Study 7.7 ■ The 25 studies define a positive stress test in several different ways. Some require greater duration and extent of ST segment depression on electrocardiogram than others. The meta-analysis researcher decides to use only studies that use the same definition of a positive stress test. Unfortunately, only 12 studies can be included in the meta-analysis.

It is important to find a common end point for a meta-analysis, but it is not essential that the end point be defined in the same way in all the studies. This is a common problem that is not generally dealt with by excluding studies. Rather, all studies with data on follow-up stress testing are included. The results of studies that use a common definition of a positive stress test can then be compared with studies that use other definitions. If the results are similar, regardless of the definition of a positive stress test, then all the studies can be combined in one analysis using their own definitions of a positive stress test. If there are substantial differences that depend on the definition of a positive stress test, then separate analyses can be performed for studies that used different definitions.

Completeness and Effect of Observation

The completeness of the investigations included in a meta-analysis depends on the completeness of the particular studies chosen for inclusion. The effect of observation also depends on the particular type and characteristics of the investigations that are included. Because of the large number of factors that can influence the quality of the assessment process, it is tempting for the meta-analysis investigator to eliminate studies that do not meet quality standards. As we have seen, some meta-analyses are conducted using only studies that meet predefined quality standards. Other meta-analysis researchers attempt to achieve this end by including only randomized controlled trials, presuming that they constitute the preferred type of investigation.

Although these are accepted approaches, others argue that both high- and low-quality studies should be included and that an analysis should be conducted to determine whether they produce similar or different results.

RESULTS (5,6)

The goals of analysis of results in a meta-analysis are the same as those in other types of investigations. We are interested in the following:

- **Estimation:** Estimating the strength of an association or the magnitude of a difference. This is often called *effect size* in meta-analysis.
- **Inference:** Performing statistical significance testing to draw inferences about the population on the basis of the data in the sample.
- **Adjustment:** Adjusting for potential confounding variables to determine whether they affect the strength or statistical significance of the association or difference.

Estimation

The strength of an association in a meta-analysis may be estimated by using any of the estimation measures used in conventional studies. Most meta-analyses in the health research literature use odds ratios. Odds ratios are often used because they can be calculated for case–control studies, cohort studies, and randomized controlled trials. When only randomized controlled trials are included in a meta-analysis a relative risk may be used as the estimate of the strength of the association.[7.4]

[7.4] Continuous dependent variables such as weight or diastolic blood pressure can also be used in meta-analysis, although they require different techniques.

Inference

Statistical significance testing in meta–analysis can use two types of techniques, often called *fixed effects model* and *random effects models*. Fixed effects models assume that all the studies come from one large population and only differ by chance. Random effects models assume that there are differences between the study populations that made a difference in outcome. It is easier to demonstrate statistical significance using a fixed effects model. That is, fixed effects models have greater statistical power. However, it is useful in meta–analysis to perform both types of statistical significance tests. If their results are nearly identical, one can be confident about combining the different studies.

When we combine a large number of studies and perform statistical significance testing, the results may be statistically significant even when the individual studies are not statistically significant. Remember from our previous discussion that when the number of participants is large, it is possible to demonstrate statistical significance even for small differences that have little or no clinical importance. Thus, in meta–analysis, it is especially important to distinguish between statistically significant and substantial or clinically important.

Learn More 7.2 discusses the most common method for displaying the results of a meta-analysis known as a forest plot.

LEARN MORE 7.2 ■ FOREST PLOT (6) ■ A forest plot is a graphic that is often used to summarize the data from a meta-analysis. It allows one to gain a side-by-side comparison of the results of each of the investigations that have been combined to produce the results of a meta-analysis. The most common measure of the strength of the relationship is an odds ratio since odds ratios allow one to use case-control, cohort studies, as well as randomized controlled trials. The odds ratio of 1.0 indicates that no association has been found. The forest plot also includes confidence intervals for each investigation.[7.5]

The following forest plot Figure 7.2 includes the key features that we expect from a forest plot. The size of the squares is proportionate to the sample size of the investigation. The summary measure indicates the result combining the studies included in the meta-analysis. When studies are divided into two groups because the results are believed to be heterogeneous, the article may include more than one forest plot.

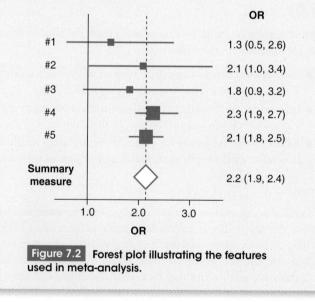

	OR
#1	1.3 (0.5, 2.6)
#2	2.1 (1.0, 3.4)
#3	1.8 (0.9, 3.2)
#4	2.3 (1.9, 2.7)
#5	2.1 (1.8, 2.5)
Summary measure	2.2 (1.9, 2.4)

Figure 7.2 Forest plot illustrating the features used in meta-analysis.

[7.5]The graph may be plotted on a natural logarithmic scale when using odds ratios or other ratio-based effect measures such as a relative risk, so that the confidence intervals are symmetrical about the means from each study and to prevent increased emphasis on odds ratios >1 when compared with those <1.

Adjustment

When there is a difference between the results of a random effects and a fixed effects statistical significance test, it suggests that there are differences between the populations from which the studies' subjects were obtained that makes a difference in the outcomes of the investigations. This is a form of confounding variable.

Adjustment in meta-analysis, like adjustment in the other types of studies we have examined, is designed to take into account potential confounding variables. In meta-analysis, adjustment also has additional goals. Adjustment aims to determine whether it is legitimate to combine the results of different types of studies. It also examines the effects of including investigations with particular characteristics in the combined results. Thus, the process of adjustment allows us to determine whether including studies with different characteristics, such as different types of patients or different approaches to treatment, affect the results. Looking at and learning from the impacts of those types of factors is what we mean by harnessing the benefits of diversity.

To combine investigations, we need to establish that the results are what we call *homogeneous*. This concept is illustrated in the following example:

Mini-Study 7.8 ■ Assume that the randomized controlled trials and cohort studies of TLC for single-vessel coronary artery disease in Table 7.2 were identified for a meta-analysis. Look at the graph in Figure 7.3, which compares the results of the study and control groups in these studies with respect to their outcome measure.

TABLE 7.2	Studies of Transthoracic Laser Coronaryplasty in Randomized Controlled Trials and Cohort Studies	
Study Number	**Adverse Outcomes**	**Study Type**
1	5/100 ST 10/100 C	RCT
2	80/1,000 ST 100/1,000 C	RCT
3	25/100 ST 20/100 C	RCT
4	2/100 ST 10/100 C	RCT
5	40/1,000 ST 120/1,000 C	RCT RCT
6	5/100 ST 20/100 C	RCT RCT
7	10/100 ST 10/100 C	Cohort Cohort
8	20/100 ST 20/100 C	Cohort
9	30/1,000 ST 90/1,000 C	Cohort
10	60/1,000 ST 150/1,000 C	Cohort

ST, study; C, control; RCT, randomized controlled trial.

(Continued)

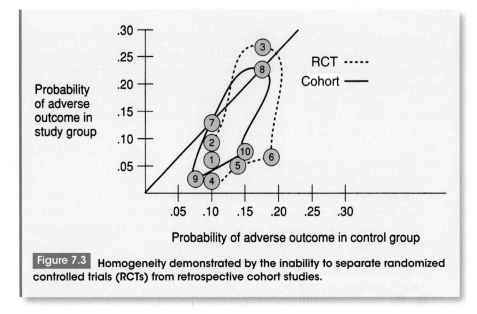

Figure 7.3 Homogeneity demonstrated by the inability to separate randomized controlled trials (RCTs) from retrospective cohort studies.

The two curves in Figure 7.3 are constructed by connecting the points represented by randomized controlled trials with one another and the points represented by retrospective cohort studies with one another. They demonstrate a homogeneous effect because the curves overlap to a large extent:

Mini-Study 7.9 ■ The data for patients with more severe disease were compared to the data for patients with less severe disease. Table 7.3 displays the data and Figure 7.4 constructs the same type of curves displayed in Figure 7.3.

TABLE 7.3	Studies of Transthoracic Laser Coronaryplasty with High and Low Severity of Illness	
Study Number	**Adverse Outcomes**	**Severity of Illness**
1	5/100 ST 10/100 C	Low
2	80/1,000 ST 100/1,000 C	Low
3	25/100 ST 20/100 C	Low
4	2/100 ST 10/100 C	High
5	40/1,000 ST 120/1,000 C	High
6	5/100 ST 20/100 C	High
7	10/100 ST 10/100 C	Low
8	20/100 ST 20/100 C	Low

(Continued)

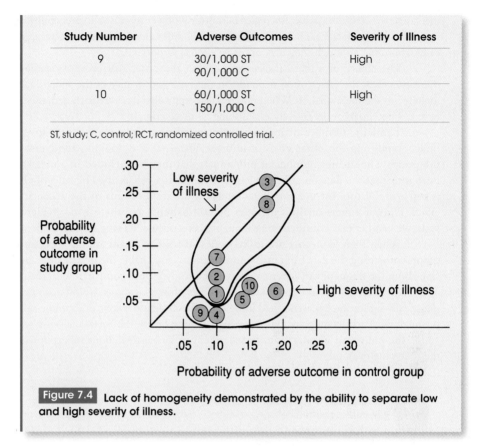

Study Number	Adverse Outcomes	Severity of Illness
9	30/1,000 ST 90/1,000 C	High
10	60/1,000 ST 150/1,000 C	High

ST, study; C, control; RCT, randomized controlled trial.

Figure 7.4 Lack of homogeneity demonstrated by the ability to separate low and high severity of illness.

A homogeneous effect allows the meta-analysis investigator to combine the two types of studies into one analysis. The next example illustrates what we mean by a heterogeneous effect.

Table 7.3 and Figure 7.4 show that when studies including patients with more severe illness are compared with studies including patients with less severe illness, the outcome measures are not homogeneous. The curve connecting the studies of patients with a high severity of illness can be separated from the curve connecting studies of patients with a low severity of illness. This is what we mean by heterogeneous. Studies of more severe illness in general tend to have a high proportion of bad outcomes in the control group. This lack of homogeneity implies that separate analyses should be conducted, with one analysis for studies of patients with low severity of illness and a separate analysis for studies of patients with high severity of illness. The results of these separate meta-analyses will demonstrate that TLC has greater efficacy for patients with a high severity of illness.[7.6]

INTERPRETATION

In a meta-analysis, the investigator often tries to determine whether contributory cause or efficacy has been demonstrated. As with other types of investigation, the interpretation begins by asking whether the definitive criteria of (1) association, (2) prior association, and (3) altering the cause alter the effect been fulfilled?

In establishing associations using meta-analysis, it is important to recognize that meta-analysis aims to increase the sample size by combining studies. This has the potential advantage of

---

[7.6] The degree of overlap in the curves needed to label the effect as homogeneous is subjective. This is an inherent limitation of the graph technique. Statistical significance testing is also available to examine the homogeneity of studies. These statistical significance tests, such as the *Q-statistic*, have low statistical power. However, a *P* value <.1 is often used to justify combining all the studies into a single meta-analysis.

increasing the statistical power. Increases in statistical power increase the probability of demonstrating statistical significance. Thus, even small but real differences may be demonstrated to be statistically significant, although they may not have clinical importance.

The ability of a meta-analysis to establish the criteria of prior association and altering the cause alters the effect often depends on the type and quality of the individual investigations included in the meta-analysis. When randomized controlled trials are included, these investigations have the potential for definitively establishing all three criteria.

The large number of individuals included in a meta-analysis may give it advantages in accomplishing the other goals of interpretation—that is, looking at adverse events and at subgroups. The greater number of individuals that may be included in a meta-analysis allows us to interpret the data on safety or harms with greater reliability. The rule-of-three in reverse is still a useful tool for helping us to interpret the implications of the absence of an adverse effect. Thus, if a meta-analysis includes 30,000 patients and there is no evidence of anaphylaxis, we can be 95% confident that if anaphylaxis occurs, its true frequency is <1 per 10,000.

When there is an increase in frequency of adverse events among those in the treatment group, combining the data from many investigations may enable the investigators to draw conclusion about the frequency of adverse events in the study groups compared with the control groups.

In meta-analysis as opposed to other types of investigations, we do not need to wait until statistically significance is established using all of the data before we can examine subgroups. When the analysis of results suggests the presence of heterogeneity, the meta-analysis researcher can examine the individual investigations to see what can be learned about subgroups, as illustrated in the following example:

Mini-Study 7.10 ■ A meta-analysis of the efficacy of a treatment for Alzheimer disease suggested heterogeneity according to the severity of the disease and the extent of family support. The meta-analysis suggested that the treatment had the greatest efficacy when used on groups with early disease who had the highest level of family support. This data were used as the basis for planning a randomized controlled trial using only patients with early Alzheimer disease who had high levels of family support.

This example illustrated the way the meta-analysis can be interpreted and used as the basis for drawing conclusions. Even when conclusions about statistical significance are not possible, the interpretation may be useful in planning future studies.

The large number of subjects included in a meta-analysis is an advantage when examining subgroups. For instance, if an exploratory meta-analysis of TLC used all 25 available studies, the investigator might be able to examine subgroups such as men versus women and repeat TLC versus initial TLC, especially if differences between these groups were hypothesized at the beginning of the investigation. If the data were available, the investigator might also examine a subgroup such as types of anticoagulation used to examine the hypothesis that this factor makes a difference in the outcome.[7.7]

In the process of interpretation of a meta-analysis, the investigators may want to consider removing *outliers*. Outliers are studies that produce results that are very different from the majority of studies. It is very tempting to merely exclude all outliers from an analysis, but this should be done only if there is very good reason. Often, in fact, additional information can be obtained by looking carefully at the outliers as part of the interpretation and asking why the results are different. This is demonstrated in the next example:

[7.7] Unfortunately, data are often not presented in a way that allows the investigator to combine the subgroups from different investigations. As with other types of investigations, even when the data are available, it is important to perform a limited number of subgroup analyses on the basis of predetermined study hypotheses.

Mini-Study 7.11 ■ Among the 25 studies of TLC, one demonstrated that the results of TLC were substantially worse than those associated with medication or surgery. This study was performed at the beginning of the TLC era, using obsolete procedures and no anticoagulation. A second outlier demonstrated that the best results for TLC were achieved using the newest technique at a medical center that has the largest volume and longest experience with TLC.

Here the exceptions help to prove the rule that TLC is an effective treatment. At other times, outliers may challenge the conclusion, producing new hypotheses for further investigations. In general, outliers should not be excluded from a meta-analysis. If one outlier is excluded, the others should also be excluded. Here, examination of these two studies supports the efficacy of TLC.

Finally, when interpreting the results of a meta-analysis, we need to reexamine the issue of publication bias. Publication bias is so important in meta-analysis that we often examine its potential impact as part of the interpretation. In doing so, we can estimate the number of studies showing no effect that would need to be missing from the meta-analysis in order for the results to no longer be statistically significant.[7.8] This number of studies is called the *fail-safe n*. The following example illustrates how to interpret the fail-safe n:

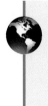

Mini-Study 7.12 ■ A meta-analysis of TLC for single-vessel coronary artery disease using all 25 studies has a fail-safe n of 100. Thus, the authors concluded that publication bias is very unlikely to affect the meta-analysis results.

It is unlikely that there exists 100 completed but unpublished studies that on average showed no difference between TLC and standard therapy. This degree of publication bias is unlikely to occur. Thus, we can be reasonably confident that if publication bias exists, it does not explain or have a dramatic effect on the conclusions.

EXTRAPOLATION

To Similar Populations

Meta-analysis is capable of providing an estimate of the average strength of an association, that is, the effect size. It can also help us with statistical significance testing, allowing us to infer efficacy in the larger population from which the study samples were obtained. Average strength of an association can be very useful when making extrapolations designed for groups of individuals. However, when trying to make decisions for a particular patient, the results of a meta-analysis may not be as useful as examining the results of one particularly relevant study, as demonstrated in the next example:

Mini-Study 7.13 ■ A patient at the medical center with the longest experience using TLC, the newest techniques, and the largest volume is being considered for TLC. The results of the meta-analysis comparing TLC with other therapies for this type of high-risk patient indicate very little difference. However, the data from this medical center unequivocally support the use of TLC for this type of high-risk patient at this medical center.

[7.8] The investigator actually calculates the fail-safe n assuming that the missing studies are, on average, the same size as the studies included in the meta-analysis, and that the studies, on average, show no effect (i.e., they have a zero difference or an odds ratio of 1).

Data available from the same institution based on similar patients are often more informative than using the average strength of an association obtained from a meta-analysis. Thus, despite the important role that meta-analysis can play in research and clinical care, it does not automatically produce the most useful results for a particular patient.

Beyond the Data

Issues of extrapolation are not limited to how well the therapy works. Issues of harm or safety also need consideration and require extrapolation beyond the data. The large number of patients that is often included in a meta-analysis can produce more reliable extrapolation about harms or safety of therapies. The assessment of safety, however, is still limited to the duration, dosage, and types of outcomes assessed by the studies included in the meta-analysis, as illustrated in the next hypothetical example:

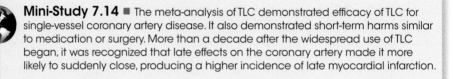

Mini-Study 7.14 ■ The meta-analysis of TLC demonstrated efficacy of TLC for single-vessel coronary artery disease. It also demonstrated short-term harms similar to medication or surgery. More than a decade after the widespread use of TLC began, it was recognized that late effects on the coronary artery made it more likely to suddenly close, producing a higher incidence of late myocardial infarction.

Studies can only draw conclusions about what they measure. The ability to assess long-term consequences requires long-term follow-up. Long-term safety or effectiveness are no better assessed by a meta-analysis than by the individual investigations that are included in the meta-analysis.

To Other Populations

Extrapolating results from a meta-analysis to practice poses the same dangerous consequences as with other types of investigations. When extrapolating to populations that are not included in the meta-analysis, it is important to recognize and make explicit the assumptions that are being made. For instance, imagine the following situation:

Mini-Study 7.15 ■ A large, well-conducted meta-analysis of TLC concluded that TLC was safe and effective and better than standard treatment for single-vessel coronary artery disease. The authors concluded that TLC should be used for treatment of coronary artery disease in two- and three-vessel disease. Subsequent studies demonstrated the superiority of TLC for single-vessel disease, but found that the extensive exposure to laser treatment needed for two- and three-vessel disease was associated with adverse events not previously recognized when using TLC to treat single-vessel coronary artery disease.

When an extrapolation is made to new situations, it is often assumed that the new circumstances will not be associated with new adverse events. In this example, this assumption was not correct. Thus, regardless of the type of investigation, the reader of the health research literature must be aware of the dangers of extrapolation to new populations and situations.

Meta-analysis has gained an important role in health research. It has helped to halt continued study of issues for which there are already adequate data. It has helped us gain more accurate measures for the magnitude of benefits and harms of therapies. By harnessing the benefits of diversity, meta-analysis has also helped us better understand what factors affect the outcomes of a therapy.

Despite the many advantages of meta-analysis, it requires the same type of attention to quality study design that is required for other types of research. In addition, because it relies on the existing literature, meta-analysis incorporates special techniques and is often limited in what it can attempt to do and what conclusions it can draw.

The classic literature review article has been dramatically restructured by the introduction of meta-analysis and its use as part of systematic reviews. If we are to obtain the maximum amount of information from the existing literature, the principles of meta-analysis must be understood and applied.

REFERENCES

1. Liberati A, Altman DG, Tetzlaff J, et al. The PRISMA statement for reporting systematic reviews and meta-analyses of studies that evaluate healthcare interventions: explanation and elaboration. *BMJ.* 2009;339:b2700. doi:10.1136/bmj.b2700.

2. Stroup DF, Berlin JA, Morton SC, et al. Meta-analysis of observational studies in epidemiology: a proposal for reporting. *JAMA.* 2000;283:2008–2012.

3. The Cochrane Collaboration. Systematic reviews. http://www.cochrane.org/about-us/evidence-based-health-care. Accessed July 25, 2011.

4. Petitti DB. *Meta-Analysis, Decision Analysis, and Cost-Effectiveness Analysis: Method for Quantitative Synthesis in Medicine.* 2nd ed. New York, NY: Oxford University Press; 2000.

5. Jenicek M. *Foundations of Evidence-Based Medicine.* Boca Raton, FL: Parthenon Publishing; 2003.

6. Fletcher R, Fletcher S. *Clinical Epidemiology: The Essentials.* 4th ed. Baltimore, MD: Lippincott Williams & Wilkins; 2005.

thePoint ✳ Visit http://thePoint.lww.com for interactive Q&A, flaw-catching exercises, searchable eBook, and more!

UNIT II
TESTING A TEST

8 | Testing a Test—M.A.A.R.I.E. Framework: Method, Assignment, and Assessment

INTRODUCTION

Testing a Test is about how we use evidence to make decisions. We will begin by using the M.A.A.R.I.E. framework to better understand research articles on tests. That is, we will look at the methods, assignment, assessment, results, interpretation, and extrapolation issues, and see how they apply to evaluation of a test. We will then apply and extend what we have learned to two increasingly common applications screening for asymptomatic diseases and the development of prediction and decision rules.

Next, we will take a look at how we can combine information from various sources to compare two or more interventions taking into account the harms and the benefits of each using the technique known as *decision analysis*. We will also look at how issues of cost can be incorporated extending the technique of decision analysis as cost-effectiveness analysis. Using what we have learned, we will step back and see how evidence can be used as the basis for evidence-based recommendations. Finally, we will explore the emerging field of translational research and see how evidence can be translated into practice. Let us begin by taking a look at how we can apply the M.A.A.R.I.E. framework to diagnostic tests.

TESTING A TEST

Using the information obtained from tests to make decisions has become an integral part of health care. Thus, it is not surprising that studies designed to measure the information provided by tests are an increasingly important form of investigation. We will examine these types of investigations by using the M.A.A.R.I.E. approach to look at method, assignment, assessment, results, interpretation, and extrapolation.

The M.A.A.R.I.E. framework is designed for use in critically reviewing research articles, including articles on diagnostic testing. Most students and practitioners encounter tests designed for diagnostic purposes in the clinical setting after the research has been completed. Learn More 8.1 looks at a framework for Testing a Test that can be used to put together the information obtained from the research to use for clinical purposes. It should alert you to the types of information that need to be obtained from research studies of diagnostic tests.

Until recently, research on diagnostic and screening tests has not been published in a consistent format, often leaving the reader with many unanswered and unanswerable questions. Recently, a set of standard and comprehensive methods for reporting investigations of diagnostic tests known as STAndards for Reporting Diagnostic Accuracy (STARD) have been adopted by many journals (1). These criteria have been incorporated into the components of the M.A.A.R.I.E. framework for Testing a Test.

The application of the M.A.A.R.I.E. framework to research on tests is illustrated in Figure 8.1.

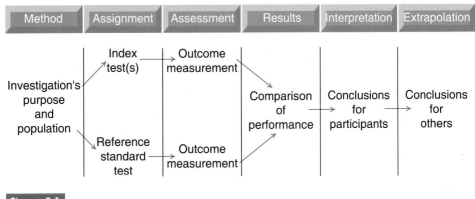

Figure 8.1   **M.A.A.R.I.E. framework for investigations of tests.**

LEARN MORE 8.1 ■ TESTING FOR DIAGNOSIS IN CLINICAL PRACTICE ■ Clinical diagnosis rests on the principle that individuals with a disease are different from individuals without the disease and that diagnostic tests can distinguish between the groups. Diagnostic testing, to be perfect, requires that (1) all test results are one of two values that we will call X or Y. (2) all individuals without the disease have one value on the test. We will call this *X*, and (3) all individual with the disease have a different value for the test, we will call this *Y*. Figure 8.2 illustrates this situation.

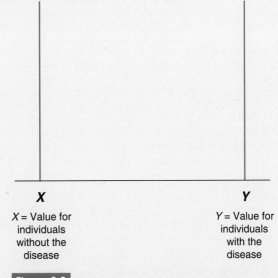

X = Value for individuals without the disease

Y = Value for individuals with the disease

Figure 8.2   **Conditions required for a perfect diagnostic test in which the test results are either *X* or *Y*.**

If this reflected the realities of clinical practice, the job of clinicians would be very easy. All clinicians would need to do is to select the right test and get the answer whether an individual has or does not have the disease of interest.

The realities of clinical practice are far more complex. In fact none of the three requirements for perfection hold up on practice. Figure 8.3 more closely reflects these realities. There is variation in all three of the requirements for perfection: the test itself, those without the disease, and those with the disease. Understanding these variations is central to the understanding the use of diagnostic tests in clinical practice.

(Continued)

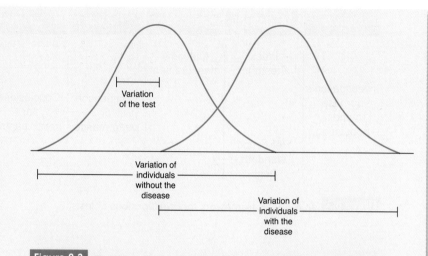

Figure 8.3 **The three types of variation that affect the clinical use of diagnostic tests.**

As suggested in Figure 8.3, the degree of variation in the results of the test itself should be small compared with the variation among those with and those without the disease. As we will discuss, we often rely on the laboratory or those conducting the test to ensure that the variation in the test itself is quite small, that is, the test results are reproducible. Nonetheless, when doubt exists repeating a test may be an important clinical step.

The usefulness of a test for diagnosis greatly depends on the degree of overlap between those with the disease and those without the disease. Figure 8.4A–C represents three possible degrees of overlap.

Figure 8.4A reflects the ideal situation, despite the variation among those with and without the disease, there is no overlap between those with and without the disease. Figure 8.4B reflects the typical situation in which there is a small but important degree of overlap. This is the most common situation and the one that we will focus on as we look at investigations of diagnostic tests. Finally, at times, Figure 8.4C may reflect the realities of the situation, where there is so much overlap that the results of the test do not add any useful clinical information. The situation displayed in Figure 8.4C may be illustrated in the following example:

Mini-Study 8.1 ■ One hundred individuals with long-standing cirrhosis of the liver underwent aspartate aminotransferase (AST) liver enzyme tests to assess their liver function. Most of these patients had AST levels within the range of normal or reference range. The authors concluded that these patients had well-functioning livers.

In this situation, those with cirrhosis have a similar range of values to those without the disease much like Figure 8.4C. The patients with cirrhosis may not have enough viable hepatocytes to generate high levels of AST. Thus, despite the fact that AST may serve as an excellent measure of liver function in many situations, when used to assess liver function among those with cirrhosis, the level of AST does not add useful information. This example emphasizes the key clinical point that a test that performs well for one purpose may not perform as well for a different purpose.

Thus, when confronted clinically with a new test, it is important to appreciate the potential variability of the test, the variability of those with

(Continued)

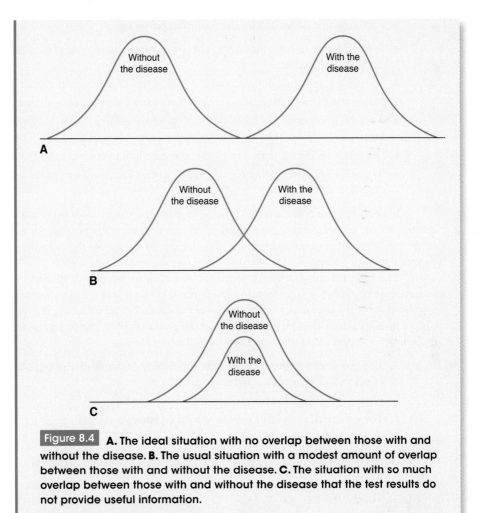

Figure 8.4 **A. The ideal situation with no overlap between those with and without the disease. B. The usual situation with a modest amount of overlap between those with and without the disease. C. The situation with so much overlap between those with and without the disease that the test results do not provide useful information.**

the disease, and the variability of those without the disease. It is especially important to recognize when the degree of overlap between those with the disease and those without the disease is so great that no useful information is provided by the results of the test.

Now let us examine each of the components of the M.A.A.R.I.E. framework beginning with the Method component.

METHOD

Purpose of Testing (2)

Testing can be seen as the collection of information to assist in decision making. When looked at this way, much of what is done in health care can be regarded as testing, from obtaining information from the history and physical examination to making decisions based on the prognosis of a disease. To understand the use of a test, we need to appreciate the multiple purposes for which a test may be used.

The same test may at times be used for more than one purpose, but its performance often depends on the specific purpose for which it is being used.

Testing may be used for at least the following purposes:

- Testing for risk factors: testing for factor(s) or other disease(s) that increase the risk of the disease of interest.
- Screening test: testing patients without symptoms for a particular disease
- Diagnostic testing: testing patients with symptoms for a particular disease
- Testing for causation: testing to establish the relationship between symptoms and disease
- Testing for prognosis: testing to predict the outcome of disease
- Testing for response: testing response to treatment including testing for adverse events associated with treatment

In order to identify the test that is being evaluated, the term *index test* is used. Thus, the first question to ask when reading an investigation on tests is: What is the purpose for investigating the index test? We will focus our attention in this chapter on testing for the purpose of diagnosis. In chapter 9 we will address the use of testing for screening and for prognosis.[8.1]

The fundamental purpose of diagnostic testing is to increase or decrease the probability that a disease or condition is present. To achieve this purpose it is essential to first make an estimate or guestimate of the probability of the disease or condition before obtaining the results of the test. This probability is called the *pretest probability* or the *prior probability*. The pretest probability or prior probability incorporates information from the following inputs:

1. The prevalence of the disease or the probability of the disease in population or groups of individuals similar to a particular patient
2. Predisposing diseases and risk factors of the individual.
3. The pattern of symptoms presented by the patient.
4. The results of previous testing

Learn More 8.2 illustrates the uses of each of these inputs into the pretest or prior probability of the disease.

LEARN MORE 8.2 ■ PRETEST PROBABILITY: WHERE DOES IT COME FROM? ■ To understand the uses of these four types of inputs imagine that we are interested in estimating the pretest probability of coronary artery disease for the following individuals:

A 23-year-old woman

A 65-year-old male

The first type of input is derived from the frequency of disease in populations or groups of indiv.iduals similar to a particular patient. This is called the *prevalence* of the disease. Prevalence indicates how common or probable the disease is in a particular population. The estimate of prevalence begins at the population level with the recognition that coronary artery disease is a very common disease in most developed countries. In addition we know that it increases with age and that the prevalence rates in females are lower than in males though the prevalence in females rapidly increases after menopause.

These two patient profiles represent very different probabilities of coronary artery disease. The 23-year-old woman has a very low pretest probability

(Continued)

[8.1] There are other possible uses of testing, including environmental testing to determine possible exposure to a risk factor such as lead and testing to provide a baseline for subsequent diagnostic testing. Baseline testing can be considered a method for substituting individual data for population data when defining a positive and a negative test, as we will discuss later in this chapter.

of clinically important coronary artery disease, well under 1%. The 65-year-old male on the other hand, has a considerably higher pretest probability of clinically important coronary artery disease, most likely more than 20% by virtue of his gender and age, regardless of any other risk factors or symptoms.

The second input into the pretest probability is predisposing diseases and risk factors of the individual. Imagine that the 65 year-old male has Type 2 diabetes. Diabetes substantially increases his probability of coronary artery disease. To consider the impact of risk factors, let us imagine the following pattern of risk factors in our 23-year-old woman and 65-year-old man.

The 23-year-old woman with a strong family history of early coronary artery disease, exercises regularly, does not smoke cigarettes, and has a blood pressure of 110/70 and an LDL level of 90 mg/dl.

The 65-year-old male diabetic has no known family history of early coronary artery disease but does not exercise regularly, is 30% over his ideal body weight, has smoked 1 pack of cigarettes per day for 45 years, and has a blood pressure of 150/95 and a LDL level of 160mg/dl.

Now we know much more about the pretest probability of disease. This information from risk factors may modestly increase the probability that the 23-year-old woman has clinically important coronary artery disease, while the presence of multiple risk factors raises the pretest probability for the 65-year-old man, most likely to the range of 50% or more.

The third input into the pretest probability is the pattern of symptoms presented by the patient. Imagine the following in our patients:
The 23-year-old woman experiences chest pains radiating to her left arm when she exercises strenuously.

The 65-year-old man with diabetes has not experienced chest pains or pressure, including when walking rapidly, which is his most strenuous form of exercise.

This information substantially raises the probability that the 23-year-old woman has clinically important coronary artery disease. For the 65 year-old man, asymptomatic coronary artery disease is still quite likely. Despite the presence of symptoms in the 23-year-old woman, she still is far less likely to have clinically important coronary artery disease than the 65-year-old man.

Notice that the pretest probability often utilizes the results of previous testing, the fourth input. Here, the blood pressure obtained on physical examination and the LDL level are used to develop a pretest probability of disease. In addition, the results of a test such as an exercise stress test may provide further information that may be used to help establish a pretest probability for additional testing.

Thus there are multiple inputs that contribute to our estimates of the pretest probability of disease. Each of these inputs requires data as well as subjective judgment. In addition, clinicians may not agree on how much weight or importance to place on each of these inputs. For instance the pattern of symptoms often receives considerable weighting when clinically estimating the pretest probability of a disease. On the other hand the prevalence of the disease may not receive the importance or weight that it deserves. Thus accurately estimating a pretest probability of a disease is an important but difficult to acquire skill.

METHOD

Study Population

The study population for an investigation of tests is defined by its inclusion and exclusion criteria. Inclusion and exclusion criteria should be defined to help ensure that those included in the investigation reflect those with and without the disease when the test is used in practice on its intended or target population.

Let us see what can happen when the participants used for investigation of a test are quite different from the people for which the test is intended:

Mini-Study 8.2 ■ A test is intended to be used to make an early diagnosis of myocardial infarction (MI). It was evaluated on patients who presented with chest pain in cardiologists' offices. The patients were included even if they had a previous MI. The results of the test indicated excellent diagnostic performance in early diagnosis of MI. When the same test was used in emergency departments on all patients with chest pain without a clear-cut explanation, the test did not perform nearly as well.

The patients being followed by cardiologists are likely to have had a previous MI or known coronary artery disease. They may also have complications of coronary artery disease such as heart failure. These patients are likely to have different symptoms and a different pattern of test results when they experience another MI compared with a population of emergency department patients with no history of MI. Therefore, it is important that the investigator defines the intended population when studying the performance of a test. If the intent is to use the test on a general population with chest pain but no previous history of coronary artery disease, it is important that the investigation of the test be conducted in emergency departments, primary care clinic, or a similar setting.

To describe the participants, the STARD criteria expect that investigators will indicate their inclusion and exclusion criteria. In addition, as we will see when we consider assignment, considerable detail is expected on the process of patient recruitment that along with the inclusion and exclusion criteria ultimately determine whether the participants are representative of the target population for whom the index test is intended.

METHOD

Sample Size

Participants in a study of diagnostic accuracy undergo the test being investigated, that is, the index test, as well as a second test. This second test is the best available or agreed-upon method for definitively diagnosing the presence or absence of the disease. This definitive test is called the *reference standard* or the *gold standard*. As we will see, the data for evaluating tests come from comparing the results of the index test with the results of the reference standard test.

We need to ask the following questions: How many participants need to undergo the index test and the reference standard test to provide adequate statistical power? That is, what is the expected sample size?

It may be surprising to learn that sample size for evaluating diagnostic and screening tests have not been agreed upon. The STARD recommendations do not make specific recommendation for the number of participants.[8.2]

Despite the absence of specific recommendations for sample size, some general guidelines are useful. For diagnostic tests in which the pretest probability is moderately high, 100 to 200 participants are usually adequate. When we are dealing with screening tests with a low pretest probability of disease, 1,000 or more participants are often required to adequately evaluate an index test being used for screening for disease.[8.3]

[8.2] Despite the absence of clearcut recommendations for the number of participants, as we will discuss in the next chapter, investigators are now expected to report the confidence intervals around their results. This has the effect of encouraging larger sample sizes.

[8.3] The issue of statistical power in evaluating diagnostic tests is different from hypothesis-testing investigations since there is no hypothesis that the index test differs from the reference standard test. The clinically relevant question is what is the confidence interval around the measurement of results such as the sensitivity and specificity? Hypothesis testing may be relevant when tests are being compared with one another. In this situation, a large numbers of participants are often required to produce substantial statistical power to demonstrate statistically significant difference between the performance

Now we have addressed the basic issues of the method component. We have focused on the purpose of the testing, the study population, and the sample size. Now we can take a look at the Assignment chapter and examine the characteristics of the participants and the conduct of tests.

ASSIGNMENT (3,4)

The assignment process defines those who are included in an investigation. For those who are included, their results on the index test will be compared with their results on a definitive, gold standard, or what is technically called a *reference standard* test. The assignment process for investigations of diagnostic tests describes the recruitment of patients, how they were assigned to comparison groups, and how the index test and the reference standard test were conducted.

Assignment: Recruitment

It is important that the investigators report how the participants included in the investigation of the test were recruited. Recruitment is the process of identifying individuals who fulfill the previously defined inclusion and exclusion criteria and turning them into participants in the investigation. Recruitment can occur through various mechanisms, from advertising to inviting all eligible patients coming to an emergency department to become participants. The mechanism used may affect the types of individuals with and without the disease who become participants.

According to the STARD recommendations, the investigator needs to indicate the beginning and end dates of recruitment as well as the setting(s) and location(s) where the data were collected. The clinical and demographic characteristics such as age, gender, spectrum of presenting symptoms, and known conditions and treatments need to be reported.

As we discussed under study population, the aim is to include in the investigation individuals with the disease who reflect the full spectrum of the disease that the investigators are trying to detect. In addition, the aim is to include individuals without the disease who might be mistakenly believed to have the disease include those with other diseases of the same organ system. The data provided on the recruitment process and on the specific individuals included in the investigation can help us determine whether these aims have been accomplished.

Assignment: Process

Investigators need to report on the process of assignment of participants. Participants may be assigned in three basic ways:

1. Identify and recruit all patients who fulfill inclusion and exclusion criteria from a setting that reflects the target population before any of them has had either the index test or the reference standard test.
2. Identify individuals with the disease and without the disease as defined by the results of the reference standard test. Those who are identified are then recruited to subsequently undergo the index test.
3. Identify individuals who have already undergone the index test and who then are recruited to subsequently undergo the reference standard test.

The first of these methods is considered the best way to assign participants. It helps ensure that the participants are representative of the target population of those with and those without

---

of two tests. Sample size for case–control studies might be used as a guide for sample size in evaluating diagnostic tests. The use of from 100 to several hundred patients with and also without the disease can serve as general guidelines for appropriate sample size for investigations of diagnostic tests, especially when the pretest probability of the disease among those who receive the test is in the range of 50%. The evaluation of screening tests requires a considerably larger sample size. Their sample size often parallels that of cohort studies or randomized controlled trials.

the disease. However, methods number 2 and 3 are often used and can each produce errors in investigations.

When using method 2, we need to ask whether those chosen reflect the full spectrum of the disease that we are interested in. It is tempting for the investigator using this approach to include only those with clear-cut disease and those in good health. When those in the gray area, such as those with other diseases of the same organ system, are not included, the results may be very different, as illustrated in the next example:

Mini-Study 8.3 ■ An investigation of a new test for prostate cancer began by identifying those with prostate cancer and age-matched men who had no evidence of prostate cancer according to the reference standard test and no evidence of other prostate disease. Those with and without prostate cancer then received the new test. The investigator found that the new test was as good as the reference standard test. When used in practice, the new test did not perform well because it was often positive for those with moderate to severe benign prostate hypertrophy.

This failure to include those with other diseases that might also be positive on the index test is called *spectrum bias.*

Method 3 is also prone to bias. When participants are identified based on having already undergone the index test, there is the possibility for what is called *verification bias.* Let us see how verification bias can occur and its potential consequences in the next example:

Mini-Study 8.4 ■ A new test for coronary artery disease was evaluated by obtaining data on all patients who underwent the new test and were then recruited to undergo the reference standard coronary arteriogram. Only a small percentage of those who underwent the new test were willing to volunteer to undergo the invasive reference standard test. The new test performed extremely well against the coronary arteriogram. When another investigator evaluated the new test by obtaining the new test and also a coronary arteriogram on all those who were eligible for an investigation, the new test, that is, the index test, did not perform well.

In this example, only those who already had undergone the new test, that is, the index test, and agreed to undergo the reference standard test are included in the investigation. Those who underwent the new test but not the reference standard test may not volunteer for various reasons. For instance, they may have had such an unequivocally negative test that they did not want to accept the potential harm of the coronary arteriogram. Alternatively, they may have had such a positive test that it was decided to act on the basis of the results of the patients' condition and the new test.

Thus, whenever patients are assigned based on having already had either the index test or the reference standard test, there is the potential for bias. Ideally, participants are recruited who meet inclusion and exclusion criteria from a population similar to the target population and have not undergone either the index test or the reference standard test. That is method number 1.

Even when method number 1 is used, the STARD statement requires reporting the number of eligible individuals who are excluded and the reasons for exclusion. Let us see how exclusion of patients might affect an investigation in the next scenario:

Mini-Study 8.5 ■ Investigators offer a new test along with a reference standard test to all patients who presented with hematuria in a primary care setting. The test requires transurethral insertion of a fiberoptic scope. Most of the patients who agreed to the test had gross hematuria, whereas most of those who met the inclusion and exclusion criteria but refused the test had microscopic hematuria. The test performed very well among those recruited for the investigation. However, when used in practice, the test failed to detect the types of pathology often associated with microscopic hematuria.

When an investigation is conducted on only a subset of the intended population of participants, it should not come as a surprise when its performance on the patients like those excluded from the investigation is not as good as on the types of patients included. Thus, it is important to understand not only the inclusion and exclusion criteria but to appreciate the types of participants that were actually included in the investigation.

Because of the importance of understanding the characteristics of participants, the STARD statement strongly encourages investigators to include a flowchart that not only indicates the characteristics of the participants but also indicates the reasons for exclusion of those who met the eligibility criteria. Figure 8.5 illustrates the type of flowchart that should be

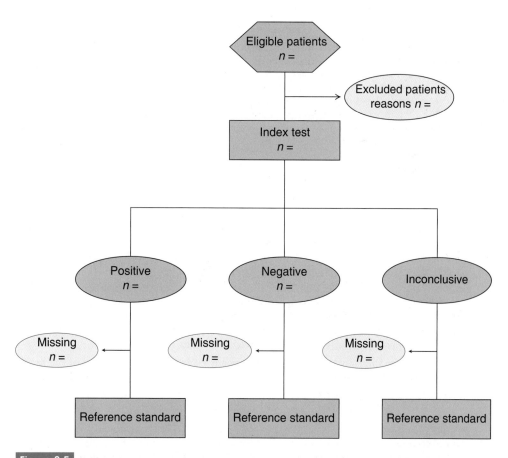

Figure 8.5 **Flow chart for displaying the recruitment and participation process.** (Adapted from STARD Initiative checklist and flow diagram. http://www.stard-statement.org/flowdiagram_maintext.htm. Accessed July 29, 2011.)

included in a journal article to provide data on recruitment, as well as the characteristics of the participants.[8.4]

Assignment: Conduct of Tests

The technical details of the conduct of the index test and the reference standard test need to be described in sufficient detail, or citations provided, to allow for replication of the investigation. According to the STARD criteria, these details should include the following:

■ Technical specifications of materials and methods used, including how and when measurements were taken

■ The training and expertise of individuals conducting and reading the test

In addition, the investigator needs to provide information on the reference standard test, indicating the rationale for its use to establish a definitive diagnosis. The selection of the reference standard test may not be straightforward. To compare the results of the reference standard test with the index test, the reference standard test needs to definitively diagnose those with and those without the disease.

To accomplish this goal, invasive tests such as biopsies may need to be used. Determining the best reference standard test can itself be an important issue, since to paraphrase Will Rogers, nothing is certain except biopsy and autopsy, and even these may miss the diagnosis. Let us see the type of problem that may be encountered in selecting an appropriate reference standard test in the next example:

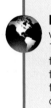

Mini-Study 8.6 ■ One hundred individuals who were admitted to a hospital with diagnostic Q waves on their electrocardiograms (ECGs) and who died within 1 hour of admission were autopsied for evidence of MI. The autopsy was used as the reference standard test for MI. Autopsy revealed evidence of MI in only 10 patients. The authors concluded that the ECG was not a useful method for making the diagnosis of an MI. They insisted on the reference standard test of pathologic diagnosis.

The usefulness of all index tests is determined by comparison with a reference standard test that has previously been shown by experience to definitively diagnose the disease under study. Autopsy diagnoses may be used as the reference standard test. However, even an autopsy may be a less-than-perfect measure of disease, as illustrated in this example. The pathologic criteria for MI may take considerable time to develop and may not be present among those who died shortly after admission. It is possible that the diagnostic Q waves on an ECG are a better reflection of an MI than pathologic changes at autopsy. The investigator should be sure that the reference standard test selected has, in fact, been shown to be the definitive standard for diagnosis.

Two specific relationships between the conduct of the index test and the reference standard test should be examined:

1. Were the investigators masked as to the results of the other test?
2. Were there any interventions that occurred between the conduct of the index test and the conduct of the reference standard test?

[8.4] Investigations of tests may be conducted by comparing one index test with a reference standard. Alternatively, an investigation may compare two or more index tests with the same reference standard. When comparing two or more tests, we need to ask how the participants were assigned to groups. It is possible to assign participants to study and control groups by observing the choices that are made in the course of health care. Alternatively, it may be possible for an investigator to intervene and assign the patients using a process of randomization. When ethical and practical, randomization is a better method because it helps ensure that the participants in each group will be similar.

Those who conduct the index test and the reference standard test should ideally be masked as to the results of the other test. That is, neither those who conduct nor those who read either test should be aware of the outcomes of the other test. Let us see how this expectation might be violated and the potential consequences in the next example:

Mini-Study 8.7 ■ A gastroenterologist was investigating a new test for gastric cancer. He properly identified and recruited the participants. He then conducted the new test during the course of an endoscopy. He compared the results of the new test with the results of the endoscopy, using the endoscopy as the reference standard test.

Although convenient, having the endoscopist perform and read both the reference standard test and the index test does not result in masking. The investigator here is aware of the results of the endoscopy when obtaining and reading the results of the new test. To avoid this problem would have required two investigators to participate in the endoscopy process, one performing the endoscopy itself and the other performing and reading the new test, each without knowledge of the other's findings.

In addition to reporting whether masking occurred, the STARD criteria expect the investigators to indicate the time interval between the index test and the reference standard test and whether any treatment was administered in the time period between conducting the two tests. The following example illustrates how the time interval and the provision of treatment between the times of the two tests might affect the results:

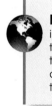

Mini-Study 8.8 ■ An investigator properly identified and recruited patients to investigate a new test for asthma. Participants were initially administered the new test. Two weeks later, after having receiving whatever treatments were provided by their attending physicians, they underwent a reference standard test. The new test did not perform as well as expected when compared with the reference standard test.

Ideally, the index test and the reference standard test should be performed within a brief period of time. In this case, the administration of treatment between the two tests may make it more difficult for the subsequent test to detect the disease. This is especially important in a disease such as asthma, where the treatment can hide the existence of the disease even when tested by a reference standard test.

Thus, the process of assignment requires the investigator and the reader to look closely at how the individuals were recruited and assigned to receive the index and reference standard tests and how these tests were conducted. Once this is accomplished, the next step is to look at the measurements made as part of the assessment process.

ASSESSMENT (5,6)

The assessment process in studies of testing, similar to the assessment process in other types of investigations, addresses the issues of measurement. When performing the measurements, we usually aim to establish whether the index test is positive or negative. Thus, we first need to examine how positives and negatives can be defined.

Definition of Positives and Negatives

The STARD statement expects the investigators to report the definition and rationale for defining positive and negative test results. As we will see, there are several methods that may be used to define positive and negative results for the index test.

When the test claims to either detect or fail to detect a condition, defining positives and negatives may be quite straightforward, such as when a test is positive or negative for growth of an organism or presence of a drug. However, this is not the situation when tests provide numerical data such as the prostate-specific antigen test, pulmonary function testing, or even such basic tests as the hemoglobin level. The investigators then need to define what they mean by a positive and a negative. This often requires the use of *cutoff lines* or *cutoff points* that separate negative from positive measurements.

To utilize a test that produces quantitative results, the authors need to report the procedure used to establish these cutoff lines. Often this entails development of what is called the *reference interval* or *range of normal*. The reference interval often divides test results into below the reference interval, within the reference interval, and above the reference interval.[8.5]

Most clinical laboratory results are reported using the concept of a reference interval. Laboratory reports often express this reference interval as, for example, 30 ± 10 or alternatively as 60 ± 40. The first reference interval should be interpreted as 20 to 40, whereas the second reference interval should be interpreted as 10 to 100.[8.6]

Let us take a look at how a reference interval is obtained using the traditional approach. Then, we will examine the limitations of this approach and outline other methods that are increasingly being used to define positives and negatives.

The reference interval values are traditionally developed using the following steps:

1. The investigator locates a particular group of individuals who are believed to be free of the disease for which the test is being conducted. This group is technically known as the *reference sample group*, but for clarity we will call it the *disease-free group*. These individuals are frequently students, hospital employees, or other easily accessible volunteers. Often they are merely assumed to be free of the disease, although at times they may undergo extensive testing to ensure they do not have the disease that the test attempts to diagnose.

2. The investigator then performs the test of interest, that is, the index test, on all the individuals in the disease-free group and plots their test measurements.

3. The investigator next calculates a reference interval or range of normal that includes the central 95% of the disease-free group. Strictly speaking, the reference interval includes the mean (average) measurement plus or minus the measurements within two standard deviations from the mean. Unless there is a reason to do otherwise,[8.7] the investigator chooses the central part of the range so that 2.5% of disease-free individuals have measurements above the reference interval and 2.5% of disease-free individuals have measurements below the reference interval.

[8.5] Here we will proceed under the assumption that a negative test result is a result that is within the reference interval and a positive result is one that is above the reference interval. Low levels on a test may or may not be of importance, depending on the nature of the test and of the disease. When low levels are associated with a disease, the same basic principles apply for defining a positive and a negative test.

[8.6] It is important to distinguish the method for presenting reference intervals from the method used to present confidence intervals. Data may at times be presented as an observed value ± the standard error, for example, 30 ± 10. In this situation, the confidence interval is approximately 30 ± 2 (10) or 10 to 50.

[8.7] One reason to do otherwise is when the distribution of the test measurements is not symmetrical. An alternative in this situation is to perform a transformation such as a logarithmic transformation, which may produce a symmetrically distribution. Use of the central 95% or the mean ± two standard deviations may then still be a useful approach. At times, levels beyond one end of the reference interval, often the lower end, may also be included in the definition of negative. For instance, low levels of uric acid or cholesterol are not considered to be outside the reference level. When this is the situation, the 5% outside the reference interval may refer entirely to those with levels above the cutoff point of the reference interval.

To illustrate the development of the reference interval, imagine that investigators have measured the heights of 100 male medical students and found numerical values that looked like those in Figure 8.6.

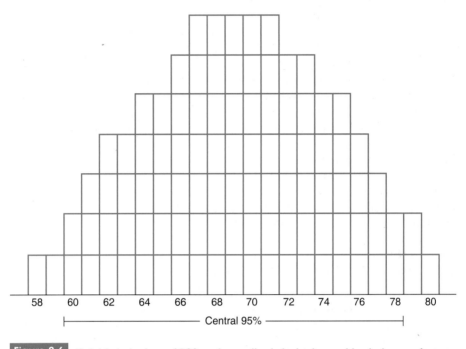

Figure 8.6 **Heights in inches of 100 male medical students used to derive a reference interval.**

The investigators would then define a reference interval that includes 95 of the 100 male medical students. Unless they had a reason to do otherwise, they would use the middle part of the range so that the reference interval for this "disease-free group" would be from 60 to 78 in (152 to 198 cm).

Let us look first at the implications of those principles for calculating the reference interval and illustrate the errors that can result from failure to understand these implications.

- By definition, 5% of a group without disease will have a measurement on a particular test that lies outside the reference interval.

As suggested by our reference interval for male medical students, individuals outside this range may not have any disease; they may simply be healthy individuals who are outside the reference interval. Thus, outside the reference interval and disease are by no means synonymous. The more tests that are performed, the more individuals there will be who do not have a disease but whose numerical values are outside the reference interval on at least one test.

Taking this proposition to its extreme, one might conclude that a "normal" person is anyone who has not been investigated sufficiently. Despite the absurdity of this proposition, it emphasizes the importance of understanding that the definition of the reference interval often intentionally places 5% of those without the disease outside the reference interval. Thus, the phrase "outside normal limits" or "outside the reference interval" must not be equated with disease, and outside the reference interval should not be labeled "abnormal."

Let us see how the impact of violating this principle in the next example:

Mini-Study 8.9 ■ In a series of 1,000 consecutive health maintenance examinations, a total of 12 laboratory tests were done on each patient even though no abnormalities were found on a history or physical examination. Five percent of the tests were outside the reference interval, a total of 600 tests. The authors concluded that these test results fully justified doing the 12-test panel on all health maintenance examinations.

A reference interval, by definition, generally includes only 95% of those who are believed to be free of the condition. If a test is applied to 1,000 individuals who are free of a condition, on average 5%, or 50 individuals, will have test results outside the reference interval. If 12 tests are applied to 1,000 individuals without evidence of disease, then on average, 5% of 12,000 tests will be outside the reference interval. Five percent of 12,000 equals 600 tests.

Thus, even if these 1,000 individuals were completely free of disease, one would expect on average 600 test results that are outside the reference interval. These merely reflects the method of determining the reference interval. Remember that test results outside the reference interval do not necessarily indicate disease and do not by themselves justify doing multiple laboratory tests on all health maintenance examinations.[8.8]

■ The reference interval used needs to be derived from individuals like those on whom it is being used in practice.

In general, the reference interval or range or normal is calculated using one particular disease-free group. Therefore, when applying the reference interval to a particular individual, we need to ask whether a particular individual has a reason to be different from those in the disease-free group.

For instance, if male medical students were used to obtain a reference interval for height, this reference interval may not be applied to women. One could not apply it to children and would have to be careful applying it to elderly individuals who tend to lose some height as they age. The type of problem that can result from using an inappropriate reference interval is illustrated in the next example:

Mini-Study 8.10 ■ A group of 100 medical students was used to establish the reference interval for granulocyte counts. The reference interval was chosen so that 95 of the 100 granulocyte counts were included in the range of normal. The reference interval for granulocyte count was determined to be 2,000 to 5,000. When asked about an elderly black man with a granulocyte count of 1,900, the authors concluded that this patient was clearly outside the reference interval and needed to be further evaluated to identify the cause of the low granulocyte count.

It is unlikely that there are many elderly black men among the group of medical students used to establish the reference interval. In fact, elderly black men have a different reference interval for granulocyte count than elderly white men. Thus, the reference interval established for the medical students may not have reflected the reference interval applicable to this elderly black man. This gentleman was well within the range of normal for an individual of his age, race, and sex. Because elderly black men are known to have a lower reference interval for granulocyte counts, this must be taken into account when interpreting the test results.

[8.8] In considering the implications of test results, it is important to realize that all levels outside the reference interval do not carry the same meaning. Numerical values well beyond the limit of the reference interval may be much more likely to be caused by disease than numerical values that are near the borderlines of the reference interval. Test results nearer the limits of the reference interval are more likely to be due to variation of the test or to biologic variation. For instance, if the upper limit of male hematocrit is 52, then a value of 60 is more likely to be associated with disease than a value of 53.

■ Changes within the reference interval may be pathologic.

Because the reference interval includes a wide variation in numerical values, an individual's measurement may change considerably and still be within the reference interval. For instance, the reference interval for the liver enzyme AST is 8 to 20 unit per L, the range of normal serum potassium extends from 3.5 to 5.4 mEq per L, and the reference interval for serum uric acid extends from 2.5 to 8.0 mg per dl.

It is important not only to consider whether an individual's measurement lies within the reference interval but also whether the individual's test result has changed over time. The concept of a reference interval is most useful when no historic data are available for the individual. When previous results are available, however, they should be taken into account, as illustrated in the next example:

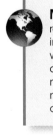

Mini-Study 8.11 ■ Among 1,000 asymptomatic Americans with no known renal disease and with no abnormalities showing on urinalysis, the reference interval for serum creatinine was found to be 0.7 to 1.4 mg per dl. A 70-year-old woman was admitted to the hospital with a serum creatinine of 0.8 mg per dl and was treated with gentamicin. On discharge, she was found to have a creatinine value of 1.3 mg per dl. Her physician concluded that because her creatinine was within the reference interval on admission as well as on discharge, she could not have had renal damage secondary to gentamicin.

A result within the reference interval does not ensure the absence of disease. Each individual has a disease-free measurement that may be higher or lower than the average measurement for individuals without disease. In this example, the patient increased her serum creatinine to more than 60%, but still fell within the reference interval. The change in the creatinine measurement suggests a pathologic process occurred. It is likely that the gentamicin produced renal damage. When historic information is available, it is important to include it in evaluating a test result. Changes within the range of normal may be a sign of disease.[8.9]

■ The reference interval must not be confused with the desirable range of test results.

The reference interval is an empirical measurement of the way things are among a group of individuals currently believed to be free of the disease. It is possible that large segments of the community may have test results that are higher (or lower) than ideal and may be predisposed to develop a disease in the future, even though the results are within the reference interval. For instance, imagine the following example:

Mini-Study 8.12 ■ The central 95% of low-density lipoprotein (LDL) cholesterol is determined among 100 American men aged 20 to 60 years who reported no evidence of coronary artery disease. The reference interval was found to be 100 to 160 mg per dl. A 45-year-old American man was found to have an LDL cholesterol of 150 mg per dl. His physician informed him that because his LDL cholesterol was within the traditionally defined reference interval, he did not have to worry about the consequences of high LDL cholesterol.

[8.9] This example also reflects the fact that older individuals have a different serum creatinine reference interval than young individuals, and women have a different creatinine reference interval than men because serum creatinine reflects the quantity of muscle mass. This example suggests that previous levels for a test may also indicate the desirable level for an individual. This is the rationale for establishing and using baseline levels that establish an individual's level before the onset of a condition or disease.

Remember that the reference interval is calculated using data collected from a group currently believed to be free of the disease. It is possible that the disease-free group consists of many individuals whose results on the test are higher (or lower) than desirable. A result within the central 95% does not ensure that an individual will remain free of the disease.

Thus, the reference interval defines the way things are, not the way they should be. American men as a group may have higher than desirable cholesterol levels. Thus, an individual with an LDL cholesterol of 150 mg per dl may well suffer the consequences of high LDL cholesterol. When research data strongly suggests a range of desirable numerical values for a test, it is permissible to substitute the desirable range for the usual reference interval. This is now standard procedure for LDL cholesterol.

The reference interval approach to defining negative and positive is not the only approach. The use of the reference interval assumes that we do not know what an individual's level should be, and therefore we need to rely on the test level as determined for others who are believed to be free of the condition.

These limitations of the reference interval suggest other methods for defining a negative and a positive result. At times each of these may be useful clinically:

- Use of a different reference intervals for different ages, gender, race, or other characteristics
- Use of an individual's own baseline level on the test at a time when they are believed to be free of the disease—that is, an individual's own desirable level
- Use of a desirable interval based on long-term follow-up of individuals with varying levels identifying the levels on a test that are associated with subsequent desirable outcomes.[8.10]

Precision and Accuracy

In addition to establishing whether the measurement obtained from an index test is positive or negative, we also need to ask whether the test is precise. Precision, or reproducibility, implies that the results are nearly identical when repeated under the same conditions. Let us see how failure to repeat the test under the same conditions can mislead us, as illustrated in the following example:

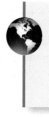

Mini-Study 8.13 ■ The precision and accuracy of a test of serum cortisol levels were evaluated by selecting 100 study subjects and drawing two blood samples from each individual. The first test was obtained at 6 a.m. and a second at noon. The authors found that, on average, an individual's second test result was twice the level found in the first test. They concluded that the large variation indicated that the test was not reproducible.

Precision, or reproducibility, implies that the test produces nearly the same results when conducted under the same conditions. In this example, the investigators did not repeat the test under the same conditions. Throughout the day and night, a physiologic cycle occurs in individuals' cortisol levels in which they are lowest in the early morning. By drawing blood at 6 a.m. and again at noon,

---

[8.10]We can use evidence that is based on subsequent outcomes to define the reference interval. This approach requires long-term follow-up rather than comparing the results of the index test to the reference standard test. Thus, it is often not a practical approach to defining positive and negative results. For research purposes, another approach is increasingly being used. Using this approach, no definition of a positive or a negative is used during the assessment component. The definition of positive and negative is established only after comparing the measurements obtained using the index test to the results of the reference standard test. In this approach, a positive result and negative result is defined later after first determining the cutoff point at which the index test's performance is the maximized using a receiver operator characteristics (ROC) curve. We will examine ROC curves in the next chapter.

the investigators were testing at different points in this cycle. Even if the test itself was completely reproducible, the different conditions of the subjects would produce variation in the test results.

Studies that examine reproducibility require that the test be read or interpreted twice. A reproducible test should produce nearly identical results when read by two readers or observers, or by the same observer when they are unaware of their own reading on the first attempt. This is called *interobserver* and *intraobserver reproducibility*.

Interobserver reproducibility is evaluated by having a second reader record their test results without knowing the results of the other reader. Intraobserver error is evaluated by having the same reader obtain results twice. The second reading occurs without the individual being told his or her own measurement on the initial test.

Let us see how these conditions may be violated when evaluating reproducibility, as illustrated in the next example:

Mini-Study 8.14 ■ An investigator studying the reproducibility or precision of urinalysis asked an experienced laboratory technician to read a urinalysis sediment, to leave the slide in place, and then to repeat the reading in 5 minutes. The investigator found that the reading performed under the same conditions produced perfectly reproducible results.

In this example, the technician knew the results of the first test and was likely to have been influenced by the first reading when reexamining the urine 5 minutes later. Determining that a test's results are reproducible requires that the second measurement be performed without knowing the results of the first measurement.

Whenever an observer's assessment is needed to obtain the results of a test, there is potential for interobserver and intraobserver variations. Two radiologists may read the same X-ray film differently (i.e., interobserver variation). An intern may interpret an ECG differently in the morning than he or she did when reading the same test performed in the middle of the night (i.e., intraobserver variation).

Reproducibility of test measurements ensure us that the measurements obtained can be relied on to be the same if and when the test is repeated. Reproducibility is sometimes called reliability because when it is present, we can rely on the measurement obtained from using the test once.

Reproducibility of an index test can be expressed quantitatively as discussed in Learn More 8.3. The STARD statement does not require a quantitative assessment of reproducibility. However the STARD criteria do require reporting the methods used and the estimates of reproducibility obtained if these were conducted.

LEARN MORE 8.3 ■ **MEASURING THE REPRODUCIBILITY OF A TEST** ■ The reproducibility, precision, or reliability of a test is measured by comparing the results obtained under the same conditions by two different observers or readers, that is, *interobserver variability or interrater reliability* as well as the results obtained by the same observer, that is, *intraobserver variability* or *test–retest reliability*. Measuring reproducibility requires first establishing cutoff line(s) that are used to define a positive and a negative test. Each set of measurements of the test can then be classified as agreement or disagreement.

Let us see how interobserver variability and interobserver variability might be measured in the following example.

(Continued)

Mini-Study 8.15 ■ A new test for dementia was evaluated for interobserver and intraobserver variation. A nursing home population of 100 with a prevalence of dementia of 50% was used. Two readers administered the new test two different times over a 1-month period. Each observer was told to score 50% of the tests positive and 50% of the tests negative to correspond with previous diagnostic assessments by neurologist. The results indicated that there was 50% agreement between the observers as well as between the readings of the same observer. The investigators were not sure whether this represented good agreement.

The 50% interobserver and intraobserver agreement represents the extent of agreement expected by chance alone. When the probability of a positive or a negative is 50%, the situation is parallel to flipping two coins. Two heads or two tails will occur 50% of the time by chance alone. Therefore, a summary measurement is needed that takes into account chance agreement. The most commonly used measurement is known as *Kappa* or the *Kappa statistic*. Kappa is defined as follows:

$$\frac{\text{Agreement observed} - \text{Agreement by chance}}{1 - \text{Agreement by chance}}$$

In this situation, Kappa can be calculated as follows:

$$\frac{0.5 - 0.5}{1 - 0.5} = 0$$

Thus, Kappa indicates that the degree of agreement does not exceed that which is expected by chance alone. Kappa may vary from 0 to 1 with 0 indicating no agreement and 1 indicating complete agreement. Poor agreement is often defined as a Kappa <0.20, substantial agreement as Kappa of 0.60 to 0.80 and 0.80 to 1.0 as nearly perfect agreement. Unfortunately, focusing only on Kappa does not give us a complete picture of the extent of agreement. Let us see why this occurs in the following scenario:

Mini-Study 8.16 ■ The new test for dementia was again evaluated for interobserver and intraobserver variation. This time 100 individuals from a community center for seniors were used with a prevalence of dementia of 10%. Two readers administered the new test two different times over a 1-month period. Each observer was told to score 10% of the tests positive and 90% of the tests negative to correspond with previous diagnostic assessments by neurologists. The results indicated that there was an 81% agreement between the observers as well as between the readings of the same observer. The investigators again were not sure whether this represented good agreement.

When most of the results are negative (no dementia) or positive (dementia), we expect a higher degree of agreement by chance alone. When the disease has a low prevalence, a guess of negative is usually correct. In fact when the probability of disease is 10%, we expect 81% agreement by chance alone. Once again in this example, the Kappa is 0 indicating no agreement beyond chance. However, in this situation where 81% agreement occurs by chance, it is difficult to obtain substantial or nearly perfect agreement since agreement by chance is already so high. Therefore, when interpreting a Kappa, it is important to take into account the prevalence of the condition.

(Continued)

> As alternative to Kappa exists know as *Phi*. Phi has the advantage
> of taking into account chance agreement but not being affected by the
> prevalence of the condition. Therefore, Phi may be a better measure when the
> prevalence of the condition is especially high or especially low.[8.11]

Learn More 8.4 provides examples of the issue of accuracy and precision as well as the use of the reference interval for two commonly used clinical tests hematocrit and uric acid.

LEARN MORE 8.4 ■ HEMATOCRIT AND URIC ACID—PRECISION AND ACCURACY PLUS REFERENCE INTERVAL

■ In Learn More 8.1, we discussed a framework for understanding tests in clinical practice. Let us apply that framework to two commonly used clinical tests hematocrit and uric acid.

Hematocrit Precision and Accuracy

The hematocrit is a measurement of the percentage of the total blood composed of packed red blood cells. Routine hematocrits are measured by either the finger stick method of assessing capillary blood or the venipuncture method. Both methods can accurately measure the relative quantity of red cells to total blood, but accuracy and precision of the techniques require attention to technical detail. Capillary blood can be expected to have a hematocrit about 1% to 3% lower than venous blood. Excessive squeezing of the fingertip can milk out extra plasma and falsely lower the hematocrit. When anemia is severe, the finger stick measurement is less accurate.

In assessing the accuracy with which the hematocrit measures the physiologic status, remember that relative and not absolute red cell mass is being tested. Misleading results are possible when dehydration or diuresis lowers the plasma volume. Individuals with reduced plasma volume may present with hematocrits higher than the reference interval. These are normal variants but may be confused with polycythemia (pathologically elevated hematocrit).

Reference Interval

The reference interval of the hematocrit is different for men and women. This is generally recognized and reported by laboratories as separate reference intervals for men and women. Less often recognized are different reference intervals for different stages of pregnancy, different ages, and persons living at different altitudes. The hematocrit usually falls during pregnancy beginning somewhere between the third and the fifth month. Between the fifth and eighth months, a reduction of 20% compared with previous levels is not unusual. The hematocrit generally rises slightly near term and should return to its previous level by 6 weeks postpartum.

Age has a pronounced effect on hematocrit, especially among children. The reference interval on the first day of life is 54 ± 10 (i.e., the reference interval is 44 to 64). By the fourteenth day, the interval is 42 ± 7. By 6 months, the reference interval is 35.5 ± 5. The average hematocrit gradually increases through the teenage years, with the average reaching 39 between 11 and 15 years of age. Adult reference intervals are 47 ± 5 for men and 42 ± 5 for women.

(Continued)

[8.11] Phi = $[(\sqrt{\text{Odds ratio}^2}) - 1]/[(\sqrt{\text{Odds ratio}^2}) + 1]$. When the odds ratio is >1, Phi = (Odds ratio − 1)/(Odds ratio + 1). Phi can vary from +1 to −1, with 0 indicating only chance agreement. Thus, the magnitude of Phi as opposed to Kappa directly indicates the extent of agreement. In addition, confidence limits can be calculated for Phi but not for Kappa, and Phi can be used when the size of the sample is small (7).

Low barometric pressure has a pronounced effect on the reference interval for hematocrits. Native residents who live at high altitudes have generally higher hematocrits. The reference interval at about 4,000 ft (1219 m), for instance, is 49.5 ± 4.5 for adult men and 44.5 ± 4.5 for adult women. Even higher reference ranges occur at higher altitudes. The reference interval for hematocrits is quite wide. Thus, if an individual begins near the upper end of the interval, as much as one-fifth of the red cell volume may be lost before anemia can be demonstrated by a hematocrit below the bottom of the reference interval. Comparisons with previous hematocrits are important in assessing the development of anemia. For any one individual, the hematocrit is physiologically maintained within quite narrow limits. Thus, changes in hematocrit may be a better diagnostic measure.

Uric Acid Precision and Accuracy

Uric acid levels in the blood can be measured precisely using automated techniques. There are several different methods, each of which gives slightly different levels. It is important to compare levels obtained by the same method. Levels of uric acid can vary over short periods. Dehydration, for instance, can rapidly and substantially increase uric acid. Uric acid blood levels accurately measure the uric acid in the serum. They do not, however, accurately assess all the important physiologic parameters of uric acid. They are not an accurate gauge of total body uric acid. Crystallized and deposited uric acid, for instance, is not included in the serum measurement. With respect to the development of gout, crystallized and deposited uric acid is often the governing consideration. In addition, uric acid serum levels are only one factor affecting the excretion of uric acid. Some individuals without a high level of serum uric acid may excrete large quantities of uric acid, predisposing them to uric acid stones.

Reference Interval

The reference interval for uric acid is quite wide; the interval varies from about 3.5 to 8.5 mg per dl in most laboratories, with some variation depending on the method used. A large number of individuals are found with values slightly above the upper reference limit and very few are found with values below the lower reference limit. Very few individuals with values only slightly above the upper reference limit develop gout. This has caused some clinicians to argue that slightly high levels of uric acid should not be treated. They are actually arguing that the upper reference interval should be increased so that the serum level of uric acid can improve performance when used to separate those who are predisposed to gout from those who are not.

Completeness

When participants are recruited based on inclusion and exclusion criteria, the aim is for all patients to undergo both the index test and the reference standard test. It is possible that participants may undergo one of the tests, usually the index test, and then fail to have the other test. This is a form of loss to follow-up that, like other forms of loss to follow-up, can bias an investigation if those lost to follow-up are different from those who remain.[8.12]

Thus, at a minimum, the investigators are expected to report the number and characteristics of those who are lost to follow-up. This is usually done as part of the overall flowchart of participation.

[8.12] The reason for the absence of a test result may not be known and the measurement may be referred to as missing. When results are missing, it is tempting to assume that the measurements are on average the same as those for other similar participants. When this is done, we say that the data is *interpolated*. Interpolation is a general term implying that data is filled in, usually between two points that are actually measured, as opposed to *extrapolation*, which implies that data is extended beyond the points actually measured. The form of interpolation referred to here makes the assumption that missing data is missing by chance and therefore the measurement would have been on average the same as the data on those we were not missing. This assumption may often turn out to be incorrect. Thus, when using interpolation, it is often important to also analyze the data by excluding participants with missing data.

In addition to the issue of completeness, test results may at times be inconclusive or indeterminant. For instance, lung scans as a test for pulmonary embolism are often reported as three potential outcomes: low probability or negative, high probability or positive, and intermediate probability or inconclusive.

A test may also be indeterminant because it was not possible to successfully complete the test for technical reasons; failure of the patient to be willing or able to fully cooperate; or various other reasons. When a large percentage of the results are indeterminant or inconclusive, this may greatly affect the value of the test, as illustrated in the next example:

> **Mini-Study 8.17** ■ A new index test for acute aortic rupture was shown to produce results very similar to the reference standard when it is positive and also when it is negative. However, over 50% of the time the test could not be completed because of its technical complexity. In addition, 10% of the patients died while waiting for the results.

Tests that have a substantial number of indeterminant values may not be as useful as they first appear. As illustrated in this example, it is important to understand not only the probability of indeterminant results but also the reasons that they occur. If the results take considerable time, they may not be helpful for an emergency condition such as ruptured aortic aneurysm even if they are eventually shown to be just as good as the reference standard test.

We have now examined how the index test is measured and are ready to see how these measurements can be compared with the reference standard test. We are ready to move on to the results, interpretation and extrapolation components of the M.A.A.R.I.E. framework in Chapter 9.

REFERENCES

1. Bossuyt PM, Reitsma JB, Bruns DE, et al. Towards complete and accurate reporting of studies of diagnostic accuracy: the STARD initiative. *Ann Intern Med.* 2003; 138(1):40–44.

2. Sackett DL, Haynes RB, Guyatt GH, Tugwell P. *Clinical Epidemiology: A Basic Science for Clinical Medicine.* 2nd ed. Boston, MA: Little, Brown and Company; 1991.

3. Grobbee DE, Hoes AW. *Clinical Epidemiology: Principles, Methods, and Applications for Clinical Research.* Sudbury, MA: Jones and Bartlett Publishers; 2009.

4. Guyatt G, Rennie D, Meade MO, Cook DJ. *Users' Guides to the Medical Literature: Essentials of Evidence-Based Clinical Practice.* 2nd ed. New York, NY: McGraw-Hill Companies; 2008.

5. Mayer D. *Essential Evidence-Based Medicine.* Cambridge, UK: Cambridge University Press; 2004.

6. Fletcher R, Fletcher S. *Clinical Epidemiology: The Essentials.* 4th ed. Baltimore, MD: Lippincott Williams & Wilkins; 2005.

7. Guyatt G, Rennie D. *Users' Guides to the Medical Literature: A Manual for Evidence-based Practice.* Chicago, IL: AMA Press; 2002.

thePoint ✳ Visit http://thePoint.lww.com for interactive Q&A, flaw-catching exercises, searchable eBook, and more!

9 | Testing a Test—M.A.A.R.I.E. Framework: Results, Interpretation, and Extrapolation

RESULTS (1,2)

The results component of the M.A.A.R.I.E. framework for Testing a Test asks about the performance of the index test compared with the reference standard, that is, gold standard test, or definitive test. The results component presents quantitative estimates of the information provided by the index test compared with the perfectly performing reference standard. Confidence intervals can be used to draw inferences from these estimates. Finally, the results need to take into account the relative importance of false positives and false negatives when evaluating the diagnostic ability of a test.

Estimates: Sensitivity and Specificity

The results component of the M.A.A.R.I.E. framework asks us to compare the index test and the reference standard test, that is, the gold standard or perfect test. The aim is to produce summary measurements or estimates of the performance of the index test compared with the what we define as the perfect or gold standard test. The basic measurements that are used to perform this important job are called *sensitivity* and *specificity*. A single summary measurement can be produced by combining sensitivity and specificity to calculate what is called *discriminant ability*. These are the estimates used in reporting the results of an investigation of tests. Let us see first how we calculate sensitivity and specificity.

Sensitivity measures the proportion or percentage of the participants with the disease as defined by the reference standard test who are correctly identified by the index test. In other words, it measures how well the index test detects the disease. It may be helpful to think of sensitivity as *positive in disease*.

Specificity measures the proportion or percentage of the participants who are free of the disease, as defined by the reference standard test, that are correctly labeled free of the disease by the index test. In other words, it measures the ability of the index test to detect the absence of the disease. Specificity can be thought of as a *negative in health*.

To calculate sensitivity and specificity, the investigator must do the following:

1. Classify each participant as being disease positive or disease negative according to the results of the reference standard test
2. Classify each participant as positive or negative according to the index test
3. Relate the results of the reference standard test to the index test, often using the following 2 × 2 table:

	Reference Standard Positive = Disease	Reference Standard Negative = Free of the Disease
Index test positive	*A* = Number of participants with the disease and index test positive = *true positives*	*B* = Number of participants without the disease and index test positive = *false positives*
Index test negative	*C* = Number of participants with the disease and index test negative = *false negative*	*D* = Number of participants without the disease and index test negative = *true negative*
	A + *C* = Total with the disease	*B* + *D* = Total free of the disease

Sensitivity = percentage of the participants with the disease as defined by the reference standard test who are correctly identified as having the disease by the index test = $A/(A + C)$ × 100% = true positives/(true positive + false negatives) × 100%

Specificity = percentage of the participants who are free of the disease as defined by the reference standard test and who are correctly labeled free of the disease by the index test = $D/(D + B)$ × 100% = true negatives/(true negatives + false positives) × 100%

To illustrate this procedure using numbers, imagine that a new test is performed on 500 participants who have the disease according to the reference standard test and 500 participants who are free of the disease according to the reference standard test. We can now set up the 2 × 2 table as follows[9.1]:

	Reference Standard Positive = Disease	Reference Standard Negative = Free of the Disease
Index test positive	**400 = true positives**	**50 = false positives**
Index test negative	**100 = false negatives**	**450 = true negatives**

Sensitivity = 400/500 × 100% = 80%

Specificity = 450/500 × 100% = 90%

A sensitivity of 80% and a specificity of 90% are in the range of a number of tests used clinically to screen for and diagnose disease such as mammography and exercise stress testing.[9.2]

Notice that the sensitivity and specificity are always defined in comparison to the reference standard test. That is, the best that an index test can achieve is to produce the same results as the reference standard test. When there is a disagreement between the index test and the reference standard test, the index test is considered wrong and the reference standard test is considered correct.

What happens if the new test is actually better than the reference standard test? If the new test is safer, cheaper, or more convenient than the reference standard test, it may come to be used in clinical practice even if its performance is considered less than perfect. Clinical experience may eventually demonstrate the new test's superior performance, even allowing the new test to be used as the reference standard test. In the meantime, the best the new test can do is to match the established reference standard test.

Estimates: Discriminant Ability

As we have seen, sensitivity and specificity are our basic measures of how well the index test discriminates between those with the disease and those who are free of the disease.

Sensitivity and specificity together provide us with the information we need to judge the performance of the index test relative to the reference standard test. Ideally, however, we would like to have one number that summarizes the performance of the test. Fortunately, there is a simple

---

[9.1] Notice that the index test being evaluated has been applied to a group of participants in whom 500 have the disease and 500 are free of the disease as defined by the reference standard test. This division of 50% with the disease and 50% free of the disease has been a common distribution used for an investigation of a new test and provides the greatest statistical power. Notice, however, that does not represent the population's prevalence of the disease except in the unusual circumstance in which the prevalence is 50%.

[9.2] The principles stressed here are most important when the sensitivity and specificity are in this range. When tests have sensitivity and specificity close to 100%, issues such as Bayes' theorem and the relative importance of false positive and false negative take on less importance. Nonetheless, even sensitivities and specificities of greater than 98% may produce large numbers of false-positive results when a disease has a very low prevalence such as 0.01% or 1% in a thousand. Issues such as safety, cost, and patient acceptance may be especially importance at very high sensitivities and specificities.

means to combine the sensitivity and the specificity to obtain a single measurement of what is called the *discriminant ability* of a test. Discriminant ability is the average of the sensitivity plus the specificity:

$$\text{Discriminant ability} = (\text{sensitivity} + \text{specificity})/2$$

Thus, in our example, the sensitivity equals 80% and the specificity equals 90%, and the discriminant ability is calculated as follows:

$$(80\% + 90\%)/2 = 85\%$$

How do we interpret discriminant ability? The discriminant ability tells us how much information the index test provides compared with the reference standard test, which by definition provides perfect information. That is, we assume that the reference standard test does a perfect job of separating positive and negative results. Perfect discriminant ability is therefore 100%. This occurs only when both the sensitivity and the specificity are 100%.

Discriminant ability provides a method to understand the information content of a test. To understand this use of discriminant ability, let us take a look at what we call a *receiver operator characteristics (ROC) curve*. The ROC curve axes are illustrated in Figure 9.1.

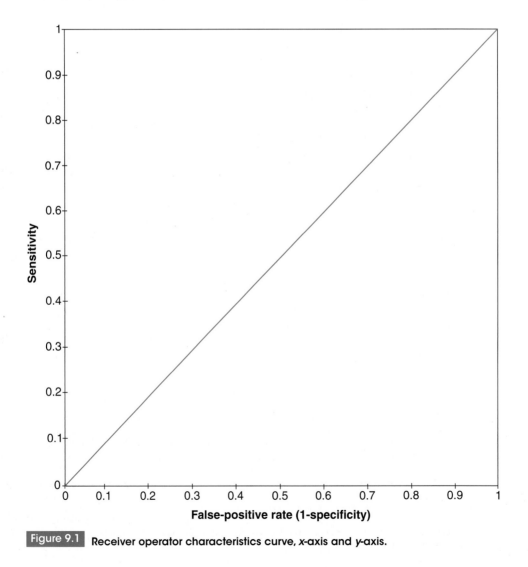

Figure 9.1 Receiver operator characteristics curve, *x*-axis and *y*-axis.

The ROC curve compares the sensitivity on the *y*-axis to 100% − specificity (i.e. the false-positive rate) on the *x*-axis. Notice that for the ROC curve, a perfect test lies at the left upper corner where the sensitivity and specificity are both 100%. Thus, the ROC curve allows us to compare the performance of a particular index test to this perfect test that lies in the left upper corner of the ROC curve.

The diagonal line that crosses from the lower left to the upper right of the ROC curve in Figure 9.1 indicates the zero information line. That is, the combination of sensitivity and specificity that provides no additional information beyond that already known before obtaining the results of the index test. If the discriminant ability is 50%, mere guessing or flipping a coin would do just as well as using the results of the index test.

Now, let us plot our sensitivity of 80% and our specificity of 90% for our index test on the ROC curve. Figure 9.2 plots this index test. It also has lines from this test to the left lower and right upper corners of the ROC curve. The area under these lines turns out to be the discriminant ability,[9.3] that is, the (sensitivity + specificity)/2.

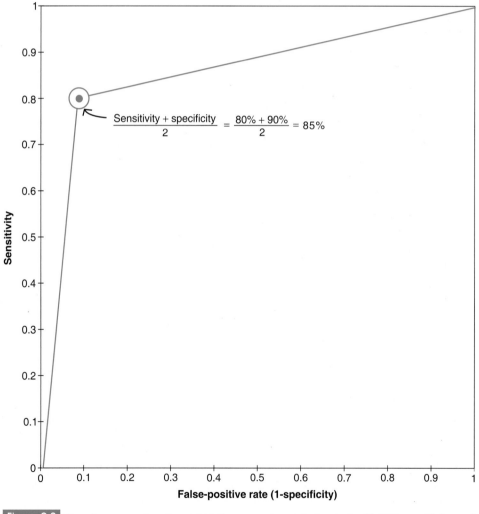

Figure 9.2 Receiver operator characteristics curve for an index test with 80% sensitivity and 90% specificity.

[9.3] To convince yourself of this relationship, draw lines connecting the "dot" to the left lower and right upper corners. Then using geometry, calculate the area under these lines. The sum of these areas equals the discriminant ability.

Here, the discriminant ability is 85%. To understand the discriminant ability, it is important to recognize that the additional information provided by the index test is the difference between the discriminant ability and the diagonal no-information line. Failure to appreciate this principle can lead to the following type of error:

Mini-Study 9.1 ▪ A new test has been shown to have a sensitivity of 60% and a specificity of 40%. The authors of the investigation conclude that although these results are less than ideal, they still indicate the new test has a discriminate ability of 50% and can therefore provide 50% of the information necessary for diagnosis. They thus advise routine use of the test.

The authors are correct that the discriminant ability equals 50%, since $(40\% + 60\%)/2 = 50\%$. However, a discriminant ability of 50% indicates that the test provides no additional information beyond what is already known. Thus, when drawing conclusions about the discriminant ability, the area under the ROC curve, we need to compare this summary measurement to 50%, not to 0%.

As we have seen, discriminant ability and the ROC curve tell us how well an index test performs. Discriminant ability can also be helpful in determining the best cutoff points to use to define positive and negative for the index test if our goal is to maximize the discriminate ability of the index test. This approach is discussed in Learn More 9.1.

LEARN MORE 9.1 ▪ **USING ROC CURVES TO SET CUT-POINTS FOR POSITIVE AND NEGATIVE RESULTS** ▪ Remember that in Chapter 8 we stressed the need to define a positive and a negative result and indicated that an additional approach is available. One increasingly common approach is to wait to choose the cutoff points for positive and negative until after the measurements of both the index test and reference standard test are known.

Using this approach to select the best cutoff point to define negatives and positives for the index test, the investigator chooses the cutoff point at which the discriminant ability will be maximized.[9.4] Thus, to determine the cutoff point, the investigators may take the following steps:

1. Choose several potential cutoff points
2. Calculate the sensitivity and specificity for each set of potential cutoff points
3. Calculate the discriminant ability for each set of potential cutoff points
4. Choose the set of cutoff points that produces the greatest discriminant ability

Thus, we have now seen that sensitivity, specificity, and their average (the discriminant ability) are the most common measures of a test's performance. Once these summary measures or estimated are obtained, we need to examine the issue of inference or how the results may have been affected by chance.

Inference

When drawing inferences from the results of an investigation of a test, we are interested in whether the results that we observe are likely to hold true in larger populations like those from which the sample was obtained. To address this question, the STARD statement recommends that investigations of tests report not only the sensitivity and specificity but also the confidence intervals around the sensitivity and specificity.

[9.4] Determining the maximum discriminant ability is the same as finding the point on the ROC curve that maximizes the area under the curve. Thus, this method may also be referred to as maximizing the area under the ROC curve.

Thus, investigations of tests are increasingly reporting the observed sensitivity and specificity and also their 95% confidence intervals. These confidence intervals tell us how much confidence we should place on the results observed in our samples. They let us know that the true values in the population from which the samples were obtained may be higher or lower than the observed values.

It is important to recognize that one factor affecting the confidence interval is the number of participants included in the investigation. Everything else being equal, the larger the number of participants, the narrower is the confidence interval. Large investigations will tend to have narrow confidence limits and will encourage us to place more confidence in their results.

Ideally, confidence intervals for tests are converted into statistical significance levels. However, we do not expect to be able to conclude that one test's sensitivity or specificity is statistically significant compared with another. Thus, for tests, we merely ask the question: What is the 95% confidence interval around the sensitivity and the specificity?

Adjustment: Diagnostic Ability

In investigations of tests, like other types of investigation, we need to ask whether there are other factors that need to be taken into account or adjusted for as part of the analysis of the results. When we discussed the measurement of discriminant ability, we assumed that a false negative and a false positive were equally undesirable. That is, we gave equal weight or importance to false negatives and false positives.[9.5]

False-negative results and false-positive results may not always be of equal importance. There are various reasons why a false negative and a false positive may not be of equal importance, for instance,

- A false negative may or may not result in harm to the patient, depending on whether the disease may be detected later at a time before there are irreversible adverse consequences.
- A false positive may or may not result in harm to the patient, depending on the probability of harm due to further testing and/or from treatment begun on the basis of a false-positive test.

To better understand what we mean by the relative importance of false-negative and false-positive results, we can examine testing for glaucoma and ask the question: What factors influence the importance of false-negative and false-positive results?

- Factors that may influence the importance of false-negative results for glaucoma include: vision loss from glaucoma is largely irreversible and may develop before it is apparent to the patient. Treatment is generally safe but not completely effective in preventing progressive visual loss. Regular repeat routine testing may still detect the glaucoma in time for treatment to prevent substantial visual loss.
- Factors that influence the importance of false-positive tests include: follow-up of initial positive results requires multiple tests and follow-up visits that may create patient anxieties and costs. Follow-up tests pose little danger of harm to the patient.

Thus for glaucoma testing, let us assume that you came to the conclusion that a false-negative is worse than a false-positive result. Let us see how this conclusion can influence the use of tests, as illustrated in the next example:

[9.5] Discriminant ability assumes that false positives and false negatives are of equal importance. Thus, when maximizing discriminant ability to set the cutoff points, one is also assuming that false positives are equal to false negatives. Thus, cutoff lines should ideally also include consideration of the relative importance of false positives and false negatives.

Mini-Study 9.2 ■ Test A for glaucoma had a sensitivity of 70% and a specificity of 90%, giving it a discriminant ability of 80%. Test B for glaucoma had a sensitivity of 80% and a specificity of 80%, giving it the same discriminant ability. The investigators concluded that these two tests were interchangeable in terms of diagnostic ability.

These two tests are interchangeable in terms of discriminant ability since each has an 80% discriminant ability. However, diagnostic ability requires us to also consider the relative importance of false negatives and false positives.

If we regard a false negative as worse than a false positive, we might prefer Test B since it has a higher sensitivity and thus fewer false negatives. This preference for Test B would result in more false positives. If, on the other hand, we regard false positives as worse than false negatives, we might favor Test A since it has a higher specificity and thus fewer false positives. Since we previously decided that false negatives are considered worse than false positives, we should prefer Test B to Test A.[9.6]

We have now examined the results component of the M.A.A.R.I.E. framework and have found that sensitivity, specificity, and their average (discriminant ability) are the measures used to judge the information obtained from an index test. We have seen that confidence intervals rather than statistical significance tests are used to report test results. We have seen that a false positive and a false negative may not be of equal importance. Now we are ready to go on to the interpretation of the results.

INTERPRETATION (3–5)

Sensitivity, specificity, and discriminant ability have been chosen as measures because they are inherent characteristics of a test that should be the same when the test is applied to a group of patients in whom the disease is rare or to a group of patients in whom the disease is frequent. That is, they provide estimates of a test's performance that should be the same regardless of the pretest probability of a disease—the probability of the disease before the test is performed. Ideally, this allows researchers in Boston, Barcelona, or Beijing to apply the same test and interpret the results of testing despite their very different populations.

Interpretation requires us to do more than ask how much information is provided by a test or which test provides the most information. It asks us to use the information to address the following questions:

- *Ruling in and ruling out disease*: Interpretation asks us to compare two or more index tests to determine which performs the best for ruling in and ruling out a disease.
- *Posttest chances of disease, or Bayes' theorem*: Interpretation asks us to combine information from what we have called the pretest probability of disease with the information from the test to draw conclusions about the chances of disease after information from the test is included.
- *Clinical performance*: Interpretation also asks us to take into account safety, costs, and patient acceptance when drawing conclusions about the use of a test.

[9.6] No attempt is made here to quantitate the relative importance of false positives and false negatives. Although possible, this process is rarely seen in the research literature. The impact of different weights on false positives and false negatives usually has its impact on the cutoff point selected between positives and negatives. The trade-off between false negatives and false positives is also affected by the number of false negatives and the number of false positives that will occur. This in turn is affected by the pretest probability of the disease. When more than one index test is being compared with a reference standard, it is important to determine whether the index tests generally have the same or different types of false positives and false negatives. This will be important when we look at strategies for combining tests.

Ruling In and Ruling Out Disease

As we have seen, the ROC curve is very useful for graphing sensitivity and specificity and visualizing discriminant ability. In addition, ROC curves can be used to visualize which test does the best to rule in and rule out a disease. Figure 9.3 illustrates how we can use the ROC curve to answer these questions. Figure 9.3 indicates with a black dot the sensitivity and false-positive rate (1-specificity) of a test to which other tests are being compared. The performance of a second test can be compared with this test by graphing the second test's results on the same ROC curve. The second test may be located in one of four locations labeled on Figure 9.3. These have the following meaning:

- Superior discriminant ability—the second test is better for ruling in and also ruling out the disease
- Inferior discriminant ability—the second test is worse for ruling in and also ruling out the disease
- Superior for ruling out—the second test is better for ruling out but worse for ruling in the disease
- Superior for ruling in—the second test is better for ruling in but worse for ruling out the disease

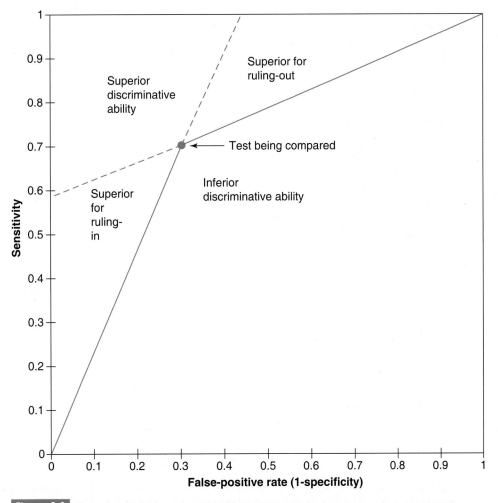

Figure 9.3 **Use of receiver operator characteristics (ROC) curve to decide which test is better for ruling in and ruling out a disease.** If a test's sensitivity and false-positive rate are represented by the black dot, then test results for other tests can be compared based on where they fall on the ROC curve.

Let us look at an example of how we can use the ROC curve:

Mini-Study 9.3 ■ Let us assume that two tests have the same discriminant ability. Test Yellow has a sensitivity of 90% and a specificity of 70%. Test Blue has a sensitivity of 85% and a specificity of 75%. Everything else being equal, which test is better to rule in the disease? Which test is better to rule out the disease?

Figure 9.4 illustrates how we can use the ROC curve. Since test Yellow is up and to the right of Test Blue, it falls within the area designated as "superior for ruling out" in Figure 9.3. This indicates that Test Yellow is better for ruling out the disease but that Test Blue is better for ruling in the disease.[9.7]

It is tempting to conclude that the better test to rule in the disease is the test with the greatest specificity and the better test to rule out the disease is the test with the greatest sensitivity. Although this is often true, there are exceptions as illustrated in Learn More 9.2.

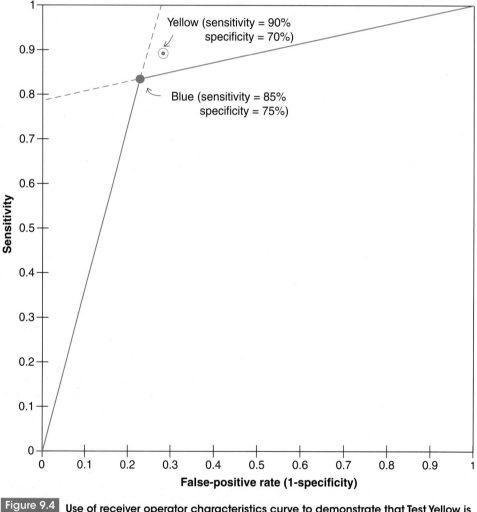

Figure 9.4 Use of receiver operator characteristics curve to demonstrate that Test Yellow is superior for ruling out the disease and Test Blue is superior for ruling in the disease.

[9.7] If you draw the lines through the Yellow test instead of the Blue test, the results will be the same though the graphic will look somewhat different. Try it out.

LEARN MORE 9.2 ▪ BEST TEST TO USE TO RULE IN AND RULE OUT A DISEASE ▪ The best test to use to rule in a disease is not always the test with the greatest specificity and the best test to use to rule out a disease is not always the test with the greatest sensitivity. Take a look at the following example:

Mini-Study 9.4 ▪ Let us imagine that Test Red has a sensitivity of 80% and a specificity of 70%, whereas Test Green has a sensitivity of 85% and a specificity of 50%. Everything else being equal, which test is the better test to rule in the disease? Which test is the better test to rule out the disease?

Figure 9.4 illustrates that Test Red is actually better both for ruling in and slightly better for ruling out the disease.[9.8] This is the situation since Test Green falls within the "inferior discriminant ability" area as illustrated in Figure 9.5.

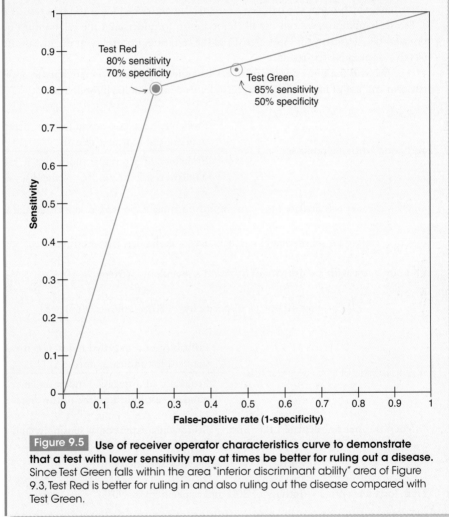

Figure 9.5 Use of receiver operator characteristics curve to demonstrate that a test with lower sensitivity may at times be better for ruling out a disease. Since Test Green falls within the area "inferior discriminant ability" area of Figure 9.3, Test Red is better for ruling in and also ruling out the disease compared with Test Green.

[9.8] This example also illustrates that likelihood ratios, which we will discuss later in this chapter, rather than either sensitivity or specificity alone are the best way to compare tests to determine which test is best for ruling in and which test is best for ruling out the disease. Use of likelihood ratios may produce results that are not intuitive. Imagine for instance that Test no. 1 has a sensitivity of 80% and a specificity of 70%. Test no. 2 has a sensitivity of 85% and a specificity of 50%. Test no. 1 has the largest likelihood ratio of a positive test and the smallest likelihood ratio of a negative test. Thus, Test no. 1 should be used to rule in and to rule out the disease, everything else being equal. It is important to remember, however, that this conclusion also assumes that other factors that affect our choice of test, such as cost, safety and patient acceptance, are equal. As we will see, this is rarely the situation.

Posttest Chances of Disease: Bayes' Theorem

In chapter 8 we looked at how the pretest probability of a disease can be estimated starting with disease prevalence and taking into account other diseases and risk factors, symptoms, and at times other test results. To interpret the results of a test, this pretest probability of disease needs to be combined with the information that is obtained from a test using what is called *Bayes' theorem*.[9.9]

Bayes' theorem is fundamental to the process of combining information on the pretest chances of the disease with information from the test of interest, that is, the index test. There are several ways to express Bayes' theorem, but one that is particularly helpful for understanding the relationship between pretest and posttest chances of the disease is the likelihood ratio form of Bayes' theorem. Therefore, we need to understand what we mean by *likelihood ratios*.

Likelihood ratios can be calculated from sensitivity and specificity. Likelihood ratios can be used instead of ROC curves to directly compare two or more index tests. They allow us to determine which one is the best test to use to rule in and which is the best test to use to rule out a disease. In addition, we can use likelihood ratio to understand the relationship between pretest probabilities, sensitivity and specificity, and the resulting probability of the disease after obtaining a positive or negative test result.

We will use our example of an 80% sensitivity and a 90% specificity to appreciate the calculation and use of likelihood ratios. First, let us define the likelihood ratios.

$$\text{Likelihood ratio of a positive test (LR+)} = \frac{\text{Probabity of a positive index test if reference standard test indicates disease}}{\text{Probabity of a positive index test if reference standard test indicates free of the disease}}$$

Often it is easier to calculate LR(+) using this formula expressed as sensitivity and specificity

$$LR(+) = \text{sensitivity}/(1 - \text{specificity}) = \text{sensitivity}/\text{false-positive rate}$$

Thus, for a test with a sensitivity of 80% and a specificity of 90%,

$$LR(+) = \text{sensitivity}/(1 - \text{specificity}) = 80\%/(100\% - 90\%) = 8$$

$$\text{Likelihood ratio of a negative test (LR-)} = \frac{\text{Probabity of a negative index test if reference standard test indicates disease}}{\text{Probabity of a negative index test if reference standard test indicates free of the disease}}$$

Often, it is easier to calculate LR(−) using this formula expressed as sensitivity and specificity

$$LR(-) = (1 - \text{sensitivity})/\text{specificity}$$

Thus, for a test with a sensitivity of 80% and a specificity of 90%,

$$LR(-) = (1 - \text{sensitivity})/\text{specificity} = (100\% - 80\%)/90\% = 0.22$$

[9.9]We have identified the factors that go into the pretest probability of the disease. Unfortunately, there is no general agreement on how to combine or weight these factors. Therefore, two clinicians may agree on each of the factors that go into calculating the pretest probability and still come to different conclusions about the pretest probability. At times, clinicians may place greater weight on information obtained from symptoms than from information obtained from other factors. This may result in underestimating the pretest probability of common diseases and overestimating the pretest probability of rare diseases.

How can we interpret these likelihood ratios? Likelihood ratios provide a direct indication of the amount of useful diagnostic information contained in a positive and in a negative test. Likelihood ratios tell us the probability that an index test will be correct compared with the probability that it will be incorrect. Thus, likelihood ratios provide a ratio alerting us to the probability of correct information compared with the probability of incorrect information. An LR(+) or LR(−) of 1 indicates that no diagnostic information is gained by knowing that the test is positive or that the test is negative.

For a likelihood ratio of a positive test (LR+), we are comparing the probability that a positive index test indicates disease with the probability that it indicates that an individual is free of the disease. A likelihood ratio of a positive test can vary from 1 to infinity, and larger is better.

A likelihood ratio of a negative test (LR−) tells us the probability that a negative index test will be incorrect compared with the probability it will be correct. For a likelihood ratio of a negative test, we are comparing the probability that a negative index test indicates disease with the probability that it indicates that an individual is free of the disease. A likelihood ratio of a negative test can vary from 1 to 0, and smaller is better.

The likelihood ratios help us understand which test is best for ruling in and for ruling out disease.

- Everything else being equal, the test with the greatest likelihood ratio of a positive test is the best test to use to rule in the disease.
- Everything else being equal, the test with the smallest likelihood ratio of a negative test is the best test to use to rule out the disease.

Likelihood ratios can help make clear the relationship between pretest probability and posttest probability. If the pretest probability of disease is known or can be estimated, Bayes' theorem allows us to calculate the posttest probabilities of a disease after obtaining the results of a test. These posttest probabilities of disease are often called the *predictive values*. The *predictive value of a positive test* indicates the probability that the disease is present after obtaining a positive result on the index test. The *predictive value of a negative test* indicates the probability that the disease is absent after obtaining a negative result on the indexed test. Thus, 1 minus predictive value of a negative test tells us the probability that the disease will be *present* after obtaining a negative result on the test.

One way to appreciate the relationship between the pretest chances of the disease, the likelihood ratios, and the posttest chances of disease is to examine the likelihood ratio form of Bayes' theorem, as discussed in Learn More 9.3.

LEARN MORE 9.3 ■ LIKELIHOOD RATIO FORM OF BAYES'

THEOREM ■ The likelihood ratio form of Bayes' theorem for a positive test results states:

> Posttest odds that the disease is present if the test is positive =
> Odds that the disease is present before the test × Likelihood ratio of a positive test

Remember that odds like probability includes those with the disease in the numerator but odds, in contrast to probability, only includes those without the disease in the denominator.

The likelihood ratio form of Bayes' theorem for a negative test results states:

> Posttest odds that the disease is present if the test is negative =
> Odds that the disease is present before the test × Likelihood ratio of a negative test

Thus, if we know or can estimate the odds that disease is present before conducting a test and we also know the relevant likelihood ratios of test, we can multiply the two and determine the odds of disease after the results of the test are known. That is, we obtain the odds of disease after the results of the test are known by multiplying the pretest odds times the likelihood ratio of either a negative or a positive test, depending on the results of the test. We still need to convert odds to

(Continued)

probabilities but as we will see, there are charts or nomograms that can do that for us.

For instance, if the probability of the disease is 50%, the odds are 1:1 (one to one). For our test, a likelihood ratio of a positive test is 8. Thus, the posttest odds = (pretest odds) (LR+) = 1 × 8 = 8. That is, if the pretest odds are 1:1 or 1, the posttest odds are 8:1 or 8. A posttest odds of 8 is the same as a posttest probability of approximately 89%.

Similarly, if the pretest probability of the disease is 50%, that is, odds are 1 and the likelihood ratio of a negative test is 0.22, then the posttest odds are 0.22. A posttest odds of 0.22 is the same as a posttest probability of approximately 18%.

Although the calculations discussed in Learn More 9.3 may be helpful in understanding the relationship between the chances of disease before and after knowing the results of a test, most people think in probabilities, not in odds. Fortunately, Bayes' theorem also allows us to start with pretest probabilities and, using the likelihood ratios we have obtained on the index test, calculate the predictive values of a positive and a negative test.

Table 9.1 displays the predictive value or posttest probability of a positive test and the predictive value or posttest probability of a negative test when using a test with a sensitivity of 80% and a specificity of 90% for pretest probabilities of 1%, 10%, 50%, and 90%. The table shows how the pretest probabilities relate to the predictive value of a positive and also the predictive value of a negative test when we use a test with a sensitivity of 80% and a specificity of 90%. This table demonstrates the dramatic impact that the pretest probability can and often does have on the predictive values or posttest probabilities of disease when the sensitivity and specificity are relatively low.[9,10]

TABLE 9.1	Relationship of Pretest Probability of the Disease to Posttest Probability for a Test with a Sensitivity of 80% and a Specificity of 90%	
Pretest Probability	Posttest Probability of the Disease If Test is Positive i.e, Predictive Value of a Positive Test	Posttest Probability of Being Free of the Disease If Test is Negative, i.e. Predictive Value of a Negative Test (Probability of the Disease)
1%	7.5%	99.8% (0.2%)
10%	47.1%	97.6% (2.4%)
50%	88.9%	81.8% (18.2%)
90%	98.6%	33.3% (66.7%)

Let us return to the examples of a 23-year-old woman and a 65-year-old man we encountered as we began the Testing a Test section. As we discussed, ruling in and ruling out disease requires more than the results of a test. It requires us to make our best estimate or educated guess regarding the probability or odds of disease before the test is conducted.

Now let us use these examples to demonstrate with numbers the impact of pretest probability on the probability of disease after the results of a test are known, or what we have called the posttest probability or the predictive value of the test. For our examples of a 65-year-old man and

---

[9,10]Note that the predictive value of a positive test and the predictive value of a negative test can be directly calculated from a 2 × 2 table if the number of individuals with and without the disease in the population are reflected in the 2 × 2 table. In this situation, the predictive value of a positive test equals the number of true positives divided by the sum of the number of true positives plus the number of false positives. The predictive value of a negative test can be calculated as the number of true negatives divided by the sum of the number of true negatives plus the number of false negatives. The predictive value of a positive test indicates the probability that the disease is present according to the reference standard test if the index test is positive. The predictive value of a negative test indicates the probability that the disease is absent according to the reference standard test if the index test is negative.

a 23-year-old woman, we will assume that a stress test has a sensitivity of 80% and a specificity of 90%. Once again, we will be estimating the posttest probability or predictive values of

- a 23-year-old female athlete with a chest pain and a family history of coronary artery disease (assuming her pretest probability of coronary artery disease is 1% and her stress test is positive).
- a 65-year-old man with chest pain and multiple risk factors for coronary artery disease (assuming his pretest probability of coronary artery disease is 50% and his stress test is now negative.)

Let us see how these results affect the posttest probabilities or predictive values. Looking at Table 9.1, we find that the following:

- the 23-year-old women with a pretest probability of coronary artery disease of 1% and a positive stress test has a predictive value of a positive test or a posttest probability of coronary artery disease of only 7.5%.
- the 65 year old man with a pretest probability of coronary artery disease of 50% and a negative test has a predictive value of a negative test or a posttest probability of *not having* coronary artery disease of 81.8% (that is, he has approximately an 18% probability of *having* coronary artery disease).

Thus, the 23-year-old woman with a positive stress test actually has a lower probability of having coronary artery disease (7.5%) than the 65-year-old man with a negative stress test (18%). Thus for many clinical tests, it is essential to focus not only on the test results, but on the pretest probability of the disease to understand the probability of disease after the test results are known.

Another way to obtain these same results is to use a nomogram that allows us to go from pretest probability using the likelihood ratio of the test result to obtain a posttest probability of disease. Learn More 9.4 illustrates the use of this type of nomogram.

Finally, 2 × 2 tables can be used to display the results of Bayes' theorem and allow you to calculate the predictive values for any pretest probability by filling in the table and using the 2 × 2 table to calculate the predictive values. This use of Bayes' theorem is illustrated in Learn More 9.5.

Clinical Acceptance

As we have seen, the likelihood ratios and the pretest probabilities of disease are the key information needed to interpret the results of a test. However, they are not the only issues. Additional issues such as safety, cost, and patient acceptance often are important, especially when we are asked to choose between tests. Data from an investigation may be helpful in answering questions such as:

- The type and frequency of adverse events associated with the test
- The frequency with which additional tests are required if the test is positive or negative, and thus some appreciation of the costs
- An estimate of the degree of patient adherence to the protocol as a measure of patient acceptance

As part of the interpretation of the test, we should be asking these types of questions. For instance, patients in the investigation may not return or complete the test, suggesting a low level of acceptance. Depending on the nature of the test, this may be due to inconvenience, discomfort, or the intrusive nature of the test.

The cost of the test is generally covered by the investigation itself and is not generally a factor in whether or not the patient participates. However, cost may affect the use of the test in clinical practice. Thus, it is helpful if the investigator reports data on the resources required, including professional time to conduct and interpret the test. This provides useful information for extrapolating to the use of the test in clinical practice.

Data on safety need to be reported, indicating side effects or adverse events associated with use of the test in enough detail to enable the reader to understand the nature and timing of the adverse events.

LEARN MORE 9.4 ■ USE OF A NOMOGRAM TO CALCULATE POSTTEST PROBABILITY OF DISEASE ■ The nomogram in Figure 9.6 allows us to obtain the posttest probability of a disease if we can estimate the probability of disease before the test is preformed (the pretest probability) and if we know the likelihood ratio of the test results.

Pretest probability % of disease	Likelihood ratio ±	Posttest probability % of disease

Figure 9.6 **Nomogram that can be used to relate the pretest probability of the disease to the posttest probabilities or predictive values using the likelihood ratios.** (Modified from Fagan TJ. Nomogram for Bayes' theorem. *N Engl J Med.* 1975;293:257.)

To use the nomogram, we do the following:

1. Estimate the pretest probability or prior probability
2. Find from the literature the likelihood ratio of a negative or a positive test, depending on the results of the test
3. Draw a straight line through these two points and extend it to the posttest probability of disease line to obtain an estimate of posttest probability

(Continued)

For the 23-year-old woman, we begin with a pretest probability of disease of 1% and obtain a positive exercise stress test. The likelihood ratio of a positive exercise stress test is 8. Thus, as illustrated in Figure 9.7, the posttest probability of coronary artery disease is 7.5%.

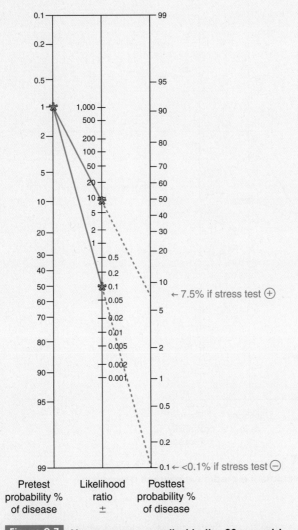

Figure 9.7 Nomogram as applied to the 23-year-old women to calculate the predictive value of a positive test.

For the 65-year-old man, we begin with a pretest probability of 50% and obtain a negative exercise stress test. The likelihood ratio of a negative exercise stress test is 0.22. Thus, as illustrated in Figure 9.8, the posttest probability of coronary artery disease is 18%.

(Continued)

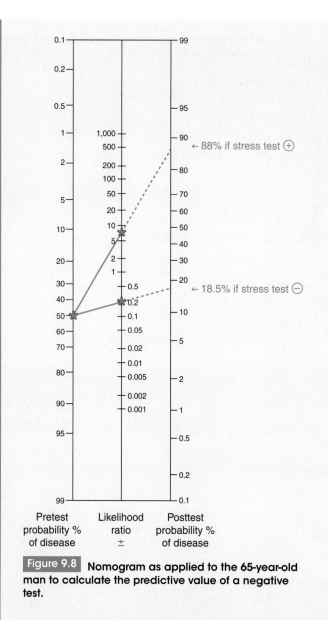

Pretest
probability %
of disease

Likelihood
ratio
±

Posttest
probability %
of disease

Figure 9.8 **Nomogram as applied to the 65-year-old man to calculate the predictive value of a negative test.**

These results are the same as we found when using the odds ratio form of Bayes' theorem. They are also the same as we would obtain if we used 2 × 2 boxes. Since we are dealing with three different ways to use Bayes' theorem, we expect all the results to be the same.

**LEARN MORE 9.5 ■ USING 2 × 2 TABLES TO CALCULATE PREDIC-
TIVE VALUES ■** Using 2 × 2 tables to calculate predictive value begins with
blank 2 × 2 tables that allow comparison of the index test results and the disease as measured by the reference standard or gold standard test. Figure 9.9
displays 2 × 2 tables for pretest probabilities of 1%, 10%, 50%, and 90%. For the
1% pretest probability situation, the 1% implies that 10 out of 1,000 individuals
have the disease. For the 10% pretest probability, the 10% implies that 100 out
of 1,000 individuals have the disease and so on. Notice that these figures are
filled in at the bottom of each 2 × 2 table, indicating the total with and without the disease.

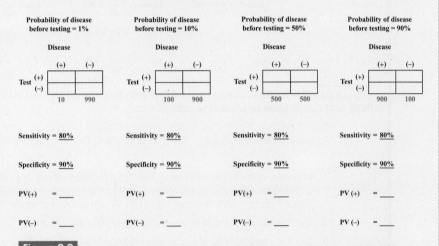

Figure 9.9 **2 × 2 table with pretest probabilities or prevalence of 1%, 10%,
50%, and 90%.**

Once the 2 × 2 tables are set up to reflect the pretest probability or
prevalence of the disease and we have identified the sensitivity and the
specificity of the test, we can use the sensitivity and specificity to fill in the
2 × 2 tables. For the 1% situation, an 80% sensitivity means that 8 out of the 10
individuals with the disease will be true positive and 2 will be false positives.
Thus, we can fill in the left upper box with 8 and the left lower box with 2.

Using the same approach, we can fill in the boxes on the right-hand
side of the 2 × 2 table for the 1% pretest probability using the specificity.
Among the 990 individuals without the disease, 90% will be true negative and
10% will be false negatives. Thus, 0.90 × 990 = 891 and 0.10 × 990 = 99. Therefore, we can fill in the right upper box with 99 and the right lower box with 891.
The 2 × 2 tables for the 10%, 50%, and 90% probability of disease before testing
can be filled in using the same method.

Figure 9.10 displays all four filled in 2 × 2 tables with the predictive values of a positive test and the predictive value of a negative.[9.11]

(Continued)

[9.11] The predictive value of a negative test asks: What is the probability that the disease is absent after obtaining a negative
test. At times, you may see this information presented instead as the *false-negative rate*. The false-negative rate is the probability that the disease is present after obtaining a negative test. Thus, the predictive value of a negative and the false-negative
rate adds to 100%.

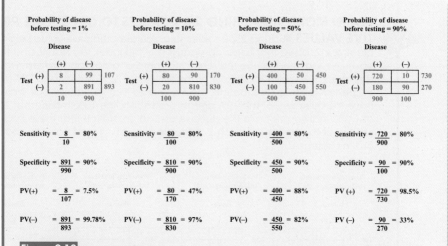

Figure 9.10 2 × 2 table filled in using a test with 80% sensitivity and 90% specificity with calculation of predictive values.

To summarize, the steps in filling in and using the 2 × 2 table are as follows:

1. Fill in the data in the row below the 2 × 2 table to reflect the prevalence of the disease in the population; that is, if the prevalence is 1%, then for every 1 person with disease, there are 99 without the disease

2. Use the sensitivity to fill in the two boxes in the left column

3. Use the specificity to fill in the two boxes in the right-hand boxes

4. Add across the top row of boxes to obtain the total number of positives

5. Add across the bottom row of boxes to obtain the total number of negatives

6. Calculate the predictive value of a positive using the data in the tops row and its sum

7. Calculate the predictive value of a negative using the data in the bottom row and its sum

It should come as no surprise that the results of the 2 × 2 table form of Bayes' theorem produce the same results as the likelihood ratio form and the nomogram form. Each form of Bayes' theorem is useful for somewhat different purposes. Hopefully, the 2 × 2 form provides you with an understanding how Bayes' theorem utilizes the pretest probability of disease plus the sensitivity and specificity to calculate the posttest probability of disease.

The following example illustrates how the issues of safety, cost, and patient acceptance may influence the interpretation of which test to use:

Mini-Study 9.5 ■ Two tests for gallstones were being compared. Test A has a slightly greater LR(+) and a slightly lower LR(−) indicating that Test A is slightly better for ruling in gallstones and also ruling out gallstones. However, Test A was more expensive, was associated with more adverse events, and resulted in more discomfort to the patient. The researchers recommended that Test A be used only when the patient's clinical condition suggested that the condition was life threatening,

The researchers' recommendation takes into account differences in cost, side effects, and discomfort. Use of tests is often determined as much by their cost, safety, and patient acceptance as they are by small differences in their ability to rule in or rule out a disease. This is especially true when the disease is not considered to be life threatening.[9.12]

Now that we have gathered as much information as possible about the meaning of the test for those in the study's population and we need to go on to ask the most important question: How should the test be used for those who were not included in the investigation? This is the process of extrapolation.

EXTRAPOLATION

Extrapolation of diagnostic test results, like extrapolation in other types of investigations, is the process of going beyond conclusions for participants in the investigation to draw conclusion about those who are not in the investigation. Extrapolation asks questions about the use of the test in other settings.

To Target Population

The aim of most investigations of tests is to draw conclusions about the use of the test in clinical practice. That is, patients in practice are the usual target population for the investigation. When asking questions about usefulness of the test in the target populations, we need to ask following the question:

> Do the conditions for the use of the test in practice differ in ways that are likely to affect its performance?

Extrapolation of test results, like extrapolation of other types of investigations, asks us to examine the assumptions that underlie the conclusions that we have drawn for the participants in the investigation. A key assumption for tests is that their sensitivity and specificity, and thus their discriminant ability will remain the same when the test is applied to new populations with lesser or greater prevalence of the disease. That is, we usually assume that the sensitivity and specificity of a test is the same regardless of the setting in which it is used.

Fortunately, this key assumption does generally hold up. However, when applying a test to a population with a very different severity of disease, its discriminant ability may not be the same, as illustrated in the next example:

> **Mini-Study 9.6** ■ Urine cytology was assessed as a method for diagnosing bladder cancer by comparing those with advanced bladder cancer and those without bladder cancer. The test was shown to have very high discriminant ability. When used in practice, the test did not perform well, missing most of the patients with bladder cancer that was still in the early stages where treatment was effective.

Extrapolation requires that we step back and take a look at the assumptions that were made in investigating the test. If the test was applied to a clinical population that substantially differs from the study's population, its performance in practice may be disappointing. Thus, the most cautious extrapolation is to clinical populations and clinical situations that are very similar to the ones used in the investigation.

[9.12] It is often not clear how to combine considerations of cost, safety, and patient acceptance, that is, how much importance or weight to place on each one. There is no standard formula, and these factors are often considered using subjective judgments.

Beyond the Data

Recommendations for the use of tests in practice often require making additional assumptions. As with extrapolation of the results of other types of investigations, we often need to extrapolate beyond the data.

The timing of tests and their frequency of use are typical issues that often require extrapolation beyond the data. Issues of frequency of use are a key issue for screening programs, but also are relevant to follow-up of a diagnosis.

Conclusions about frequency of follow-up testing are often extrapolations beyond the data since they are not made on the basis of actual patient follow-up. Conclusions regarding frequency of follow-up testing are often made on the basis of current understanding of the course of a disease, as well as the available interventions. When these underlying assumptions change, it is important to be aware of the need to reconsider the frequency of follow-up, as illustrated in the next example:

> **Mini-Study 9.7** ■ Testing for prostate cancer recurrence was advised every 6 months for 5 years based on clinical experience indicating that recurrence was generally slowly occurring and rarely if ever recurrs after 5 years. A new, very successful treatment for early recurrence was developed, leading to the conclusion that more frequent follow-up was needed and the follow-up testing should extend for 10 years.

Thus, the use of tests in clinical practice is subject to change over time, depending on several factors including the available treatment options. Testing always needs to be seen as a means to an end. When the options for treatment change, we often need to reconsider the use of testing.

To Other Settings or Populations

The occurrence of extrapolations to other settings or populations can be obvious, such as when we apply the results obtained in one country to a country with a very different spectrum of disease. It can be more subtle as illustrated in the next example:

> **Mini-Study 9.8** ■ A test for acute cholecystitis was recently developed, and its diagnostic performance evaluated in a carefully conducted study of a spectrum of patients with symptoms compatible with cholecystitis. Patients in the investigation received the new test within 24 hours of the initial presentation with symptoms. The new test was found to improve upon the diagnosis of acute cholecystitis compared with other standard tests. To make the test practical clinically, the authors recommended using the test within 72 hours after the patient's initial onset of symptoms compatible with cholecystitis.

The investigators' recommendations indicate an approach to implementation that is different from the one they investigated. The participants were tested within 24 hours of the onset of symptoms. When extrapolating to clinical practice, they have recommended that the test be performed within 72 hours of onset of symptoms. Although this may be a necessary accommodation to the realities of clinical practice, it is important to recognize that the population being tested may now be very different. In making this extrapolation, the investigators are assuming that delay in testing will not affect the performance. This assumption may or may not hold true.

Extending the time period for referral beyond that in the investigation may affect both the types of patients that are referred and the performance of the test. Extending the time of use may lead to the application of the test to quite different populations in quite different setting. The time extension may lead to far more widespread use of a test, and the performance of the test may not meet expectations. With testing, as with other types of investigations, extrapolation may put us out on a limb and leaves us in limbo. Recognizing the occurrence of extrapolation is a key to appreciating its potential consequences.

We have now examined the application of the M.A.A.R.I.E. framework to an investigation of diagnostic testing. To review and apply the M.A.A.R.I.E. framework to Testing a Test, take a look at the following questions to ask in Testing a Test.

Questions to Ask When Testing a Test

These Questions to Ask can be used as a checklist when reading research articles on diagnostic testing.

Method—The investigation's purpose and population

1. **Purpose:** What is the intended purpose of the investigation?
2. **Study population:** What are the inclusion and exclusion criteria?
3. **Sample size:** What is the sample size?

Assignment—The participants and the tests

1. **Recruitment:** How are the participants recruited?
2. **Assignment process:** Does the assignment process avoid spectrum and verification bias?
3. **Conduct of tests:** How are the index test and reference standard test conducted?

Assessment—Measurement of the outcomes for the index test(s) and reference standard test

1. **Definition of positives and negatives:** How are a positive and a negative result defined for the index test(s)?
2. **Precision and accuracy:** How precise (reproducible) are the index test(s)?
3. **Completeness:** How complete and unequivocal are the test results?

Results—Performance of the index test(s) compared with the reference standard

1. **Estimates: sensitivity, specificity, and discriminant ability:** How well do the index test(s) perform among those with and without the disease as defined by the reference standard?
2. **Inference:** What are the confidence intervals around the estimates?
3. **Diagnostic ability:** How well do the test(s) perform taking into account the relative importance and characteristics of those with false positives and false negatives?

Interpretation—Conclusions for the participants in the investigation

1. **Ruling in and ruling out disease:** Which index test performs better for ruling in and for ruling out a disease?
2. **Posttest chances of disease (Bayes' theorem):** How well do the test(s) perform in diagnosing disease when pretest probability of the disease is taken into account?
3. **Clinical acceptance:** Is there data on patient acceptance, cost, or safety that needs to be taken into account when deciding whether or when to use the test(s)?

Extrapolation—Conclusions for those not included in the investigation

1. **To target population:** Do the conditions for the use of the test in practice differ in ways that is likely to affect its performance?
2. **Beyond the data:** Have the investigators gone beyond the data to draw conclusions on the timing of tests or the frequency of use etc.?
3. **Other settings or populations:** Have the investigators indicated how the index test(s) should be implemented in other settings or populations?

REFERENCES

1. Mayer D. *Essential Evidence-based Medicine*. Cambridge, UK: Cambridge University Press; 2004.

2. Sox HC, Blatt MA, Higgins MC, Marton KI. *Medical Decision Making*. Boston, MA: Butterworth-Heinemann; 1988.

3. Fletcher R, Fletcher S. *Clinical Epidemiology: The Essentials*. 4th ed. Baltimore, MD: Lippincott Williams & Wilkins; 2005.

4. Guyatt G, Rennie D. *Users' Guides to the Medical Literature: A Manual for Evidence-based Practice*. Chicago, IL: AMA Press; 2002.

5. Greenberg RS, Daniels SR, Flanders WD, Eley JW, Boring, JR. *Medical Epidemiology*. 4th ed. New York, NY: Lange Medical Books; 2005.

thePoint ✳ Visit http://thePoint.lww.com for interactive Q&A, flaw-catching exercises, searchable eBook, and more!

10 Screening—Prediction and Decision Rules

Screening for asymptomatic disease as well as prediction and decision rules are two increasingly important applications of the principle of testing that we examined in Chapters 8 and 9. In this chapter, we will take a look at each of these applications of testing principles.

SCREENING (1-3)

Criteria for Successful Screening

Screening is a special form of testing that aims to detect specific diseases in individuals who are asymptomatic for that disease. The goal of screening for a disease is to identify asymptomatic individuals who have the disease in order to intervene to improve outcome.[10.1]

When evaluating a screening test, it is helpful to utilize a series of ideal criteria for justifying screening. Although few screening tests fulfill all of the following criteria, these criteria provide an ideal standard against which particular screening tests can be compared:

1. Substantial morbidity and mortality: The disease or condition often leads to death or disability.
2. Early detection improves outcome: Early detection is possible and improves outcome.
3. Screening is feasible: A high-risk group can be identified and tested using a testing strategy with good diagnostic performance.
4. Screening is acceptable and efficient: The testing strategy has acceptable harms, costs, and patient acceptance.

Let us see how we can use these criteria to evaluate the use of screening tests.

Substantial Morbidity and Mortality

The importance of selecting diseases for screening that produce substantial morbidity and mortality is the key starting point for screening. Morbidity may include disabilities such as blindness or strokes, or extended period of costly health care such as kidney dialysis or treatment for coronary artery disease. Despite the importance of identifying conditions for screening that produce substantial morbidity and/or mortality, this condition may be ignored, as illustrated in the following example:

Mini-Study 10.1 ■ Screening for asymptomatic hemorrhoids is being considered all adults. The condition is found to have a high prevalence. However, screening was not recommended since asymptomatic hemorrhoids was also found to result in little morbidity or mortality.

[10.1] Asymptomatic implies that the individual does not have symptoms of the disease for which the screening test is being used. They may have other diseases and/or other symptoms. The term *screening* may be used with other somewhat different meanings. Tests may be used in the presence of symptoms when the clinician wishes to test for various physiological measurements or a range of possible diseases. Screening may also refer to a panel of tests designed to differentiate the cause of a clinical pattern, such as drug screening in the presence of clinical manifestations of intoxication. Screening for asymptomatic disease should also be distinguished from *case finding*. Case finding usually, but not always, refers to identification of an individual with a communicable disease with the intention of locating and treating their contacts.

Despite the high prevalence of asymptomatic hemorrhoids, the low morbidity and mortality makes it a poor candidate for screening. A common condition that poses little harm to individuals is not a good candidate for screening.

Early Detection Improves Outcome

The evidence that supports the ability to detect disease at an early stage often comes from studies that compare the stage of disease among individuals diagnosed through screening with those whose disease was diagnosed in the usual course of health care. The probabilities of detecting disease in early stages through screening and through the usual course of health care may be compared. If there is a higher probability of detecting early disease with screening, the results suggest early detection is possible through screening of asymptomatic individuals, as illustrated in the next example:

 Mini-Study 10.2 ■ An investigation of the diagnosis of breast cancer through monthly self-examination and yearly clinical examination was compared with the diagnosis of breast cancer using these methods as well as yearly mammography among women 50 years of age and older. The investigation demonstrated that the use of mammography increased the probability that the diagnosis of breast cancer would occur at an earlier state of the disease.

Achieving early detection, however, is not necessarily the same as detecting disease that will go on to cause morbidity or mortality. It is possible that the disease detected by screening may never become clinically important, as illustrated in the next example:

Mini-Study 10.3 ■ A new test is able to detect thyroid cancer in 20% of all men older than 80 years. Cancers detected in these men using the new test are generally found to be microscopic foci that are at an earlier stage than thyroid cancers diagnosed during the course of health care. The investigators are enthusiastic about the possibility of early detection of thyroid cancer and argue that this test is likely to be useful in screening for thyroid cancer in men older than 80 years.

The ability to detect cancer early is not the same as the ability to detect cancers that are likely to go on to become clinically important. Older men may die with thyroid cancer rather than die from thyroid cancer. The goal of early detection is not just to identify cancer early, but also to identify those cases that need effective therapy to prevent progression to clinically important disease.

Screening should not be recommended unless an intervention is available that can improve the outcome of patients detected by screening. Thus, unless there is therapy, or other effective interventions, that is more effective when used early in the disease, there is generally no reason to conduct screening for disease. Thus, the ability to detect disease at an early stage is not enough to fulfill this second criterion for screening. Effective treatment must be available and be more effective when used during the asymptomatic phase.[10.2]

The benefit of screening is ideally demonstrated using a randomized controlled trial that randomizes patients to a screening group and a usual medical care control group.[10.3]

[10.2] At times, screening may be worthwhile for other reasons. It may be worthwhile to detect communicable disease in order to prevent spread even if no effective treatment is available.

[10.3] Even when using a randomized controlled trial, it is necessary to follow up those diagnosed with the disease. They should be monitored not just until they are diagnosed, but until they have had an opportunity to develop the adverse outcome we hope to prevent. That is because a randomized controlled trial that demonstrates improvement in early outcome is not always sufficient. The outcome in the screened group should remain better than groups undergoing the usual methods of diagnosing the disease, even years after the disease is detected.

Often, however, it is not possible to perform randomized controlled trials with long-term follow-up. Thus, we often rely on studies that compare the outcome of groups that have been screened with that of groups that have not been screened by conducting cohort studies. These studies may provide important data that suggest the ability of screening to successfully improve the outcome.

Cohort studies of screening, however, are susceptible to misleading results because of *lead-time bias*. This bias results from comparing the time from diagnosis to an outcome, such as death, between those diagnosed through screening and those diagnosed in the usual course of health care. The potential for lead-time bias is illustrated in the next example:

> **Mini-Study 10.4** ■ An X-ray screening program to detect lung cancer was performed among a group of smokers who were asked to participate. Their outcomes were compared with the outcomes of individuals in a control group whose lung cancer was diagnosed in the usual course of medical care. The study and control groups' individuals were matched for age and number of pack-years of cigarette smoking. The screened group had a greatly improved survival 1 year after their diagnosis of lung cancer compared with the survival 1 year after diagnosis among the unscreened control group.[10.4]

Even if the treatment for lung cancer has no effect, we would expect the results for the screened group to be better. By detecting the disease earlier, screening with chest X-rays moves back the time of diagnosis. As illustrated in Figure 10.1, unfortunately, screening with chest X-rays has not moved forward the time of death. The increase in time between diagnosis and death may be entirely due to lead-time bias; that is, the screening had led to early detection without improved prognosis.

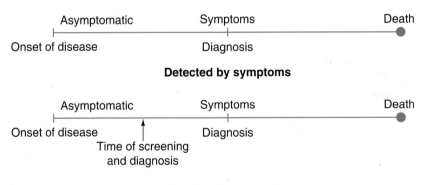

Figure 10.1 Lead-time bias in which earlier diagnosis by screening does not alter outcome.

There is a second reason why comparing screened and unscreened populations using a cohort study to assess their outcome may not produce convincing evidence of an improved outcome among those screened. This is known as *length bias*. As illustrated in Figure 10.2, length bias

---

[10.4] In recent years, spiral computed tomography (CT) scanning has shown promising results for early detection and treatment. It may now be possible to find lung cancers at a stage where cure is still possible. The fact that spiral CT is able to detect far smaller lung cancer may mean that it can detect lung cancer at a stage in which early detection is not only possible, but can improve outcome. Despite the success of spiral CT, it needs to be recognized that a large number of false positives will occur.

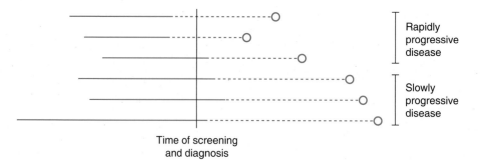

Figure 10.2 **Length bias demonstrating why more slowly progressive cases of disease may be detected by screening.** Solid lines indicate preclinical phase; dotted lines, clinical phase; and circles, death or other end point.

occurs when there are two different types of a disease, one of which is slowly progressing and one of which is rapidly progressive such as slow-growing and rapidly growing cancer.

When screening is performed initially, most cases that are detected will be slow growers. This is because slow growers remain in the presymptomatic or asymptomatic stage for a longer period of time and thus constitute most of cancer cases detected by screening. Fast growers, on the other hand, remain in the presymptomatic stage for a shorter period of time and constitute a smaller proportion of cases of cancer detected by screening. When length bias results in detecting mostly slow growers with a good prognosis, it appears that screening has done its job of improving outcome. Unfortunately, all that has happened is the identification of a group with good prognosis who have a better outcome than a group with poor prognosis made up mostly of rapid growers.[10.5]

Length bias, like lead-time bias, can be prevented by the use of large randomized controlled trials since we can assume that the study and control groups have the same proportion of slow growers and rapid growers. Let us take a look at an example that illustrates the advantage of a randomized controlled trial:

Mini-Study 10.5 ■ A study of prostate cancer among men older than 70 years compared the time between diagnosis and death for men screened for prostate cancer with those who were diagnosed in the course of medical care. Prostate cancers have a wide range of prognosis depending on the rate of growth of the cancer. The investigator found that screening produced impressive increases in the time between diagnosis and death compared with diagnosis among those who are not screened. When a randomized controlled trial was conducted, the increased longevity for the screened group and the unscreened group was nearly identical.

This example illustrates the potential for length bias whenever we are dealing with disease with a range of rates of progression. Conducting randomized controlled trials of screening may at times be the only effective way of taking length bias into account.

For diseases or conditions that cause substantial morbidity or mortality and where early detection improves outcome, we would ideally like to be able to provide screening to detect asymptomatic disease. However, before this can be advocated, two additional criteria should be fulfilled: Screening is feasible and screening is acceptable and efficient.

[10.5] Length bias assumes that disease that slowly progresses in the presymptomatic stage will remain slowly progressive once it enters the symptomatic phase. Length bias can be partially taken into account by studying groups that have previously undergone screening, thus removing from the group most of the long-standing cases of the disease.

Screening Is Feasible

Need for a High-Risk Group and More Than One Test

As we have seen, Bayes' theorem tells us that the pretest probability of a disease usually has a very strong relationship to the probability of disease after the results of the test are obtained. Thus, we need a screening strategy that allows us to identify a group at high enough risk of the disease and a testing approach that has a good enough diagnostic performance.

When performing screening, we are usually testing presymptomatic or asymptomatic individuals. Thus, we cannot rely on their symptoms to help us estimate the pretest probability of disease. Instead, we need to rely on the prevalence of the disease itself and the presence of risk factors to help us identify groups with adequately high pretest probabilities of disease.

Without being able to identify individuals who have one or more risk factors for the disease, we would often be starting with a very low pretest probability. In Chapter 9, we illustrated the posttest probabilities or predictive values when using a test with 80% sensitivity and 90% specificity on a population with 1%, 10%, 50%, and 90% probability of the disease before conducting the test. The 1% example was used to illustrate the pretest probability when risk factors for a common disease are present in a population to be screened. In this situation, it was evident that one test alone would not be adequate for diagnosis. Learn More 10.1 illustrates what may happen when the prevalence of the disease is even lower such as 1 per 1,000, which might represent the prevalence of the human immune deficiency virus (HIV) in a low risk or general population.

LEARN MORE 10.1 ■ TESTING FOR HIV ■ When the pretest probability is considerably lower than 1% for instance in the range of 1 per 1,000, successful screening is very difficult to achieve. This is the situation even when a test with high sensitivity and high specificity is used, as illustrated in the next example:

Mini-Study 10.6 ■ Suppose that the pretest probability of HIV is 1 per 1,000 in a low-risk population. Assume that we have available an excellent test for HIV antibodies with 99% sensitivity and 98% specificity. Let us see what happens when we use this test on a population of 100,000 with a pretest probability of disease of 1 per 1,000. This is illustrated in the following 2 × 2 table.

	Disease (+)	Disease (-)	Total
Test (+)	99 = True positive	1,998 = False positive	2,097
Test (-)	1 = False negative	97,902 = True negative	97,903
Total	100	99,900	

The prevalence or pretest probability of HIV of 1 per 1,000 is reflected by the 100 with the disease compared with the 99,900 without the disease in the 2 × 2 table above.

The posttest probability or the predictive value of a positive test can be calculated directly from this 2 × 2 table as follows:

Predictive value of a positive test = true positives/(true positives + false positives)
99/2,097 = 0.047 = 4.7%

Notice that even after we have obtained a positive test, the probability of disease is still less than 5%. Thus, even when screening with an excellent test, it is usually important that we apply our tests to groups of individuals who have pretest probabilities of disease considerably greater than 1 per 1,000.

(Continued)

One approach that has been used is to continue to attempt to improve the sensitivity and specificity of HIV testing. If the sensitivity and specificity can be raised to greater than 99%, then the predictive value of a positive test might be high enough to use in a low-risk population with a pretest probability in the range of 1 per 1,000. This has been called *universal testing*.

Even if screening tests can achieve these levels, it is important to recognize that these tests detect antibodies for the disease. Antibodies may not appear for 4 to 6 weeks or even longer after exposure and subsequent infection with HIV occurs. Unfortunately, during the period before the antibodies appear, the virus is rapidly proliferating. This is the period of the highest probability of transmission. Therefore, the usual antibody tests may be the least helpful when they are most needed.

A possible alternative to screening with antibody tests is to screen with antigen tests that detect either the DNA or RNA of the virus. These tests are currently expensive, but new approaches may make it feasible to test for HIV antigens to detect early disease. New approaches to early detection and early intervention are being extensively investigated as ways to address the continuing epidemic of HIV.

HIV screening illustrates the importance of using tests with very high sensitivity and specificity. It also underscores the limitation of even the very best tests that may fail to detect the disease at the stage when intervention is most effective.

As we have seen, we need to identify risk factors for disease that allow us to characterize a group of individuals who have an adequately high pretest probability of disease. Age is the most common risk factor because many diseases predominantly occur among particular age groups, such as premature infants or those older than 60 years. Other risk factors may be identified by such criteria as sexual history (e.g. HIV), past illness (e.g., ulcerative colitis), occupational exposure (e.g., benzene), family history (e.g., premenopausal breast cancer), and ethnicity or race (e.g., sickle cell trait).

Even if a high-risk group can be identified with perhaps a 1% pretest probability of disease, it is still usually necessary to use at least two tests to diagnose the disease. If we apply our excellent test with 99% sensitivity and 98% specificity to a group of 10,000 with a 1% pretest probability of a disease, the predictive value of a positive test is obtained as follows:

	Disease (+)	Disease (-)	Total
Test (+)	99	198	297
Test (-)	1	9,702	9,703
Total	100	9,900	

The posttest probability of the disease after obtaining a positive test, that is, the predictive value of a positive test, is as follows:

$$99/297 = 0.33 = 33\%$$

The posttest probability or predictive value of a positive test is still less than 50%. This probability is certainly not adequate to make a diagnosis. Thus, in screening the use of a second test is nearly inevitable because even with an excellent screening test and a relatively high-risk population, most of the initial positives are actually false positives. Therefore, we need to consider the implications of using more than one test or combining tests to develop a testing strategy.

Strategies for Combining Tests

There are two basic strategies for combining two tests. Using the first strategy, we label the results positive if the first test is positive and if a second test administered after the first is also positive. This sequential strategy may be called *positive-if-both-positive*. With the second strategy for combining two tests, we may perform two tests simultaneously or in parallel and label the results positive if either (or both) of the test results are positive. This strategy may be called *positive-if-one-positive*.

With the sequential positive-if-both-positive strategy, we usually administer the second test only to the individuals who are positive on the first test. The advantage of this strategy is that it requires second tests on only a small percentage of individuals. Thus, when feasible, the positive-if-both-positive strategy is usually the most desirable approach to screening.[10.6]

With the sequential or positive-if-both-positive strategy, a group that has been identified with two consecutive positives generally has a very high probability of disease. This is because the posttest probability of disease after performing the first test can often be used as the pretest probability of disease for the second test. The calculation of posttest probability using sequential testing is discussed in Learn More 10.2.

LEARN MORE 10.2 ■ SCREENING USING SEQUENTIAL

TESTING ■ In screening for asymptomatic disease, tests often need to be combined, as we have seen one test is rarely enough to definitively diagnose a disease. The most common way to combine tests is to use one test and then use a second test only if the first test is positive.

When using test #1 followed by test #2, Bayes' theorem may allow us to calculate the posttest probability (or odds) of the disease if two or more sequential tests are positive. We do this by assuming that the posttest probability (or odds) after obtaining the results of the first test can then be used as the pretest probability (or odds) for test #2 and so on. Using the likelihood ratio form of Bayes' theorem, we can express this relationship as follows:

(Pretest odds)(LR (+) of test #1)(LR (+) of test #2) =
Posttest odds of disease if both tests positive

Unless the results of using this strategy for combining tests are actually examined as part of an investigation, we need to make an important assumption when using this formula. We need to assume that a false positive on one test does not increase or decrease the chances of a false positive on the other test. This is known as the *independence assumption*. At times, the use of the posttest probability of test #1 as the pretest probability of test #2 will produce less favorable than expected results if the two tests produce the same types of false-positive or false-negative results, as illustrated in the next example:

Mini-Study 10.7 ■ Two screening tests for bladder cancer were found to have a high likelihood ratio of a positive test. Test #1 was performed first, and test #2 was performed only if the first test was positive. The investigators used Bayes' theorem to calculate the probability of bladder cancer. The investigators were surprised at the large number of patients who were positive on both tests but did not turn out to have bladder cancer.

It is possible that test #1 and test #2 produce false positives for the same types of situations. In other words, the results of the two tests may not be independent of each other; a false positive on one test may indicate a greater than chance probability of a false positive on the other test. Perhaps the presence

(Continued)

[10.6] Combining tests using sequential testing is not limited to screening. Often two or more tests are often needed for diagnosis even in the presence of symptoms.

of inflammation or other conditions produces false positives for both tests. When this is the situation, the posttest probability of one test cannot be used as the pretest probability of the second test. If two tests are not independent of each other, then combining them one after another will produce disappointing results. The best way to get around this problem is to actually investigate the ability of this sequential strategy to screen for and diagnose bladder cancer.[10.7]

As discussed in Learn More 10.2, we usually assume that the two tests are not prone to detect or to miss the same types of cases of disease. We call this the independence assumption. The independence assumption is violated when two tests are actually measuring the same phenomenon, and therefore the tests tend to have the same types of false-negative and false-positive results. If the independence assumption does not hold true, then the posttest probability of disease after obtaining two positives will often be less impressive than expected, as illustrated in the next example:

Mini-Study 10.8 ■ A testing strategy for gastric cancer included an upper gastrointestinal (GI) X-ray film performed first. A technician then performed an endoscopy without biopsy if the upper GI test result was positive. The investigators expected that those with two positive results would have a very high probability of gastric cancer and the patient could then undergo biopsy by a gastroenterologist. The results of the study, however, demonstrated that this strategy was little better than using either test alone.

These results are not surprising because the results of upper GI X-ray examination and endoscopy provide nearly the same type of information. They both rely on the gross anatomy. Thus, the results of the two tests are not independent, and individuals with two positive results will have a less than expected probability of having gastric cancer.[10.8]

Now let us take a look at the simultaneous, parallel, or positive-if-one-positive testing strategy. The positive-if-one-positive strategy may be implemented by having all individuals initially undergo both tests. For instance, when screening for colon cancer, testing stool for blood as well as using a flexible sigmoidoscopy is an example of a positive-if-one-positive strategy. This strategy is most useful when the two tests tend to detect different types of disease. For instance, flexible sigmoidoscopy is better for detecting left-sided colon cancers, whereas stool blood testing is better for right-sided colon cancer. The positive-if-one-positive strategy, however, is only useful when the tests detect different types of disease. If the tests detect the same type of disease, using two tests may merely increase the cost without increasing the diagnostic performance, as illustrated in the next example:

[10.7] Another issue that comes up when using the sequential approach to screening is which test to use first. One of the more confusing issues in screening using the positive-if-both-positive strategy is which test to use first. A common misconception is to use the test with the greater sensitivity first. Everything else being equal, the better test to use first is the one with the greatest likelihood ratio of a positive test since this results in fewer second tests. As we discussed and illustrated in Chapter 9, the test with the greatest sensitivity is not always the test with the greatest likelihood ratio of a positive test. When the test results are independent and the goal is to maximize the predictive value of a positive test after obtaining two positive results, it does not matter which test we use first. You can see this by taking a look again at the likelihood ratio form of Bayes' theorem. We get the same results whether we multiply the LR(+) of test #1 times the LR(+) of test #2 or alternatively we multiply the LR(+) of test #2 times the LR(+) of test #1. However, if we first use the test with the higher LR(+), we will have fewer second tests to perform. Thus everything else being equal, we might first use the test with the greatest likelihood ratio of a positive test since this results in fewer second tests being conducted. Often everything else is not equal, and we need to consider other factors including the harms, costs, and acceptability of the two tests in deciding which test to perform first. Therefore in practice, the least expensive and/or safest test is generally used as the first test in the screening process.

[10.8] In general, tests that rely on different mechanisms of disease detection—such as exercise stress testing, thallium stress testing, and catheterization—will produce results that are more independent of each other than tests that rely on the same type of data such as gross anatomy.

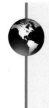

Mini-Study 10.9 ■ Mammography and sonography are being studied to determine whether a strategy that uses both of these tests on all women older than 50 years will improve the diagnosis of breast cancer. It was found that mammography detected 90% of the cancers, whereas sonography detected 60% of the cancers. The investigators expected to be able to detect nearly all breast cancers using both tests. They were disappointed when the results showed that performing the two tests did little better than using mammography alone.

If both mammography and sonography detect the same type of breast cancer, then administration of both tests will produce results that are no better but more costly than administration of mammography alone. Thus, the need to utilize tests that produce different types of false positives and false negative is important for simultaneous testing as well as sequential testing.

Screening Is Acceptable and Efficient

Before a feasible testing strategy can be put into practice for general use, it is important to consider whether it is acceptable. Issues of acceptance may relate to the patient's willingness to undergo the procedure. Colon cancer screening, for instance, faces problems with patient acceptance even though it has been shown to be fulfilling other criteria, as illustrated in the next scenario:

Mini-Study 10.10 ■ A demonstration screening program for colon cancer provided free sigmoidoscopy examination for all patients who volunteered. The examination required cleansing enemas, special dietary preparation, and telephone registration. Little privacy was provided during the examination. The investigators could not understand why there were very few volunteers.

Issues of patient acceptance may be overcome as procedures become routine and as clinical skills and patient-centered delivery of care increase. The acceptance of screening, however, also needs to take into account potential harms and costs.

The harms due to screening include adverse events associated with the procedures that may range from colon perforation from sigmoidoscopy or colonoscopy to the anxiety produced by false-positive results. In addition, the harms associated with false positives as well as with true positives need to be considered, as illustrated in the next example:

Mini-Study 10.11 ■ A screening test to identify patients with a high probability of a stroke was shown to successfully identify high-risk patients. The follow-up testing that was needed, however, produced a substantial number of adverse events among those with true-positive screening tests as well as among those with false-positive tests.

Thus, the harms of screening need to be evaluated in light of the full diagnostic work-up for positive results, not merely based on the harms due to the screening test itself.

In addition to considerations of safety and patient acceptance, issues of cost need to be taken into account; that is, a screening program needs to be efficient in terms of use of resources.

An important element in the overall cost of a screening strategy is the frequency of screening. The frequency of screening is an important issue often examined in the health research literature. Screening frequency can greatly influence the cost of screening large groups of patients. The longer the interval between screenings, the more people can be screened using the same resources.

Screening a previously unscreened group and then rescreening them a second time can be expected to produce very different results. The first time a group is screened, it is possible to detect disease that has been present for an extended period of time as well as disease that has developed recently. If there is a long presymptomatic stage, the initial screening may detect a large number of individuals with the disease. Assuming these individuals are identified and treated, subsequent testing will only detect cases of the disease that have developed during the intervening period plus hopefully the small number of cases that were initially missed. Thus, we would generally expect subsequent screening to identify a much smaller number of individuals with the disease. Failure to appreciate this principle may result in the following error:

> **Mini-Study 10.12** ■ An initial screening program for breast cancer in the only women's health clinic in one community resulted in a 1% frequency of breast cancer among the women screened. The screening was continued for every eligible patient visiting the clinic. Over the next several years, the frequency of breast cancer detected fell dramatically. The investigators concluded that the frequency of breast cancer was rapidly declining in the community.

The reduction in the frequency of breast cancer detection may not reflect what is really happening in the community. Rather, it may predominantly reflect the fact that repeat testing mainly detects the newly developed cases of a disease rather than detecting new as well as long-standing cases. Most of the long-standing cases have been detected and hopefully successfully treated after the first screening.[10.9]

The time interval between tests must also consider the course of the disease. Thus, screening for slow growing cancers may not need to be performed as often as more rapidly growing cancers. Ideally, the longer the presymptomatic stage, the less frequently screening needs to be performed. However, determining the frequency of screening based exclusively on knowledge of the natural history of a disease may not be a very reliable method, as illustrated in the next example:

> **Mini-Study 10.13** ■ One reviewer who evaluated the results of the Papanicolaou (PAP) smear concluded that PAP smears should be done every 6 months to be sure that all new cases of disease are detected at an early stage. Another reviewer recommended screening patients every 5 years, arguing that cervical cancer is very slow growing and thus requires no more frequent screening.

Many screening tests depend on the adequacy of the sample obtained. In clinical practice, the PAP smear may not perform as well as in clinical studies because the sampling technique used in practice may inadequately sample the endocervical junction where cervical cancer is believed to originate. If this happens and the recommended interval is 5 years, then it can be 10 years or more before an adequate sample is obtained. Thus, in addition to the natural history of the disease, it is also important to consider the realities of testing in a clinical setting when evaluating the frequency of screening.

An additional factor affecting the frequency of screening, and thus the costs, relates to the types of individuals who seek screening tests in clinical practice. When screening depends on patients to initiate a visit, there are often two types of patients: those who are screened repeatedly and those who rarely receive screening. This may result in *self-selection bias*. Repeating screening tests at frequent intervals, which detects mostly new cases, leads to rapidly diminishing returns. Ensuring that those who rarely receive screening are included among those screened may produce far greater benefits. The trade-offs are illustrated in the next example:

[10.9] This is different from length bias because it occurs even if all disease had the same natural history. Notice that the first time screening is performed in a population, the number of cases of disease reflects the prevalence of the condition. If screening is repeated at a later time, the number of cases reflects the incidence of the disease since the previous screening plus the missed cases.

Mini-Study 10.14 ■ An organizer for a pediatric lead screening program needed to choose between testing patients every time they came in for follow-up or conducting home visits. Home visits would allow one test for every child, even those who never made an appointment. The investigators found to their surprise that they could identify far more individuals with elevated lead levels by conducting home testing in which they tested every child once.

Often those who fail to seek care are the ones who need screening the most. Factors that increase the risk of disease may be closely linked to factors that keep patients from seeking care. Social and economic factors often result in this self-selection bias.

Screening for asymptomatic disease has become an important preventive intervention in clinical practice. Its success, however, depends on being able to fulfill four ideal criteria: substantial morbidity and mortality, early detection improves outcome, feasible screening strategy with good diagnostic performance, and an acceptable and efficient testing strategy. Learn More 10.3 discusses two widely used screening tests and the extent to which they fulfill these ideal criteria.

LEARN MORE 10.3 ■ **SCREENING FOR HIGH BLOOD PRESSURE AND BREAST CANCER** ■ To better understand the application of the four ideal criteria for screening, let us look at examples of two widely used screening tests. We will examine screening for a risk factor, high blood pressure, and a disease, breast cancer, to understand how well screening for these conditions fulfills each of the four ideal criteria for screening.

Screening for high blood pressure is among the most commonly used screening tests in clinical practice; its use approaches universal testing. High blood pressure has been well established as a contributory cause of vascular disease, including coronary artery disease, strokes, and kidney disease, thus producing substantial morbidity and mortality. Large well-conducted randomized controlled trials have established that early detection is possible and can improve outcome.

The feasibility of screening for high blood pressure assumes that the condition has a high-enough prevalence in most populations to warrant universal screening with a test of high-enough sensitivity and specificity. Routine blood pressure testing has a substantial number of false positives and an occasional false negative. The frequency of false-positive results has been a difficult issue for many years. Procedures for follow-up testing of those with elevated levels of blood pressure on route testing now may include 24-hour blood pressure monitoring to separate true positive from false positives.

Reasonable levels of patient acceptance and safety and cost of blood pressure testing permit widespread screening. It is important to recognize, however, that there are adverse effects of follow-up testing including the cost and adverse effects of diagnostic work-ups such as those that include an intravenous pylogram and the cost and adverse events associated with medications.

Screening tests rarely, if ever, completely fulfill the four ideal criteria for screening. Screening for high blood pressure comes close.

As a second example, let us look at screening for breast cancer. Breast cancer is the second most frequent cause of cancer mortality in women, and because it occurs at relatively young ages, it produces the largest number of years of life lost among women due to cancer. Thus, the criterion of substantial morbidity and mortality is fulfilled.

The second criterion that early detection improves outcome has been well established based upon randomized controlled trials especially, but not

(Continued)

exclusively, among women 50 years of age and older. A feasible testing strategy has been developed using age to define a group at high-enough risk. Mammography, despite its marginal sensitivity and specificity has become the primary screening technique. Efforts to improve screening using other techniques such as magnetic resonance imaging (MRI) continue to be investigated. So far, the increased number of false-positive scans from MRIs has limited their use to women at especially high risk.

Finally, patient acceptance has increased in recent years as mammography has become routine and a large majority of women now undergo mammography at least when it is fully covered by insurance. Newer mammographic methods with reduced radiation exposure have made mammography acceptable in terms of safety issues. The cost of breast cancer screening has been acceptable since the increased cost has been considered worth the increase benefit.

Thus, the use of mammography for screening for breast cancer has become standard clinical practice. The fact that screening using mammography does not completely fulfill the four ideal criteria for screening has led to continuing investigations to define who should be screened and to evaluate new technologies with the potential for better diagnostic performance.

PREDICTION AND DECISION RULES (4-6)

Prediction and decision rules are tools based on principles of testing that are increasingly being used to improve decision making. Prediction and decision rules require the development of a prediction score, which aims to predict outcome. Cutoff lines for the prediction score are then set converting the prediction score into a test that can be used as the basis for decision making, that is, a prediction and decision rule.[10.10] There are a large number of potential uses of prediction and decision rules in medicine and in public health as discussed in Learn More 10.4.

LEARN MORE 10.4 ■ USES OF PREDICTION AND DECISION RULES ■ Institutions such as hospitals and nursing homes are increasingly being judged on the outcomes of their care taking into account the severity of illness or what is called the *case mix* of their patients. Prediction scores may be used as part of this process. This is based on the assumption that increased severity of illness requires increased use of resources and should therefore receive greater reimbursement. Thus, an institution that treats newborns with a lower average APGAR score might be reimbursed at a higher rate than institution that treat newborns with a higher average APGAR score.

Prediction score may also be used as part of clinical research to determine whether groups or cohorts of individuals have equal or nearly equal prognosis. Prediction scores known as *propensity scores* are increasingly being used to compare prognoses between groups as part of clinical research.

Prediction and decision rules may also be useful for making public health decisions that affect large number of individuals. For instance, the level of *Escherichia coli* or coliform growth in a water supply might be used to predict the risk

(Continued)

[10.10] There are various terms used in the research literature to describe what are here being called prediction scores and prediction and decision rules. Prediction score has been called prediction rule. Clinical decision rules may be used instead of prediction and decision rule. The term *prediction and decision rule* is used here to emphasize the two components of prediction of outcome and use to make decisions.

of diarrheal disease. The score might then be used as the basis for the decision to increase chlorination or at a higher level of risk to stop distribution of the water.

Clinicians are most interested in prediction and decision rules that are applied to decision making on an individual or patient-by-patient basis. There are various purposes for which prediction and decision rules can be applied to individual patients. In addition to the APGAR, we can illustrate the spectrum of purposes using the following examples.

- Prediction and decision rules may assist clinicians in identifying when to provide preventive interventions. For instance, a prediction and decision rule may recommend whether or not to treat an asymptomatic patient to prevent or delay the development of a complication of HIV infection.

- Prediction and decision rules are increasingly being used to decide on hospital admissions versus outpatient treatment and on admission to specialized units such at the NICU for high-risk infants, the coronary care unit for patients with chest pain or the intensive care unit for patients with pneumonia.

- Prediction and decision rules may be used as an adjunct to diagnosis aiming to recommend when to use expensive tests such as an MRI for back pain or when to use common but rarely helpful tests such as X-rays to evaluate an ankle injury.

- Finally, prediction and decision rules are being used to recommend the best timing for treatment of patients with life-threatening diseases such as acute leukemia.

Let us take a look at what is needed to fully develop a prediction and decision rule recognizing that this full process is a substantial endeavor that is rarely reported as a single research investigation. We can use the M.A.A.R.I.E. framework to examine the steps needed for a clinically successful prediction and decision rule. We can think of these steps as follows:

Method—A prediction and decision rule aims to develop and validate a model in which a mathematical formula is used to predict an outcome, which subsequently forms the basis for recommending an action or decision.

Assignment—A *derivation cohort* or subset of individuals from an existing database is used to develop an initial prediction score, which can then be converted using cutoff line(s) into a test called a prediction and decision rule.

Assessment—The initial prediction and decision rule is initially validated using a different subset of individuals from the same database called a *validation cohort* to provide initial validation of the prediction and decision rule.

Results—The prediction and decision rule is further validated using a process called *external validation*, which evaluates the prediction and decision rule using additional databases. The components of the prediction and decision rule may also be reviewed to see whether improvements can be made before conducting a controlled trial.

Interpretation—The implementation of a controlled trial of the prediction and decision rule, ideally a randomized controlled trial, in a clinical setting similar to the one in which the prediction and decision rule is designed to be used. The performance of the prediction and decision rule is compared with clinical judgment and/or to other prediction and decision rules.

Extrapolation—A demonstration of the use of the prediction and decision rule in clinical practice in order to understand its clinical performance and clinical acceptance, that is, its effectiveness in practice.

Prediction and decision rules aim to produce a model incorporating several factors that predict an important outcome and use this score as the basis for making decisions. Today, this modeling uses mathematics to estimate the probability of outcomes ranging from morbidity to mortality to cost and then to use these predictions to recommend a decision or action. The basic concept, however, is not new. Prediction and decision rules have been used for at least a half-century by clinicians since Virginia Apgar developed the APGAR score.

Let us begin by taking a look at the APGAR score. We will then use the M.A.A.R.I.E. framework to take a look at what would need to be done if the APGAR score were being developed today.

The APGAR score was developed by first identifying factors that clinicians believed were predictors of how well newborn infants would do with a special interest in identifying high-risk infants. The APGAR score attempts to predict the newborn's short-term prognosis based on the following five variables or factors:

Activity (muscle tone)

Pulse

Grimace (reflex irritability)

Appearance (skin color)

Respiration

Each of these factors is scored on a scale of 0 to 2 with 2 being the best or most favorable score. These factor scores are then directly added together to produce an overall score with a maximum of 10 and a minimum of 0. This constitutes the APGAR score.

Today what we will call prediction and decision rules are being used for various purposes ranging from prevention to diagnosis to therapeutic recommendations. Regardless of the specific purpose, the goal of a good prediction and decision rule is to be able to predict outcome based on what is called a *prediction score* and then to utilize the prediction score to divide patients into groups in which different actions are recommended. Let us see how we distinguish between a prediction score and a prediction and decision rule using the APGAR as follows:

Mini-Study 10.15 ■ An APGAR score is calculated on newborns scoring them on a scale of 0 to 10. Those with a score below 5 are admitted to a neonatal intensive care unit (NICU), those with a score of 5 to 7 are admitted to a unit providing extra observation, and those with a score of 8 to 10 are admitted to a standard hospital unit.

Here the APGAR score is the prediction score, which can be seen as the quantitative results of a test. The use of this test result, like other tests, requires a cutoff line. Here the cutoff lines have been set at below 5 and above 7. The cutoff lines are then used as the basis for a recommendation on where to admit the newborn. Therefore, the prediction score is used as the basis for implementing a prediction and decision rule.

Prediction scores are formulae that aim to predict outcomes such as the probability of a diagnosis, a good response to treatment, short-term or long-term prognosis or costs. They do this by combining data from several factors or tests ranging from history and physical examination to commonly used laboratory tests. These factors must be available at the time a decision is made. The APGAR for instance combines five factors, all of which can be rapidly obtained by a clinician very soon after birth.

Notice that in the APGAR, all the factors are scored on the same scale with a maximum of 2 and a minimum of 0. In addition, all the factors are given the same weight or importance. That is, the scores are added together to produce the overall APGAR score. Specific cutoff lines are chosen by a process very similar to that used for defining a positive or negative for a diagnostic test.

Let us see how a prediction and decision rule might be developed today. We will walk through the steps in developing a new prediction and decision rule that we will call APGAR-II. In doing this, we will use the MAARIE framework.

Method—The Question, the Target Population, and the Comparison

The method component of prediction and decision rules sets the stage for the subsequent components by requiring us to ask the following questions: What is the question being addressed? To whom will the results be targeted or applied? To what will the results be compared?

The question to be addressed and the use of the results are very closely related so we will consider them together using the development of APGAR-II as our example.

The first step in the developing APGAR-II is to identify the question that the prediction and decision rule is addressing and the use of the results. Clarifying the use of the rule is essential since a prediction and decision rule may work very well for one purpose but not for another, as illustrated in this following example:

Mini-Study 10.16 ■ The APGAR-II score was developed as a prediction and decision rule to recommend whether newborns should be admitted to the neonatal intensive care unit (NICU). It worked very well for that purpose. However, when the APGAR-II was used as a basis for deciding whether a neonate with a low APGAR-II score required immediate airway assistance, the APGAR-II did not do a good job of prediction.

We should not be surprised when a prediction and decision rule performs well for one purpose but not another. The key to successful use of these rules is to define the purpose for which they will be used and investigate them for that specific purpose for instance as the basis for making admission decisions.

The final question to ask in the Methods section is To what will the results be compared? Before beginning development of a prediction and decision rule, it is important to clarify how the rule will be judged. That is, to what will it be compared? It is possible to compare the results of a prediction and decision rule to a policy of admitting everyone, no one, or to use clinical judgment on a case-by-case basis to determine who should be admitted. Alternatively, one prediction and decision rule may be compared with another prediction and decision rule. Let us see how this question would apply to the development of APGAR-II:

Mini-Study 10.17 ■ The APGAR-II is designed as a prediction and decision rule to be used as basis for deciding on NICU admission of newborns. The current procedure relies on the clinical judgment of clinicians.

In general, the comparison should be with the currently accepted method of making the decision. Thus, the investigators would want to compare the decisions recommended by the APGAR-II with the decisions actually made by clinicians. In this situation, they may also want to compare the decision of the APGAR-II with the decision recommended by the APGAR score.

Assignment—Derivation of Prediction Score and Measuring Performance

Once the aim of the prediction and decision rule is clear and the comparison has been established, the next component is the assignment process that derives the prediction score and the initial prediction and decision rule from an existing database. This database will be used for what is called *derivation* in the assignment component as well as *initial validation* of the prediction and decision rule in the assessment process.

Prediction and decision rules begin by developing what is known as a *prediction score*. Prediction scores become prediction and decision rules when cutoff line are developed and the resulting categories are used to make decisions. Thus, the development of a prediction and decision rule starts by creating a prediction score and determining how well it performs in predicting important outcome(s).

The ideal database for deriving an APGAR-II prediction score needs to be very large, perhaps including data on 20,000 to 50,000 newborns. In addition, the database needs to include a large number of factors that can be considered as potential predictors. Each of these potential prediction factors should include individuals with a full range of clinically relevant levels. Let us see what we mean by an adequate database in the next example:

> **Mini-Study 10.18** ■ Investigators identified a database collected by obtaining data on all newborns in a large state over a 1-year period. Over 50,000 births were included and over 30 potential prediction factors were included in the database reflecting all the data that were routinely collected at the time of birth. Data are also available indicating where each newborn was admitted, that is, to the NICU, a special care unit or a standard unit and the outcome in terms of morbidity and mortality.

This is an ideal type of database since it includes a large number of newborns and a large number of potential predictors.[10.11] The availability of all the data collected at birth implies that the database includes all of the objective data that were available to clinicians, which is important if the investigator later wishes to compare the performance of the rule with that of clinicians.

In addition, the use of all patients in a large geographic area makes it likely that the population is representative of all patients on whom the rule might be used and includes a full range of values for each of the potential predictors. For instance, if the extent of prenatal care is an important predictor, then it is important that the database include newborns with little or no prenatal care as well as newborns with complete prenatal care. Finally, in order to develop a prediction and decision rule, it is important that the decision as to where the newborn was admitted and their outcome be included in the database.

The next step in deriving and validating the prediction score is to divide the data from the initial database into groups. The most straightforward approach is to randomly divide the data into two groups, one called the *derivation cohort* and the other called the *validation cohort*. The derivation cohort is used to derive and measure the performance of the prediction score. The validation cohort can then be used to determine whether the results can be repeated using a second sample from the same database.[10.12]

[10.11] The minimum size of databases for derivation and validation may be estimated by the following rule of thumb. The sample size needs to include at least: (100) × (number of independent variable in the prediction score/proportion of adverse outcomes expected). For instance, if the database has 30 independent or predictor variables and 10% of the newborns are expected to need NICU care, then the minimum size of the database can be calculated as 100 × 30/0.1= 30,000.

[10.12] Dividing the cohort into two groups may result in smaller than desirable groups for derivation and validation. Other statistical methods are available for this purpose that reuse selected individuals. Two of these methods are called jackknifing and boot strapping.

Let us seen how this process of deriving a prediction score using a derivation cohort works in the following example:

> **Mini-Study 10.19** ■ Using the database including all newborns from a large state, the investigator created a derivation and validation cohort. Using the derivation cohort, they performed a regression analysis to determine which combination of the 30 variables did the best job of predicting outcome. They identified eight variables that substantially contributed to prediction and also incorporated interactions between these variables when the interaction had a substantial impact on the ability to predict outcome. Among the eight variables, respiratory status was given a weight of three times that of other factors. Factors such as birth weight and activity level were given intermediate importance. Once they had developed the prediction score, the investigators selected cutoff lines for the score, which they used to recommend admission to the NICU, a special care unit or a standard hospital unit. In a carefully conducted comparison, the APGAR-II was found to perform better than the APGAR score.

This process of developing a prediction score differs in several ways from the one described for the derivation of the APGAR score. First, notice that unlike the process previously described for the development of the APGAR score, these investigators do not begin by making their best guesses as to which factor will be important in prediction. Rather they look for a database with a wide range of potential prediction factors and let the data tell them which factors are the best predictors.

Second, the prediction score, unlike the APGAR, may have a large number of variables, and they do not all receive equal importance or weight. Here respiratory status is given the greatest weight. Finally, the large number of variables and complicated weights attached to each variable means that the APGAR-II, unlike the APGAR score, cannot be easily remembered or easily calculated. A computer program may be needed to allow timely use of the information.[10.13]

How do we judge the success of a prediction score? Prediction scores like diagnostic tests are compared with perfect performance, that is, perfect prediction of outcome. The goal, rarely achieved, is 100% *discriminant ability* or perfect prediction. The discriminant ability may be calculated as the area under the receiver operator characteristics (ROC) curve. In parallel with diagnostic tests, the discriminant ability tells us the percentage of a perfect test for prediction, which can be obtained from the prediction score under investigation.

As we discussed with quantitative tests, in converting a prediction score to a test, that is, a prediction and decision rule, the investigators need to establish cutoff line(s). Setting cutoff lines requires a trade-off between false-positive and false-negative results. Often the investigators place different value or importance on a false-negative result compared with a false-positive result. When this is the situation, the investigator may want to set the cutoff lines to minimize false negatives (or at times false positives) as seen in the following example:

[10.13] In addition to including the factors that best serve as predictors, the investigators need to consider whether to include interaction terms. Interactions between factors are quite common in clinical situations. At times, the interactions are strong enough to warrant inclusion in a prediction and decision rule. This is especially true when the interaction is strong enough to frequently change the recommendation. Investigators may be hesitant to include interaction terms in prediction and decision rules because they complicate the calculations and make the rule more difficult to explain. Nonetheless, when the best possible predictions are needed, interaction terms need to be considered. In the development of prediction scores, interaction do not need to be statistically significant as is often the situation when considering whether to include interaction terms in a regression analysis. Rather the criterion for the inclusion of an interaction term in a prediction score is whether it has a substantial impact on the ability to predict outcome. Therefore, you should expect to see more interaction terms included in prediction scores than is generally the situation using regression analysis.

Mini-Study 10.20 ■ When reviewing the performance of the APGAR-II, the investigators concluded that it had greater than 95% discriminant ability. Thus, APGAR-II was able to correctly identify the best site of care for newborns most of the time. However, when it was incorrect, the newborn usually would have been admitted to a less intensive level of care and experience a greater probability of morbidity and mortality. The investigators decided to alter the cutoff lines and now found that errors that occurred resulted in admission to a more intensive site of care. Using the new cutoff lines, the discriminant ability was approximately the same.

Cutoff lines for prediction scores like those for diagnostic tests are not set in stone. The process of setting cutoff lines is a trade-off between false-positive and false-negative results. The investigators here may have preferred some unnecessary NICU admissions to minimize the morbidity and mortality even recognizing the increased cost. When we discussed this issue for diagnostic tests, we used the term *diagnostic ability,* as opposed to discriminant ability, to indicate that the relative importance of false negatives and false positives has been taken into account.[10.14]

Prediction scores are subjected to an additional measure of performance that is not required for diagnostic tests. In order to consider using a prediction score in clinical practice, it should perform well in predicting important outcomes not only in the average case as measured by its discriminant ability but in unusual cases as well. Good prediction on average is easier to achieve than good prediction for the unusual individuals who are at especially high or especially low risk. Thus, in addition to the discriminant ability, which measures how well the prediction score performs on the average case, a measure known as *calibration* is used to measure performance.

Calibration measures performance for those at especially high and also especially low risk compared with the average individual included in the data. The rarely achieved perfect calibration has a value of 1 indicating that prediction score performs just as well in the unusual case as in the average case.

Figure 10.3 displays ideal calibration. The observed performance of the prediction score, as reflected in the dotted line, is the same for the high-risk and low-risk individuals as for those at the mean or average. Figure 10.4 displays poor calibration. It reflects a common situation in which the

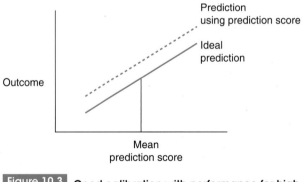

Figure 10.3 Good calibration with performance for high- and low-risk individuals being equal to the performance for the average individuals.

[10.14] Discriminant ability for a prediction and decision rule may be expressed as R^2, the percentage of variance explained by the regression equation. ROC curves may be used to assist in setting cutoff lines just as with tests. They are also useful in presenting the results since they tell us the discriminant ability of the test, that is what percentage of the variance is explained by the test results. ROC curves, however, are generally constructed under the assumption that a false positive and a false negative are of equal importance. When this is not the situation, as is often the case, then the cutoff line may need to be adjusted and a new discriminant ability or percentage of variance explained calculated taking into account the relative importance of false positives and false negatives.

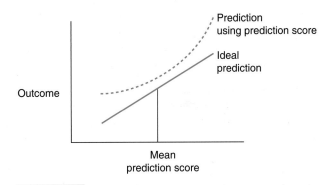

Figure 10.4 **Poor calibration with performance for high- and low-risk individuals being worse than performance for the average individuals.**

prediction score performs best for the average individual and does not perform as well for either low-risk and high-risk individuals.[10.15]

Thus, an ideal prediction score has a discriminant ability of 100% even after taking into account the relative importance of false negatives and false positives. In addition, an ideal prediction score has a calibration close to 1 indicating that it performs nearly as well on high and on low risk individuals as on the average individual. As with diagnostic tests, ideal performance is rarely achieved. Given promising performance of the prediction and decision rule as measured on the derivation cohort, the next step is to see whether its performance can be reproduced or validated using the validation cohort from the same database.

Assessment—Initial Verification of the Prediction and Decision Rule

The validation cohort is used as the initial challenge to determine whether the results obtained using the derivation cohort hold up. The simplest method for creating a validation cohort is to randomly divide the large database into two parts and use one part as the derivation cohort and the other as the validation cohort. When the size of the database is not large enough to divide into two equal cohorts, a growing number of sophisticated techniques are available to allow the investigator to more efficiently use the database.

Let us see what we mean by good validation in the next example:

Mini-Study 10.21 ■ The performance of the APGAR-II in the validation cohort is compared with its performance in the derivation cohort based on the cutoff lines established as part of the derivation of the prediction and decision rule. The investigator found that the prediction and decision rule had nearly the same discriminant ability and calibration in the validation cohort as it had when used in the derivation cohort. The investigators were very pleased with the initial validation of the APGAR-II.

The validation cohort here does provide initial support or validation for the prediction and decision rule. Notice, however, that the comparison here is with the prediction and decision rule derived from the derivation cohort. The rule's performance here is only comparing the deriva- tion cohort with the validation cohort, both of which come from the same database. It does not

---

[10.15] Calibration may be measured by the use of the standardized mortality rate (SMR), which is one way of determining how well the prediction and decision rule performs for unusual cases versus average ones. A good prediction score should have a large R^2 ideally approaching 100% reflecting good discriminant ability and an SMR of approximately 1 reflecting good calibration.

in-and-of-itself tell us whether the rule performs well compared with clinical judgment or the original APGAR. Thus, we can look at this process of initial validation as a form of internal validity.

Results—External Validation both Narrow and Broad Validation[10.16]

One hopes that the discriminant ability and the calibration using the validation cohort are just as good as those found in the derivation cohort. This initial validation, however, is just the beginning of the hoops that a prediction and decision rule must jump, though, before it can be accepted for clinical use.

Even before a prediction and decision rule is actually investigated in clinical practice, it needs to be tried out on additional existing databases. This is necessary since a trial of a prediction and decision rule in a clinical setting is a major undertaking that can do more harm than good. If the clinical decision is made on the basis of an unexpectedly poorly performing rule, wrong diagnoses can be made and/or poorer than expected outcomes can occur. Thus, the goal of the results component for a prediction and decision rule is to prepare for a clinical trial by applying the rule to new databases and looking for improvements that can be made in the rule. Once these results are in, it will be possible to determine whether the prediction and decision rule is ready for a clinical trial.

Before a prediction and decision rule is ready for a clinical trial, it is important to establish what we will call *external validity*. External validity implies that the prediction and decision rule has been evaluated using new databases both similar to the initial database as well as a database coming from different population(s). Successfully applying the rule to a similar population results in what has been called *narrow validity*. Successfully applying the rule to a population that is different from the database used for the initial derivation and initial validation has been called *broad validity*.

Let us see how narrow and broad validation might be performed in the following example of the use of APGAR-II:

Mini-Study 10.22 ■ A narrow validation of APGAR-II was conducted by using the same state's database of all newborns except now the data were collected 3 years later. Broad validation was performed by applying the APGAR-II to a national database of newborns who were admitted under Medicaid. Both of these databases indicated that on average the APGAR-II performed as well or better than the original APGAR.

Use of the same database from a subsequent year is a common method for performing narrow validation. It helps assure the investigators and readers that prognosis is not changing over time in a manner that invalidates the prediction and decision rule. Broad validation using a relevant perhaps high-risk group of patients helps ensure that the rule can be applied broadly to these patients.

In addition, narrow or broad validation may also indicate that there are alternative prediction factors that will serve approximately as well as the ones used in the original prediction and decision rule. This may be seen as an advantage by the investigator since it may provide a choice of prediction factors to include in the rule, as illustrated in the next example:

Mini-Study 10.23 ■ As part of the external validation, the investigators examined additional prediction factors. They demonstrated that the APGAR-II performed just as well when difficulty of labor was measured using a clinical score rather than requiring measurement from fetal monitoring.

[10.16] There are other approaches to organizing the levels of validity that differ from the one used here including a commonly used one that completely separates internal and external validity.(5)

Some factors may be cheaper or easier to collect or more acceptable to clinicians than others. A rule that does not require fetal monitoring may reduce the cost and make the rule easier to use. For clinicians who do not routinely use fetal monitoring, it may also increase the acceptance of the prediction and decision rule if and when it is advised for use in clinical practice. Whenever there is a choice of which factors to use, the investigator needs to consider those factors that improve the performance and ease of use. Thus, factors that are objective and can be reproducibly collected have an advantage over subjective and less reproducible factors.

Together the narrow and broad validations provide the investigator with a much better idea of the reproducibility of the predictions. In addition, it gives the investigator an opportunity to improve upon the rule in ways that aim to improve not only its performance but also it ease or cost of use and/or its clinical acceptance.[10.17]

Having made an effort to establish external validity and improve on the prediction and decision rule as part of the results component, the investigator is ready to proceed to the interpretation component.

Interpretation—Implementation of a Controlled Trial

Ideally, the APGAR-II is now put to the test of a randomized controlled trial in which the study group uses the prediction and decision rule as the basis for the decision, whereas the control group uses the currently accepted decision-making process and/or another prediction and decision rule. Once approved by an Institutional Review Board, the randomized controlled trial might compare proceed as follows:

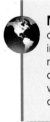

Mini-Study 10.24 ■ A consortium of hospitals organized a randomized controlled trial of the use of the APGAR-II score compared with the APGAR score in a settings that reflected the APGAR-II's intended use. Two thousand consecutive newborns are randomized to use the APGAR or the APGAR-II as the basis for the decision to admit to the NICU, a special care unit, or the standard care unit. The well-conducted investigation found that the APGAR-II had a higher discriminant ability than the APGAR and the difference was statistically significant.

Randomized controlled trials should ideally be conducted in a setting that is representative of the setting in which they will be used. They should also use as a comparison clinical judgment or other prediction and decision rule that represents the current method of decision making. It is important to be explicit about the comparison group. In this study, the investigators clearly indicate that the APGAR-II is being compared with the APGAR.

A randomized controlled trial of a prediction and decision rule should meet all the usual standards and procedures for conducting a randomized controlled trial including randomization of patients, double blinding when possible, objective assessment of outcomes, and an analysis that includes adjustment for differences between groups even when these differences are due to chance. A substantial and statistically significant difference between the APGAR and the APGAR-II groups is the best method for demonstrating the superior performance of the APGAR-II.

A randomized controlled trial may not be ethical or feasible. In this situation, as in other types of studies, a well-conducted prospective cohort study may need to be substituted for a randomized controlled trial.

[10.17] As part of the validation process, it is also important that the investigators examine the cases in which the rule does not perform well. This is key to improving the performance of the prediction and decision rule. For instance, with the APGAR, it was recognized that repeating the score after 5 minutes improved performance especially for those at highest risk.

Extrapolation—Evaluation of Clinical Application

The performance of the prediction and decision rule in a randomized controlled trial or a well-conducted prospective cohort study is important, but it does not guarantee the performance or acceptance of the rule in clinical practice. The acceptance of a prediction and decision rule may be resisted because it includes quite different factors than those currently used in the decision-making process. New prediction factors may be introduced and/or existing ones may not be included.

It is not unusual for some commonly accepted factors to have little or no predictive value especially after other related factors are included. Conversely, previously unrecognized predictor variable may turn out to be quite useful in prediction. These types of factors may influence clinical acceptance of a prediction and decision rule, as illustrated in the next example:

> **Mini-Study 10.25** ■ The APGAR-II, unlike the APGAR, did not use appearance or activity (muscle tone) as prediction factors because after taking into account other variables, these factors did not add substantially to the ability to predict. APGAR-II added six other new factors including capillary oxygen saturation and measurements from prenatal monitoring. Clinicians were not easily convinced that the new measurements should be used to replace the tried and true APGAR score despite the fact that the APGAR-II had been compared with the APGAR in a randomized controlled trial and was found to be superior.

Even when, or perhaps especially when, prediction and decision rules have been integrated into clinical practice, change may be difficult. Clinicians like most people often believe that one should "leave well enough alone" and "when it's not broke don't fix it." Prediction and decision rules, even the well-developed ones that have been shown to improve outcome, often face this barrier to implementation especially when they take on a decision-making process of long standing with a well-respected reputation.

It is clear that even the best of prediction and decision rules may not be enthusiastically accepted. Some of the reasons for lack of success in clinical applications are in the hands of the investigators. Others are clearly beyond the control of the investigators. Clinicians will often need to learn more about the derivation and validation of prediction and decision rules before they can be expected to embrace their use in general or in specific circumstances.

Issues of administrative and financial barriers to use can also be serious impediments to use even among those who accept and support the use of prediction and decision rules. Acceptance of prediction and decision rules may be facilitated when they can be computerized and delegated to those with less clinical training or experience. Insurance coverage for this process and evidence that use of the rule is accepted widely enough to provide legal protection for bad outcomes may encourage widespread use of a prediction and decision rule. Ultimately, the success of the rule is likely to depend on how well it has derived, validated, modified, and studied in clinical practice. Let us look at the issues of clinical application in the following hypothetical example:

> **Mini-Study 10.26** ■ On the basis of the randomized controlled trial, the investigators tried to convince their local hospital physicians to adopt the APGAR-II as routine procedure. When they advocated this approach, the physicians initially resisted saying the rule was too complex. After the major insurer of their patients agreed to pay to computerize and to pay for use of the rule, the physicians reluctantly agreed to use the rule for all newborns as long as they would not be legally liable for decisions that produced a poor outcome.

Even a successful randomized controlled trial of a prediction and decision rule by no means ensures its performance or acceptance in clinical practice, although it is a key step. The primary resistance of these clinicians to the use of the rule, however, was based on very practical considerations of complexity, reimbursement, and legal liability. Let us take a look at a possible fate of this prediction and decision rule in the next scenario:

Mini-Study 10.27 ■ A month after the demonstration of use of APGAR-II was begun, the use of the rule was discontinued when it was recognized the rule was being ignored and the APGAR was being calculated and used as the basis for admission decisions.

A wide range of issues may present barriers to application of prediction and decision rules. These barriers may be overcome if the rule is truly a major improvement over the usual method of decision making. Computerizing the decision-rule, providing insurance coverage, and accepting the use of the rule as a community or national standard can aid in clinical acceptance of a prediction and decision rule. These issues, however, are only relevant after there is substantial evidence that the rule performs well in clinical practice.

The complex steps required today for acceptance of a prediction and decision rule help to ensure that the prediction and decision rule is truly an improvement before it is accepted for widespread clinical use. The dramatic differences between the development and acceptance of the APGAR score and our hypothetical APGAR-II illustrated how much things have changed in clinical medicine since Virginia Apgar developed her prediction and decision rule in the 1950s.

Today prediction and decision rules are being used for a wide range of clinical decisions. They may be able to improve upon judgments of clinicians especially when it comes to judging prognosis. Despite the importance of clinical experience, prediction and decision rules have advantages over the use of the clinical judgment of individual clinicians. Clinicians, like all human beings, are not able to informally manipulate the large number of variables and accompanying weights that can be and are included in prediction and decision rules. Clinical experience with prognosis is limited by selective referral, selective follow-up, and selective recall. Prediction and decision rules aim to circumvent all of these limitations.[10.18]

REFERENCES

1. Weiss NS. *Clinical Epidemiology: The Study of the Outcome of Disease.* 3rd ed. New York, NY: Oxford University Press; 2006.

2. Morrison AS. *Screening in Chronic Disease.* 2nd ed. New York, NY: Oxford University Press; 1992.

3. Fletcher R, Fletcher S. *Clinical Epidemiology: The Essentials.* 4th ed. Baltimore, MD: Lippincott Williams & Wilkins; 2005.

4. Reilly BM, Evans AT. Translating clinical research into clinical practice: impact of using prediction rules to make decisions. *Ann Intern Med.* 2006;144:201–209.

[10.18] It is important to remember that the success of a prediction and decision rule relies on incorporating measured or objective data into decision making. When clinicians successfully utilize information by making subjective assessments of such factors as the will-to-live, nutritional status, or family support, they may be able to improve upon the predictions made by prediction and decision rules. These factors may complement the use of the prediction and decision rules in clinical practice.

5. Laupacis A, Sekar N, Stiell IG. Clinical prediction rules. A review and suggested modifications of methodological standards. *JAMA*. 1997;277:488–494.

6. McGinn TG, Guyatt GH, Wyer PC, Naylor CD, Stiell IG, Richardson WS; Evidence-Based Medicine Working Group. Users' guides to the medical literature: XXII: how to use articles about clinical decision rules. *JAMA*. 2000;284:79–84.

thePoint ✳ Visit http://thePoint.lww.com for interactive Q&A, flaw-catching exercises, searchable eBook, and more!

11 Decision and Cost-Effectiveness Analysis: M.A.A.R.I.E. Framework—Method, Assignment, and Assessment

INTRODUCTION (1,2)

Decision making in health care and public health has traditionally relied on subjective judgments, expert opinions, and nonquantitative decision making. Today, we increasingly rely on quantitative methods. Potential interventions, from prevention to palliation, are subjected to measurements of outcome that take into account the desirable outcomes (benefits), the undesirable outcomes (harms), and the financial costs. Thus, decision making has become the art and science of balancing the benefits and harms, and considering the costs. Benefits, harms, and costs have become the measures of medicine.

Why has this change occurred? In balancing benefits and harms and considering costs, it has become increasingly clear that qualitative and subjective decision making is affected by inherent limitations in how our brains process information.

Not being computers, we have limited ability to store and manipulate information and can be biased in how we structure our decision-making processes. These might be classified as limitations in data handling and limitations in data framing.

Data-handling limitations relate to our limited ability to simultaneously consider and utilize large quantities of information. To address these limitations, we often use simplified approaches or rules of thumb called *heuristics* to assist in our decision making. For many activities, including such complicated activities as diagnosis, these rules of thumb work remarkably well. However, when simultaneously examining and selecting between the available options for intervention that incorporate data on benefits, harms, and costs, our simplifying rules of thumb often reveal their limitations.

Quantitative decision making aims to overcome these limitations by using quantitative measurements rather than qualitative conclusions and by objectively combining these measurements rather than subjectively drawing conclusions. There are several potential advantages of quantitative decision making over subjective, nonquantitative decision making, including the ability to:

- Simultaneously compare three or more options
- Objectively consider events with low probability
- Explicitly state which factors are being taken into account in making a decision
- Identify the reasons for disagreements
- Identify factors that have the most influence on the preferred option
- Identify specific needs for better data

For these and other reasons, quantitative decision making is growing in importance in health care and public health. As we will see, quantitative decision making often has advantages in objectively structuring decision making and identifying areas that are critical to selecting between options. We will also see, however, that quantitative decision making also has inherent limitations that we need to recognize when reading the rapidly growing decision-making research literature.

Decision-making investigations may be used as the basis for making evidence-based recommendations or guidelines. However, these recommendations or guidelines usually require additional considerations beyond those that can be quantitatively considered in a decision-making investigation.

The process of quantitative decision-making research can be quite complex. Nonetheless, the investigations that use quantitative methods for decision making can be reviewed using the M.A.A.R.I.E. framework. Figure 11.1 illustrates the application of the M.A.A.R.I.E. framework to decision-making investigations.

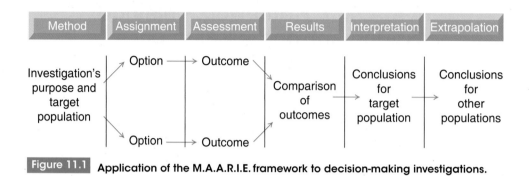

Figure 11.1 Application of the M.A.A.R.I.E. framework to decision-making investigations.

A decision-making investigation often requires the investigator to do the following:

1. **Model the decision:** This requires defining the alternatives that are being considered and the paths that eventually lead to potential outcomes. Decision-making investigations require the researcher to identify which options are being compared and what outcomes are being considered.

2. **Incorporate probabilities:** The investigator must determine which probabilities to use for measuring the favorable and unfavorable outcomes. These probabilities may come from the research literature, but they may need to be "guesstimated" based on expert opinion.

3. **Incorporate utilities:** A measurement of the value or degree of importance placed on each of the favorable and unfavorable outcomes is required. As we will see, these preferences are measured using what are called *utilities*.

4. **Incorporate costs:** As the cost of health care has increased along with the number of available options, researchers are also increasingly expected to measure and compare the financial consequences of each option being considered.

Thus, the health research literature now includes more than investigations that measure the probability of good outcomes or benefits and bad side effects or harms. Increasingly, decision-making investigations aim to measure or quantify the entire process of decision making. These decision-making investigations aim to model the decision-making process, to measure each of the components, and at times to offer recommendations or guidelines based on the research. Decision-making investigations now appear in most major clinical health care, health care management, and public health journals.

In examining decision-making investigations, we will focus on two hypothetical examples:

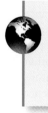 **Mini-Study 11.1** ■ The first example examines three alternatives for treating single-vessel coronary artery disease. Conventional treatment is a combination of medications, angioplasty, and surgery. There are also two new treatments. One treatment is called transthoracic laser coronaryplasty (TLC). The other is a new drug called Cardiomagic. We will be looking at how we can compare these alternatives to decide which is the most effective for treatment and which is the most cost-effective.

The second example examines options for approaching a disease that we will call Paresis A. We will examine the following situation:

Mini-Study 11.2 ■ Paresis A is a common contagious disease of childhood that is usually self-limited. However, a small percentage of children who experience the illness develop paralysis, and a few develop life-threatening complications. Long-term paralysis and late complications can occur. The conventional treatment for Paresis A has been only supportive treatment, which we will call the do-nothing approach. Recently, an expensive vaccination has become available to prevent Paresis A. We will discuss how we can compare the results of the vaccine to the do-nothing approach.

These types of decision-making investigations require a wide variety of information drawn from multiple sources. Thus, they can be very confusing to read and understand. However, decision-making investigations, like the other types of studies that we have examined, can be understood by using the M.A.A.R.I.E. framework.

METHOD (2,3)

Study Question and Study Type

Decision-making investigations differ from other types of investigations that we have examined because they generally do not begin by stating a study hypothesis. Rather, they begin by defining a study question and then identifying the options that will be considered to address the study question. Thus, the investigator does not begin by hypothesizing which option is best. Rather, the investigator's study question should be to fairly identify and compare the options using predefined criteria.

Various study questions can be addressed by decision-making investigations. The specific type of decision-making investigation used should depend on the question being addressed.

Let us begin by outlining the common types of decision-making investigations. Then it should be possible for you to determine whether the study type is appropriate to the study question.

Decision-making investigations can be divided into two general types. The first type includes efforts to consider benefits and harms—that is, favorable and unfavorable health effects. This type of investigation is often called a *decision analysis*.[11.1]

The second type of decision-making investigation is called *cost–effectiveness analysis*. Cost–effectiveness analysis will be used as a general term that includes all types of decision-making investigations that consider costs and relate them to a measure of favorable and adverse outcomes.[11.2]

Both decision analysis and cost–effectiveness analyses can be subdivided into several different types of investigations, depending on the factors that are considered.

Decision Analysis

One type of decision analysis in the literature is an *outcomes profile*.

Table 11.1 shows the favorable and unfavorable outcomes with TLC and Cardiomagic. This profile provides considerable data that may be helpful in making decisions. However, it does not in and of itself lead to preference for one option over another. The outcomes profile actually raises a series of questions that need to be considered in making decisions that can be incorporated into more complex investigations.

[11.1] The term *decision analysis* is often used even more generically to refer to all decision-making investigations that use a quantitative approach to decision making under conditions of uncertainty. In this context, all investigation types discussed here, including those that incorporate costs, can be considered decision analyses. In addition, the term *decision analysis* has been used more narrowly than we use it here to imply the use of a decision tree as the method for modeling the options being considered.

[11.2] As we discuss later in this chapter, the term *cost–effectiveness* is also used to describe one particular type of decision-making investigation in which the investigator is interested in comparing different alternatives for obtaining the same outcome. In this special type of investigation, the results are stated as additional costs per additional outcome. The term *effectiveness* as used in cost–effectiveness has a somewhat different meaning than when used in the "Studying a Study" unit of this book. Effectiveness in the context of cost–effectiveness combines the favorable and adverse outcomes. When we viewed outcomes previously, we regarded effectiveness as including only favorable outcomes. Considerations of adverse outcomes or safety were discussed separately. Thus, in decision-making investigations, we should regard the term *effectiveness* as implying net effectiveness.

TABLE 11.1	Favorable and Unfavorable Outcomes with TLC and Cardiomagic
TLC Outcomes	**Cardiomagic Outcomes**
Successful 96%	Successful 80%
Unsuccessful 3.9%	Unsuccessful 19.8%
Death 0.1%	Blindness 0.2%

Let us examine Table 11.1 to see what information is provided and what is left out. First, note that the outcomes profile provides estimates of the probability of favorable and adverse outcomes. In an outcomes profile, however, the timing of the events is not necessarily made explicit. In addition, in an outcomes profile, there is no attempt to combine or summarize the impact of favorable and adverse outcomes or long-term and short-term impacts. This process is left to the reader. An outcomes profile does not really provide a conclusion and may not allow us to determine which the best alternative is. Therefore, we may consider an outcomes profile to be a preliminary, partial, or incomplete decision-making investigation.

An outcomes profile may provide enough information to make a decision if it is clear that both the harms and the benefits of a therapy such as TLC are more favorable than the harms and benefits of Cardiomagic. It is important to recognize, however, that the outcomes of TLC and Cardiomagic are not directly comparable. Looking at the adverse effects of these two treatments requires us to compare two outcomes: death and blindness. These have very different implications. We may need to quantitate the importance of outcomes such as death and blindness and incorporate these measurements into a decision-making investigation if we wish to compare TLC and Cardiomagic. In decision-making investigations, incorporating the relative importance of an event is accomplished by measuring utility.[11.3]

A utility is designed to measure the preference of a decision-maker for a particular health outcome or state of health. As we will see, there are various methods for measuring utilities and considerable controversy about which is best. Regardless of the method chosen, the aim is to measure utilities on the same scale as probabilities. By doing so, it is possible to combine probabilities and utilities.

Thus, our goal is to measure the utilities of blindness and death on the same numerical scale. In addition, our goal is to combine the measurements of utilities that we obtain for blindness and death with the probabilities that they will occur.

Remember that probabilities are measured using a scale of 0 to 1, which is often converted to percentages from 0% to 100%. On this scale, there are no measurements greater than 1 or less than 0. The utility scale generally defines 0 as immediate death and 1 as full health or an individual's state of health in the absence of manifestations of disease or other health-related conditions.

Once utility and probability are measured on the same scale, the probability can be multiplied by the utility to produce what is called an *expected utility*. We can consider expected utility to be the probability of an outcome that takes into account its value or utility. The calculation of expected utilities is an essential step in performing a decision-making investigation that attempts to compare options and draw conclusions. Thus, an investigation that measures utilities and combines them with probabilities is called an *expected utility decision analysis*.

The possibility that death may occur raises an additional factor to consider in a decision-making investigation. At times, we may want to consider the expected number of years of life

---

[11.3] At times, outcomes profiles may be adequate for decision making when one option is clearly better than another, regardless of the utility that is placed on each outcome. In decision-making investigations, when one alternative is clearly more favorable than another, the alternative with the better outcomes is said to be *dominant*.

[11.4] If the investigator is dealing with a women's disease, then life expectancy by age and gender should be used. Similarly, if the author is dealing with a disease generally limited to black (such as sickle cell anemia), use of life expectancy by age and race would be appropriate. As discussed in the next chapter, the relevant life expectancy is not always the life expectancy derived from population data. For diseases that substantially reduce life expectancy, the appropriate life-expectancy measures take into account life expectancy for a particular disease as well as life expectancy defined by age and possibly gender and race.

gained as the result of preventing or delaying death. To accomplish this we use a measure known as *life expectancy* which as we will see is our standard measurement of average remaining life span. For situations in which an intervention prevents or delays death we can use life-expectancy measures, expressed from the average age of the individuals being treated, to estimate the average number of years of life gained by an intervention.[11.4]

Life expectancy or years of life gained can be incorporated into decision-making investigations along with probabilities and utilities. When this is done, the investigator often multiplies the probabilities times the utilities times the life expectancy to produce a measurement known as *quality-adjusted life years* (QALYs). As we will discuss, a QALY is the fundamental unit of measurement or effectiveness used in many quantitative decision making investigations.[11.5]

Decision analyses that use QALYs to take into account probabilities, utilities as well as life-expectancies represent what many experts consider a fully developed decision analysis. We will call this form of decision analysis a *QALY decision analysis*.

We have now defined three types of decision analyses as follows:

1. **Outcomes profiles:** This type of investigation merely states the probabilities of the known favorable and adverse outcomes from each of the alternatives being considered.

2. **Expected utility decision analyses:** This type of investigation combines the probabilities and utilities of each favorable and each adverse outcome and summarizes the results as overall expected utilities. Thus, expected utility decision analyses, as opposed to outcomes profiles, summarize the outcomes of each alternative and allow them to be directly compared.

3. **QALY decision analyses:** Like expected utility decision analyses, these allow direct comparison of alternatives, taking into account the favorable and adverse outcomes. However, QALY decision analyses go beyond expected utility in that they incorporate life expectancy.

Cost-effectiveness Analysis

Cost–effectiveness analyses, in contrast to decision analyses, incorporate costs as well as considerations of favorable and adverse outcomes. Cost–effectiveness analyses, like decision analyses, can be divided into several types.

As with outcomes profiles, cost–effectiveness analysis may simply measure or describe the various costs as well as the probabilities of the potential outcomes. The reader then needs to combine these outcomes to reach conclusions. This type of investigation is called a *cost–consequence analysis*. The data from a cost–consequence analysis might look like that in Table 11.2.

TABLE 11.2	Possible Data from a Cost-Consequence Analysis for Paresis A
Paresis A Vaccine	
Outcomes	Successful immunization 97%
	Unsuccessful immunization 2.9%
	Complications 0.1%
Costs	$50 per use

[11.5] QALY is the standard but not the only method for incorporating utilities and life expectancy. A method known as *Health Adjusted Life Expectancy (HALE)* is gaining recognition for combine life expectancy and quality of life measures at the population level. HALE is gaining acceptance for cost–effectiveness analysis in public health, for instance, when comparing population-wide investments. However, HALE cannot be used when examining the impact of a particular disease or condition. Another measure known as *Disability Adjusted Life Years* or DALY is useful when comparing different reasons for mortality and morbidity. DALYs gained my be used as the unit of effectiveness for population based decision making studies. QALYs are the standard measure used in a fully developed decision analysis or cost–effectiveness analysis.

Cost–consequence analyses are really partial analyses because they do not generally allow us to directly compare two or more alternatives. To compare alternatives, the investigators need to bring in outside data or judgments.

A second type of cost-effectiveness analysis has unfortunately been called a *cost–effectiveness analysis*. Using this term to describe a specific type of cost–effectiveness analysis can be very confusing. To minimize confusion, we will call this type of analysis a *cost-and-effectiveness study*.

A cost-and-effectiveness study looks at the costs required to produce an additional unit of desired outcome. For instance, imagine the following situation with Paresis A:

Mini-Study 11.3 ■ The cost of the new Paresis A vaccine including the total costs of providing the vaccine and treating any complications is $15,000 per case of Paresis A prevented.

This type of investigation compares the cost per additional desired outcome. It does not ask about the value of the outcome or the average years of life gained for the people treated. That is, cost-and-effectiveness studies do not incorporate utility or life expectancy. This type of cost–effectiveness analysis can be used to compare alternative ways of achieving one particular outcome such as a disease prevented or a life saved. However, most comparisons of intervention options produce more than one outcome which differ in their utilities and life expectancy gained or lost. Therefore it is often desirable to take into account utilities as well as life-expectancy.[11.6]

Thus, a full cost-effectiveness analysis incorporates considerations of utility and life expectancy as well as cost. This type of cost–effectiveness analysis is called a *cost–utility analysis* or a *cost–effectiveness analysis using QALY* as the measure of effectiveness. Let us see what we mean by a cost–utility analysis:

Mini-Study 11.4 ■ Paresis A vaccine was found to reduce the cost by $2,000 per quality-adjusted life year saved when it was compared with the conventional approach. The investigation took into account the utility of the outcomes as well as the life expectancy of people who experienced favorable and adverse outcomes.

This form of cost–effectiveness analysis represents a fully developed analysis. It allows us to compare any alternative, taking into account all the relevant costs and health outcomes including the probability and utility of favorable and adverse outcomes, as well as the life expectancy. Cost–utility analyses are increasingly considered the method of choice for most decision making in health care. They allow us to directly compare alternatives and determine the costs relative to the health consequences.

Cost-Benefit Analysis

At times, however, the question posed in an analysis goes beyond comparing the costs and health consequences of an intervention. Decision making may at times require looking at trade-offs between money spent on health and money spent on other important outcomes such as environmental protection, economic growth, or education. To make these types of comparisons, it is necessary to translate effectiveness as well as costs into monetary terms.

The form of analysis that converts effectiveness as well as costs into monetary terms is known as a *cost–benefit analysis*. Let us examine how a cost–benefit analysis might look:

[11.6] At times, the key issue for an analysis is the relative costs. The effectiveness of two options may be comparable, and the investigation is directed only at considering costs. This type of cost-and-effectiveness study is called a *cost analysis*.

> **Mini-Study 11.5** ■ An analysis was conducted to compare the economic costs and consequences of providing insurance coverage for paralysis vaccine with the alternative of providing college scholarships. The analysis assumes that one QALY could be converted to $50,000. The investigation found that coverage of paralysis provided a $2 benefit for every $1 cost. The alternative of paying for college tuition provided a $3 benefit for every $1 cost. Thus, paying for college tuition was considered the better alternative.

Note that cost–benefit analyses must make the conversion of QALY into dollars or other currency. This is a big step, since it requires us to place a monetary value on a year of life. Thus, this type of analysis remains controversial. Fortunately, it is not often necessary to directly compare health expenditures with other uses of money. Therefore, cost–benefit analyses are not frequently seen in the health research literature.

We will not examine cost–benefit analyses. However, as the example suggests, the conversion from a cost–utility study to a cost–benefit study is mechanically simple even though it represents a major intellectual leap. The key is determining the proper monetary value to place on a year of life. Once the monetary conversion of QALYs to dollars or other currency is agreed upon, that monetary figure merely replaces each QALY.

Thus, decision-making investigations can be classified based on the factors that they take into account as follows:

- **Decision Analysis**

    Outcomes profile: Probabilities of favorable and unfavorable outcomes

    Expected utility decision analysis: Probabilities and utilities of favorable and unfavorable outcomes

    QALY decision analysis: Probabilities, life expectancy gained, and utilities of each outcome

- **Cost–Effectiveness Analysis**

    Cost–consequence analysis: Costs and probability of favorable and unfavorable outcomes

    Cost-and-effectiveness study: Costs to gain an additional unit of desired outcome such as a life saved

    Cost–utility analysis: Costs to gain a QALY, the unit of outcome that incorporates probabilities, utilities and life expectancy gained

- **Cost–Benefit Analysis**

    Costs compared with health outcomes that are converted to a monetary value

Target Population

As with all investigations, it is important to define the target population, the population to which the results will be applied. This is important because it tells us the following three things:

1. The type of individuals who are being included and excluded
2. The type of sources that can be used to provide the necessary data
3. The types of extrapolations to similar populations that will be possible if the results favor one of the alternatives

The population that is the target of the decision-making study ideally should guide the investigator to the type of data to use. Unfortunately, data may not be available from the target population. To understand the implications of the choice of data, let us return to our coronary artery disease example and ask which population's data should be used to address the following study question:

Mini-Study 11.6 ■ We are evaluating the costs and effectiveness of three types of treatments for single-vessel coronary artery disease: Cardiomagic, TLC, and conventional treatment.

When obtaining data to address the effectiveness or cost–effectiveness of the three alternative treatments, it is important that the data come from individuals with single-vessel coronary artery disease. These treatments may also be used on patients with more extensive disease. Such individuals are likely to be older and have other related arterial disease. Thus, data derived from a population of patients with severe coronary artery disease would not be the type of data that should be used in addressing the study question. Now let us look at our other hypothetical situation:

Mini-Study 11.7 ■ We are evaluating the costs and effectiveness of a new vaccine for Paresis A, a common contagious disease of childhood that is usually self-limited, but can produce short- and long-term complications.

When obtaining data to address the costs and effectiveness of this vaccine, the data should be obtained from a population like the one on which it will be used. It would not be useful to obtain data from a population of severely ill children, especially if they had a high frequency of complications and required large expenditures if they did develop complications. Similarly, it would not be useful to obtain data from a population in which a high level of natural immunity already existed, and therefore the fully developed disease was rarely experienced.

Thus, when examining a decision-making investigation, the reader must ask, "From what population (or populations) were the data obtained?" and "Is the population appropriate to the study question?"

Perspective

To evaluate whether appropriate data were included in an investigation, it is important to consider the study *perspective*. Perspective asks about how broadly we should look when measuring the effectiveness and the costs of an alternative. Let us examine some of the possible perspectives by returning to the use of Paresis A vaccine. We could view the costs and effectiveness of the vaccine from at least the following perspectives:

- The patient who receives the vaccine and pays out of pocket
- The insurance company that pays for the vaccine as well as the short-term costs of treating Paresis A
- The government insurance system that pays for the care for individuals who develop Paresis A
- The society that, through one payment mechanism or another, receives the effectiveness and pays the costs of the administration of the vaccine and of the disease

The first three perspectives can be viewed as *user perspectives*. They reflect different ways for recipients or payers to view the costs and effectiveness of the vaccine. In theory, an investigation could be conducted from the perspective of the user of the investigation.

The fourth perspective is a *social perspective*. A social perspective implies that we are interested in the impact of the effectiveness and the costs regardless of who obtains the benefits, who suffers the harms, or who pays the costs. The choice of perspective guides the investigator in determining what should be included or excluded in the measurement of benefits, harms, and costs. Therefore, we can look at perspective as parallel to the inclusion and exclusion criteria used in other types of investigations.[11.7]

[11.7] The perspective of the decision-making investigation should be distinguished from the identity of the decision-maker. For instance, a clinician may make a recommendation by attempting to view the situation from the perspective of an individual patient, an institution, or even society as a whole.

In general, decision-making investigations should use the social perspective. Other perspectives may also be used for additional analyses. There are two basic reasons for using the social perspective. First, it is the only perspective that never counts an adverse outcome for one individual as a favorable outcome for another individual. Similarly, the social perspective is the only perspective that never counts a financial loss to one individual as a financial gain for another individual. Thus, social perspective is the only perspective that considers all the favorable and adverse outcomes and all the costs regardless of where they fall in society.

The perspective chosen should apply equally to the benefits, the harms, and the costs. If different perspectives are used for each, we cannot fairly compare or summarize the relationship between net effectiveness and costs. Use of the social perspective thus considers all the favorable and adverse outcomes regardless of who they affect and all the costs regardless of who pays the bills. Using the social perspective allows us to compare net effectiveness and costs in a consistent manner and to compare the results of one investigation with those of another.

As is often the case in study design, we do allow investigators to have it both ways. It is legitimate to conduct a decision-making investigation from the perspective of a potential user. If this is done, however, it is recommended that the investigation begin with a presentation from the social perspective. The social perspective is usually considered the ideal perspective for conducting a cost–effectiveness analysis. When a cost–effectiveness analysis is conducted from other perspectives, the results are often compared with those obtained using the social perspective. The use of the social perspective in cost–effectiveness analysis has been called the *reference case*.

It is also important to recognize that many readers of a cost–effectiveness analysis do not look at the issue from a social perspective but rather from one or more user perspectives. Ideally, the data are presented in such a way that it is possible for readers who want to take a user perspective to selectively use the data to reach their own conclusions.

Recognizing the perspective used in an investigation is especially important when we try to extrapolate the results to individuals or situations not included in the study.

In summary, when reading a decision-making investigation, we first need to address the three basic questions of study design.

- What is the study question, and is an appropriate study type being used to address the study question?
- What is the target population?
- What is the study perspective?

Having addressed these questions, we can turn our attention to assignment and see what we mean by a decision-making model. In the remainder of our discussion of decision analysis and cost–effectiveness analysis, we will examine net effectiveness, that is benefits minus harms, using probabilities, utilities, and life expectancy. In addition, we will measure costs as well as net effectiveness from the social perspective.

ASSIGNMENT (2–4)

Options

The process of assignment in a decision-making investigation involves modeling, diagramming, or otherwise structuring the decision options. The selection of the options to consider is under the investigator's control. As the reader, it is very important to review which options have been selected and, conversely, which potential options have not been included.

First, let us examine what we mean by modeling the decision-making process. To conduct a decision-making investigation, the investigator needs to select what is called a *decision-making model*. A decision-making model outlines the steps the investigator will follow in the decision-making and the *final outcomes* that occur. By final outcomes, we mean the outcomes that may occur at the completion of the decision option.[11.8] With TLC and Cardiomagic, the decision-making model may be described as follows:

> **Mini-Study 11.8** ■ TLC and Cardiomagic will be compared. Either TLC or Cardiomagic may be chosen, but not both. The outcomes of TLC are successful, unsuccessful, and death. No other therapy may be used if TLC is unsuccessful. Alternatively, Cardiomagic may be chosen. The outcomes of Cardiomagic are successful, unsuccessful, and blindness. If Cardiomagic is unsuccessful, surgery will be performed. The outcomes of surgery are successful, unsuccessful, and death. No other intervention will occur.

A common method for diagramming the decision-making process is a *decision tree*. A decision tree graphically depicts the decision options and the choices that must be made to implement each option. The decision tree also depicts the events that occur through a chance process, outside the control of the *decision-maker*. The term *decision-maker* intentionally evades the question of who is making the decision. Thus, at times, the decision-maker may be a clinician, a patient, an administrator, and so on.

Let us use our example of TLC and Cardiomagic to demonstrate the essential components of a decision tree.

Figure 11.2 represents a decision tree outlining the choice between TLC and Cardiomagic for patients with symptomatic single-vessel coronary artery disease. Note the following: First, there are two and only two options to choose from—TLC and Cardiomagic. The choices of TLC and Cardiomagic are the decision options. Second, note that there is a square connecting the two decision options. This square is called a *decision node*. A decision node is connected with each of the decision options. The decision-maker must choose one of the available decision options. Once the choice of option is made, the decision tree depicts the subsequent course of events.[11.9]

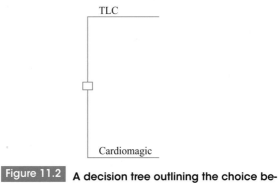

TLC

Cardiomagic

Figure 11.2 **A decision tree outlining the choice between TLC and Cardiomagic for patients with symptomatic single-vessel coronary artery disease.**

In the decision tree for TLC depicted in Figure 11.3, we see only events that subsequently occur by chance.

[11.8] The term *final outcome* is not in common usage. It is being used here to distinguish the outcomes at the right end of the decision tree from intermediate outcomes. In decision analysis, the outcomes at the right-hand side of the decision tree are the outcomes of interest. Thus, death is death and full health is full health regardless of the process of getting there. Decision analysis focuses on final outcomes not the process of getting there.

[11.9] Decision trees may be far more complex than those illustrated here. For instance, choice nodes may again appear later in a decision tree, implying that the decision-maker will need to make a subsequent decision as part of implementing a specific option.

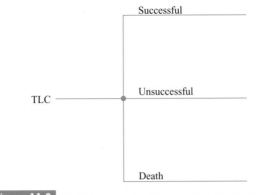

Figure 11.3 **Decision tree for TLC depicting three branches of the decision tree indicating events that occur by chance.**

For TLC, one of three final outcomes occurs: successful, unsuccessful, or death. Any individual can experience only one of these outcomes; that is, the outcomes are considered mutually exclusive.[11.10]

These three final outcomes are connected by a *chance node*. Chance nodes are represented by a darkened dot or circle. The final outcomes are indicated to the right of the chance node.

Figure 11.4 displays the option to use TLC and also the option to use Cardiomagic. Cardiomagic, unlike TLC, may be followed by surgery if it is unsuccessful. Thus, in the Cardiomagic alternative, there are two chance nodes. The first reflects the fact that the outcome can be successful, unsuccessful, or blindness. The second chance node shows that the surgery following unsuccessful Cardiomagic will be successful, unsuccessful, or will result in death.

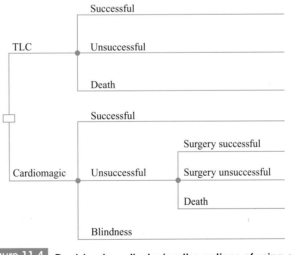

Figure 11.4 **Decision tree displaying the options of using either TLC or Cardiomagic.**

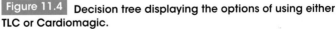

[11.10] The mutually exclusive assumption may at times make the decision tree less than a true reflection of reality. In reality, any individual can experience both an unsuccessful procedure and an adverse effect. An outcome in which more than one outcome occurs can be included as an additional potential outcome. Often, combined outcomes are not included. Fortunately, at least from the social perspective, the unusual occurrence of more than one outcome often has little overall effect on the recommendations derived from the analysis. However, for the individual experiencing both an unsuccessful procedure and an adverse event, this is a particularly poor outcome.

Relevant Options and Realistic Outcomes

Now let us see what our decision tree has and has not achieved. When looking at a decision tree, we need to ask whether the options being considered are relevant to the study question. We also need to ask whether the outcomes are realistic—that is, do they include the final outcomes that are important in practice.

When looking at a decision tree, the first question to ask is Were the relevant options considered? Notice that there is no option to use conventional treatment such as surgery, angioplasty, or medications. Furthermore, observing the natural course of events without intervening is not included as an option. Whether or not these options should be included in a decision tree depends on the question being asked and the current state of knowledge. The choice between TLC and Cardiomagic may be appropriate if one of these must be selected for a particular group of individuals or both of these have been clearly shown to be superior to the other available options. When another option is considered, it should generally be included in a decision tree.

The other key question to ask in examining a decision tree is Does the decision process include the final outcomes that are important in practice; that is, do they reflect realistic decision making? This question is more complicated than it first appears since all decision trees simplify the real decision-making process. Decision trees generally leave out unusual events, especially if they are not directly related to the therapy. For instance, a procedure that requires hospitalization may result in side effects unrelated to the therapy itself. Hospitalization may increase the chances of developing hospital-acquired pneumonia or experiencing a medication error, yet a decision tree is not generally expected to incorporate these types of events.

In addition, as we have already seen, a decision tree often skips potential options. For instance in the decision tree for our example, it was not permitted to stop after unsuccessful Cardiomagic treatment results. The greater the number of chance nodes, the more data that are needed to complete the decision tree. Thus, these types of simplification are usually necessary and acceptable to make the decision-making model manageable.

The ideal way to construct a decision tree is to think of all possible final outcomes of the options being considered and to display a decision tree that reflects all of these possible outcomes. This process will usually produce a large number of unusual outcomes and a number of similar outcomes. The researcher then combines outcomes that are similar and decides whether certain outcomes are so unusual or so inconsequential that they can be deleted from the decision tree. This very common practice is referred to as *pruning the decision tree*.[11.11]

Time Horizon

In order to include an option in a decision-making investigation it is important to determine how far into the future the outcomes will be considered. This is known as the *time horizon* or analysis horizon. The timing of occurrence of potential outcomes is an important consideration in structuring the options in a decision-making investigation.[11.12] Some events occur immediately, and others may take years to occur. Some events may occur only once, whereas others may recur in the near or distant future. Whether or not to include events that occur in the future depends on the study's time horizon.

The time horizon is the follow-up period that determines which outcomes are included in the model. The time horizon tells us how far into the future to look for favorable or unfavorable

---

[11.11] In addition, the reader must ask the bigger questions of whether the approach used in outlining the decision tree is a realistic reflection of clinical or public health decision making. Remember that the decision tree used here implied that the choice was between TLC and Cardiomagic. However, if there is an alternative to use Cardiomagic first and if it is not successful to use TLC, then the decision tree does not reflect realistic decision making.

[11.12] When examining a decision tree and considering the options, it is also important to identify the *time frame* of the analysis. The time frame is the period during the course of the disease when it is possible to use the intervention. Here, TLC and Cardiomagic are being used at the time when single-vessel coronary artery disease has become symptomatic. If the time frame of the analysis had extended to an earlier period in the course of the disease before symptoms had developed, it may have been possible to select preventive interventions. Thus, the choice of time frame can be very important in selecting decision options.

outcomes. The investigation may be interested only in short-term outcomes, such as hospital mortality, long-term outcomes such as late recurrences, or even consequences for the next generation. Notice that the TLC decision tree that we used only considers the immediate outcomes. However, what if TLC could damage the coronary arteries and increase the probability of late complications? If this is the case, a decision tree for TLC with a longer time horizon would need additional chance nodes displaying additional outcomes.

Ideally, the time horizon should extend throughout the life of the individuals who receive the intervention option. When shorter time horizons are used, the reader should ask Was the time horizon long enough to include all important favorable or adverse outcomes?

The choice of appropriate time horizon may itself be quite complex. With genetic interventions, the appropriate time horizon may extend to future generations. The time horizon may also be important in determining the proper structure of a decision tree, including which complications to consider. For instance, if the time horizon is extended long enough, the disease may recur; that is, the treated coronary artery may experience restenosis or disease may develop in additional arteries. It is possible to construct more complicated decision trees incorporating recurrences and applying techniques known as *Markov analysis* to incorporate recurrent events into decision trees. Markov analysis allows the development of complex models in which one individual can potentially move back and forth through stages of disease over extended periods.

The assignment process in decision-making investigations can be thought of as structuring the decision-making model. An important technique for displaying or diagramming a decision model is a decision tree.[11.13] Having created the decision-making model, the next step in the process is to look at how the data in the model were obtained. This issue is addressed in the assessment process.

ASSESSMENT (5–7)

The assessment process in decision-making investigations requires the investigator to obtain information from various sources and to plug these pieces of information into a decision-making model that adequately describes the decision-making process. To better understand this process, let us see what need to be done to complete our decision tree on TLC and Cardiomagic.

A decision tree is a particularly attractive technique for diagramming decision-making because it allows the investigator to incorporate not only probabilities, but also utilities, life expectancies, and even costs. We will look at how we incorporate these measurements, beginning with probabilities.

Probabilities

So far we have looked at the components of method and assignment. In our coronary artery disease example, we have described the choices to be considered (TLC and Cardiomagic) and the meaning of decision nodes and chance nodes. Assume that TLC and Cardiomagic are the appropriate choices to consider and that TLC and Cardiomagic cannot be used together. Let us refer again to our decision tree before we proceed to look at what is needed to complete the decision tree. Figure 11.5 includes the probabilities of each potential outcome of TLC and Cardiomagic. Notice that the three potential outcomes of TLC and their probabilities are successful (0.96), unsuccessful (0.039), and death (0.001). The probabilities total 1 for each option. Figure 11.5 also outlines the potential outcomes and probabilities for Cardiomagic: successful (0.80), unsuccessful (0.198), and blindness

---

[11.13] Decision trees are not the only technique that can be used to diagram a decision-making investigation. *Influence diagrams* can be used. These display the relationships between events and the factors believed to be relevant to decisions. If appropriately constructed, influence diagrams may be converted to decision trees, which may make complex decision trees, easier to display and understand.

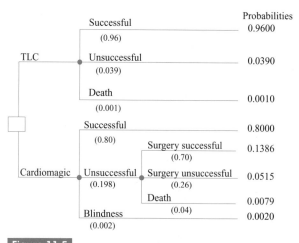

Probabilities

Successful — 0.9600
(0.96)

TLC

Unsuccessful — 0.0390
(0.039)

Death — 0.0010
(0.001)

Successful — 0.8000
(0.80)

Surgery successful — 0.1386
(0.70)

Cardiomagic   Unsuccessful   Surgery unsuccessful — 0.0515
(0.198)   (0.26)

Death — 0.0079
(0.04)

Blindness — 0.0020
(0.002)

Figure 11.5 Decision tree including the probabilities of each potential outcome.

(0.002). Calculating the probabilities of the final outcome for Cardiomagic requires us to combine probabilities. We do this by multiplying together the two probabilities. We will discuss this process further see a little later in this chapter.[11.14]

If possible, probabilities should be obtained from studies found in the research literature. Often, however, these estimates are not available and educated guesses must be used instead. When educated guesses are used to obtain probabilities, they may be referred to as *subjective probabilities*.

When using subjective probabilities, it is important to recognize that it is very difficult to accurately estimate probabilities, especially when the probability is very high (99% or more) or very low (1% or less). Thus, this problem often arises with estimates of the probability of adverse effects. In these situations, it is a common practice either to overestimate the probability, magnifying the chances of death for instance, or to underestimate the probability and therefore ignore the possibility of a rare side effect such as blindness or death.

The reader of decision-making literature needs to closely examine how the probabilities of rare but serious events were measured. When they are based on educated guesses or subjective judgments, these probabilities are especially prone to errors that need to be taken into account in the analysis.

Utilities

It is possible to directly compare the successful and unsuccessful outcomes of TLC and Cardiomagic using probabilities alone. However, it is not possible to directly compare the consequences of death and blindness using only probabilities. Thus, to complete the decision tree, it is also necessary to include a measure of the relative value or importance of death and blindness. This is performed using utilities.

Figure 11.6 includes utilities for all the final outcomes. Success is given a utility of 1, which implies that the individual returns to full health. Death is given a utility of 0, which represents the lowest possible utility. Blindness is given a utility of 0.5, which implies that it is considered to be halfway between full health and death. We will examine methods for measuring these utilities and their implications in greater detail later in this chapter. For now, we examine how utilities are incorporated into the decision tree.

[11.14] Overall probabilities are calculated based on the *independence assumption*. This assumption implies that the probability of success at surgery is not influenced by whether or not Cardiomagic was successful. At times, the independence assumption may not hold in decision-making situations. It is possible that a factor that led to failure of Cardiomagic also influences the probability of unsuccessful surgery.

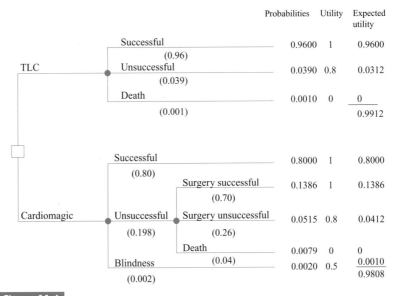

Figure 11.6 Decision tree displaying probabilities and utilities for all outcomes.

When utilities are used in a decision-making investigation, they must be measured on the same 0-to-1 scale as probabilities.[11.15] Using the same scale allows us to combine probabilities with utilities. This is performed by multiplying probabilities and utilities to obtain *expected utilities*. Expected utility can be viewed as a probability that takes into account the utility of the outcome. In expected-utility decision analysis, the expected utilities are compared. Let us see how the expected utilities would be calculated for TLC and Cardiomagic by looking at Figure 11.5.

The expected utilities of each outcome are obtained by a process known as *folding back the decision tree*. With this process, we calculate the probability of each of the final outcomes that may occur in the decision process. Once the probability of each final outcome is calculated, we multiply the final probability by the utility of that outcome. For the Cardiomagic option in our example, the following final outcomes may occur: (1) successful, (2) unsuccessful then successful surgery, (3) unsuccessful then unsuccessful surgery, (4) unsuccessful then death from surgery, and (5) blindness.

Outcomes 2, 3, and 4 require combining two probabilities to obtain the probability of the final outcome. For instance, the probability for unsuccessful Cardiomagic followed by successful surgery is obtained by multiplying the probability of being unsuccessful with Cardiomagic (0.198) by the probability of experiencing successful surgery (0.70). This equals to 0.1386, which is the probability of the final outcome.

Figure 11.5 displays the probabilities and utilities of the final outcomes. These probabilities are multiplied times their utility to produce the expected utilities for each potential final outcome of TLC and Cardiomagic, the two decision options.

One more step must be completed before we can directly compare the final outcomes of the TLC and Cardiomagic options. This step summarizes each of the options by adding together the expected utilities relevant to each option. This process is known as *averaging out the expected utilities*. In averaging out the expected utilities for TLC and Cardiomagic, we would perform the following calculations:

$$\text{TLC expected utilities} = 0.9600 + 0.312 + 0 = 0.9912$$
$$\text{Cardiomagic expected utilities} = 0.8000 + 0.1386 + 0.0412 + 0 + 0.0010$$
$$= 0.9808$$

[11.15] The question often arises as to who should be asked to assess utility. Should the investigator ask people who are already blind and have thus gained experience with blindness, or should we ask those who may become blind as a result of choosing the alternative to use Cardiomagic? The literature tells us that people who have already experienced a condition tend to score it with a slightly higher utility than those who have not experienced the condition. That is, people who have experienced blindness tend to adapt to its limitation and don't find it quite as bad as those confronted with potential blindness. The difference, however, is not great and studies of utilities may use either people who have experienced or those who have not experienced the condition to obtain measures of utility.

Now we have folded back and averaged out to calculate overall expected utilities. For an expected-utility decision analysis, these numbers represent the last step. They reflect a completed decision tree. This decision tree leads us to the conclusion that TLC is a better choice than Cardiomagic since it has a greater overall expected utility.

As we have already discussed, utilities need to be measured on a scale of 0 to 1, the same scale used to assess probabilities. Utilities, unlike probabilities, are inherently subjective; they depend on how they are viewed by each individual. Each individual measures utilities differently. Thus, there is no right utility.

What, then, are we measuring when we attempt to measure utilities? When decision-making investigations are conducted from the social perspective, the investigator is attempting to measure the average utility for individuals who are potentially affected by the outcome. Learn More 11.1 takes a look at how we can measure utilities.

LEARN MORE 11.1 ■ MEASURING UTILITIES ■ There are several techniques used to measure utilities, each of which measures a slightly different phenomenon. Currently, there is no consensus on which is best.[11.16]

The most straightforward method for measuring utilities is called the *rating scale* method. Using the rating scale method, individuals indicate their own utility for blindness using a linear scale from 0 to 1, as seen in the following example:

Mini-Study 11.9 ■ Imagine your quality of life if you became permanently and completely blind. Indicate on the following scale the relative worth of blindness. Notice that the scale extends from 0, which stands for immediate death, to 1, which stands for your state of full health.

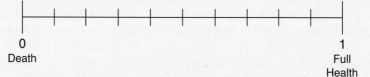

0
Death

1
Full
Health

How did you score the utility for permanent and complete blindness?

When the scores of individuals are averaged, the utility of permanent and complete blindness is usually approximately 0.50. However, there is great variability from individual to individual. Perhaps you scored permanent and complete blindness as carrying a utility as high as 0.80 or as low as 0.20. This type of variability is not unusual. In addition, it is not always obvious why one individual perceives a condition as carrying a high utility and another perceives it as carrying a low utility. At times, an individual's profession, age, or current state of activity may explain how they rate a condition's utility. More often, however, a large difference exists between similar individuals without obvious explanation. Usually the best way to estimate a condition's utility is to ask the individual.

Estimates of average utility are often quite similar from population to population, but greatly differ from individual to individual within a population. Thus, it is important to recognize that wide and unpredictable variation in utilities from person to person often exists and must be taken into account if the decision analysis is used for individual decision making.

[11.16] The technique demonstrated for directly scoring utilities on a scale of 0 to 1 is known as the *rating scale* approach. There are a growing number of other methods for scoring utilities. The *time trade-off* and *reference gamble methods* are commonly used. There is considerable controversy over the best method to use. None of the currently available methods are ideal. The time trade-off method asks the decision-maker to determine the percentage of their remaining life span that they would trade-off for a return to full health (a utility of 1). It incorporates considerations of life expectancy and discounting. The reference gamble methods ask the rater to choose between a secure outcome at a specific utility and a gamble that will bring them to either full health (a utility of 1) or alternately will produce death (a utility of 0). Reference gamble methods thus incorporate risk-taking into the measurement. The rating scale measurement has the advantages that it can be used to measure the quality of health at one point in time without incorporating issues of life expectancy, discounting for time, or risk-taking attitude.

The 0 to 1 scale used to measure utility creates issues at both ends of the scale. At the upper end, 1 is considered full health for the individual. For many medical conditions, it is impossible to bring an individual to full health. This is especially so for those with severe disabilities. Thus, when comparing an intervention designed for disabled people with one designed for people who can potentially be brought to full health, the disabled are at a disadvantage in terms of the extent of improvement that is possible as measured by utilities. An intervention may have a greater potential for improving the utility score among the potentially healthy compared with the disabled. To understand why this may be the case, consider the use of Cardiomagic in the following situation:

> **Mini-Study 11.10** ■ Cardiomagic is being evaluated for use in otherwise healthy middle-aged men compared with its use in middle-aged men on dialysis. Despite its comparable probabilities of success, no success, and blindness, the procedure was found to produce greater expected utility when used on otherwise healthy individuals.

When dialysis patients return to their previous state of health, they do not return to a utility of 1. Rather, they return to the state of health for a dialysis patient who is doing well. This explains the greater expected utility when Cardiomagic is used on otherwise healthy individuals. When dialysis patients return to their previous state of health, their utility may only increase to approximately 0.6 compared with a previously healthy individual whose health may return to a utility of 1. As suggested by this example, decision-making investigations have been criticized as having a bias against the disabled.

There are also problems at the lower end of the scale. In most decision-making investigations, 0 is defined as death. Considerable research and everyday experience tell us that, for many individuals, there are conditions worse than death. Prolonged vegetative states, severe mental incapacity, and intractable pain are typically viewed as having a utility worse than death. To use a scale that is the same as the one used for probabilities, it is not possible to incorporate negative utilities. It is possible to set immediate death as greater than 0 and to set 0 as a state worse than death. Despite the possibility of using this type of scale, it is rarely seen in the decision-making literature.[11.17]

Life Expectancy

The questions addressed so far may be the only issues addressed in a decision-making investigation. If so, the investigation is an expected-utility decision analysis. That is, it considers only the probability of favorable and unfavorable outcomes and the utilities attached to these final outcomes.

When a decision analysis incorporates life-expectancy measures, the results are usually presented using QALYs as the measurement of effectiveness. Learn More 11.2 examines what we mean by life expectancy and how it can be used as part of decision analysis.

> **LEARN MORE 11.2** ■ **USE OF LIFE EXPECTANCY IN DECISION ANALYSIS (6)** ■ Life expectancy obtained from population data utilizes the probability of death at each age in a particular year to produce a snap shot of the mortality experience of that population in a particular year. Life expectancies at any age can be calculated using what are called *cross-sectional life tables*.
>
> Cross-sectional life tables are created beginning with a hypothetical cohort of 100,000 individuals born in a particular year such as 2012. The calculations

(Continued)

[11.17] There is an additional problem inherent in the utility scale. The utility scale is linear—that is, the difference between 0.00 and 0.01 is the same as the difference between 0.50 and 0.51 or between 0.80 and 0.81. However, 0.00 is death and 0.01 implies continued life. Life and death are not measured on a continuous scale; they are discrete either/or conditions. Thus, it is important to recognize that the scale used to measure utilities cannot truly reflect the true situation, especially at the lower end of the scale.

utilize the probability of death at each age to calculate the number of individuals who are expected to survive each subsequent year. To do this, they use the probabilities of death that has been reported at each age in the year of the life table such as 2012. Thus, the life expectancy derived from cross-sectional life tables makes the big assumption that the probabilities of death at each age in 2012 will remain unchanged in the future. That is, they assume that nothing will change, a very big assumption. To the extent that the probabilities of death at different ages change, hopefully for the better, the calculated life expectancy will not be a good estimate of future longevity especially in the long term as illustrated in the following example:

Mini-Study 11.11 ■ Life expectancy for U.S. males obtained in the 1940s reflected the high rates of death from coronary artery disease especially among middle-aged men. For those born in the 1940s, a substantial percentage would have been expected to die during the first decade of the 21st century. The investigators were surprised to find that most of those born in 1940 were still alive.

Advances in prevention and treatment have greatly changed the expected life span. Fortunately, the average life span of those born in the 1940s has far exceeded the life expectancy as calculated from the cross-sectional life tables of the 1940s. Most men born in the 1940 are still alive in the second decade of the 21st century.

The term *life expectancy* sounds like it allows us to predict the future. Since the ability to predict future rates of death is limited so is the ability of calculations of life expectancy to predict the future. Nonetheless, life expectancy is often the best measure available for estimating longevity for use in decision analysis. When we are dealing with individuals who are representative of a general population, we can often obtain their life expectancy based upon their age and perhaps their gender and/or race as illustrated in the next example:

Mini-Study 11.12 ■ Life-expectancy for the average recipients of Paresis A vaccine made from a cross-sectional life table for 2012 indicated that the life expectancy for 2-year-olds was 80 years.

When a treatment is recommended for all or nearly all 2-year-olds, then we can use this life expectancy at age 2.[11.18]

When we are addressing groups of individuals with a disease, we also need to take into account the reduced longevity which can be expected due to their disease as illustrated in our single vessel coronary artery disease example:

Mini-Study 11.13 ■ The average individual with single vessel coronary artery disease is estimated to be 64 years old. Life expectancy for 64-year-olds obtained from a cross-sectional life table is estimated to be 18 years. For those without successful treatment, however, the average life span or life expectancy has been shown to be only 5 years.

Decision analysis often requires life expectancies that take into account the potentially life-threatening disease(s) of patients. These life expectancies may be

(Continued)

[11.18] Notice that the life expectancy for 2-year-olds may be slightly longer that the life expectancy at birth, which is often referred to as the life expectancy. Those who survive to 2 year have survived the causes of death during the first 2 years of life. Thus, they can be expected to live slightly longer than the average newborn. This discrepancy increases as the age increases. Thus, by age 80, life expectancy may extend for another decade or more.

> obtained from another type of life table called *longitudinal life tables,* which can be obtained from a cohort study or randomized controlled trial of those with the disease.
>
> Life expectancy for those with a disease is a combination of the impact of their age-specific mortality rate and their disease-specific mortality rate. A commonly used method for combining these factors is known as the *declining exponential approximation of life expectancy (DEALE).* The DEALE adds together the impacts of age-specific and the disease-specific mortality rates. It assumes that these two impacts are independent of each other. This assumption has been found to be generally accurate among those older than 50 years but increasingly less accurate at younger ages.
>
> The use of life-expectancy data derived from population data and group data from studies such as randomized controlled trials limits the direct application of decision analysis to individual patients. The results of decision analysis, even those incorporating individual utilizes, should be regarded as reflecting the average experience of patients. Individual patients may have a prognosis substantially better or worse than the average patient.

Now, let us see how we can incorporate life expectancy into the decision-making process using the following data[11.19]:

Mini-Study 11.14 ■ In examining the options, assume that the average individual being considered for treatment is 64 years old. Further assume that if the treatment is successful, they will return to having an average life expectancy of 18 years. If unsuccessful, assume that they will have a life expectancy of 5 years. Death produces a life expectancy of 0.

To see how these life-expectancy measures can be incorporated into the decision analysis process, let us take a look at Table 11.3.

The QALYs for each final outcome are obtained by multiplying the probability of each final outcome, the utility of each final outcome, and the life expectancy of the average individual who experiences the final outcome. Adding the QALYs together, we can average out and obtain the following results:

$$TLC = 17.44 QALYs$$

$$Cardiomagic = 17.12 QALYs$$

Once again, we can conclude that TLC is a better choice.

The measurements used to obtain life expectancy for a decision analysis can be very complex. To accurately incorporate the impact of disease on life expectancy, we need to combine life-expectancy measures using data based on age, gender, and race with data based on disease-specific survival.[11.20]

[11.19] This approach to lining up life-expectancy measures along with utilities and probabilities as the outcomes of a decision tree is rarely used in the literature. It does, however, illustrate key issues. It also points out the need to define what is included in a utility. If life expectancy is included as a separate measure, utilities should not incorporate consideration of longevity. Unfortunately, this distinction is not always made in the literature.

[11.20] As indicated in Learn More 11.2, one such approximation is known as the *DEALE*. DEALE assumes that the life expectancy at a particular age is equal to 1 divided by the sum of the probability of survival on the basis of age, race, and gender (obtained from a cross-sectional life table) plus the probability of survival as a result of disease (obtained from a longitudinal life table). The use of DEALE would imply that the reduction in life expectancy due to the need for dialysis is the same regardless of whether the patient is 65 or 35 years old. That is, the need for dialysis might shorten average life span by 10 years. A recent, more accurate approximation is known as Gama Mixed-Exponential Estimate (GAME).[8] GAME takes into account the often observed declining mortality from a disease over time. DEALE assumes that the impact of the disease continues without decline over time, thus resulting in an underestimation of life expectancy.

TABLE 11.3	Quality-Adjusted Life Years (QALYs) for TLC and Cardiomagic			
	Probability	**Utility**	**Life Expectancy**	**QALYs**
TLC				
Successful	0.9600	1	18	17.28
Unsuccessful	0.0390	0.8	5	0.16
Death	0.0010	0	0	0
Total QALYs				17.44
Cardiomagic				
Successful	0.8000	1	18	14.40
Successful after surgery	0.1386	1	18	2.49
Unsuccessful after surgery	0.0515	0.8	5	0.21
Death after surgery	0.0079	0	0	0
Blindness	0.0020	0.5	18	0.02
Total QALYs				17.12

The implications of reduced life expectancy for those with disease are illustrated in the following example:

Mini-Study 11.15 ■ A decision-making investigation is being conducted to determine whether use of TLC or Cardiomagic is better for dialysis patients with coronary artery disease whose average age is 50. The average 50-year-old is assumed to have a life expectancy of 30 years.

The average 50-year-old may have a life expectancy of 30 years based on a population's life-table data, but those on dialysis may have a much shorter life expectancy regardless of the success or failure of treatment of their coronary artery disease. Thus, the life expectancy that must be incorporated into each outcome of a decision tree is the life expectancy of the average individual on dialysis. That is, if we are dealing with dialysis patients, the relevant life expectancy may be 10 years instead of 30.

The impact of life expectancy is even more dramatic when the goal is to compare two very different treatments—one aimed at young people and the other aimed at an older population. For instance, consider the following:

Mini-Study 11.16 ■ QALY decision analysis examined the favorable and unfavorable outcomes of treating single-vessel coronary artery disease with TLC or Cardiomagic in individuals with an average age of 64. It compared these results with the prevention of Paresis A by using a vaccine in children at age 2. The prevention of Paresis A was shown to produce considerably more QALYs than the treatment of single-vessel coronary artery disease.

When comparing a treatment or a preventive intervention that is applied to very different age groups, it is important to recognize that a successful intervention among children results in a far greater improvement in life expectancy than an equally successful intervention among 64-year-olds. Thus, many more QALYs result from successful efforts to prevent Paresis A in children compared with treatment of coronary artery disease among 64-year-olds. Decision-making investigations that incorporate life expectancy, that is, when using QALYs, tend to favor the young. This tendency may or may not be justifiable, but the reader must recognize this tendency, especially when comparing different types of treatments aimed at different age groups.

Costs

Costs are not generally incorporated directly into a decision tree. Rather the decision tree is used to calculate the effectiveness, and costs are then compared with effectiveness.[11.21]

To appreciate the costs that must be considered in a cost–effectiveness analysis, let us return to our example of Paresis A:

> **Mini-Study 11.17** ■ Paresis A is a common contagious disease of childhood that is usually self-limited. However, a small percentage of children who experience the illness develop the complication of permanent paralysis, and a few develop life-threatening complications. Long-term paralysis and late complications can occur. The conventional treatment for Paresis A has been only supportive treatment, which we will call a do-nothing approach. Recently, an expensive vaccination designed to prevent Paresis A became available. A rare complication of the vaccine is development of a form of paralysis that is similar but usually less severe than the disease itself.

We will see how we can compare the costs of the vaccine with the do-nothing approach. When assessing the costs of an intervention, it is necessary to consider the types of cost discussed in the next three sections.[11.22]

Short-term Health Care Costs

Health care costs include the cost of delivering the service and treating the short-term complications. For the conventional treatment of symptoms and complications, the costs include visits for health care and the cost of providing hospitalization and treatment. For Paresis A vaccine, this would include the costs of the vaccine and the associated costs of delivering the vaccine, as well as costs of treating the short-term complications that develop as a result of administering the vaccine. It would also include the costs of health care for those who developed paralysis despite use of the vaccine.

In general, short term can be thought of as costs that occur within a year of the intervention.

Short-term Nonhealth Care Cost

Nonhealth care costs include the time and expense to access care by the patient, as well as for anyone else who must provide paid or unpaid services. These especially include the costs of

---

[11.21] Occasionally, costs are directly incorporated into a decision tree as an outcome measure. When this is done, the outcome should be called *expected value* rather than *expected utility*.

[11.22] These categories attempt to present the concepts incorporated into the recommendations of Gold et al.[2] The separation of short-term and future health care costs is presented to clarify an important distinction for the reader. The use of 1 year for short term implies that no discounting for harms, benefits, or costs is needed. The omission of the use of the term "direct" is an attempt to avoid confusion with other uses of this term, such as the use of *direct* and *indirect* to indicate program cost and institutional costs, respectively. Both of these costs are included in the concept of direct as used in cost–effectiveness analysis. Note that this section does not attempt to define the methods used for actually measuring costs. The accuracy of the measurement of costs is an important issue, but one that is beyond the scope of this section. However, it is important to distinguish between costs and prices. Costs aim to measure resource use, as opposed to prices that are affected by additional factors, especially in health care.

providing care outside the healthcare system, even when this care is provided by family members without charge.

For the conventional approach, there are no costs of obtaining the vaccine, but there will be considerable costs of taking care of the illness and the short-term complications.

For Paresis A vaccine, these costs include the time required from the parent or other caregiver to obtain the vaccine and time required to care for short-term complications of the vaccine or the disease if the vaccine is not successful.

Long-term Health Care Costs

Long-term health care costs can theoretically be separated into costs that are and are not related to the disease or the treatment which is the target of the intervention such as Paresis A or coronary artery disease. The related costs of caring for long-term consequences of the disease or its treatment should be included in a cost–effectiveness analysis. In general, unrelated long-term health care and nonhealth care costs related to other diseases or conditions are not included.[11.23]

For conventional treatment, the long-term health care costs include the long-term cost of caring for those who experience the disease and survive the short-term life-threatening effects.

For Paresis A vaccine, related long-term health care costs include the costs of providing ongoing care for all those who experience the complications of the vaccine and the costs of long-term treatment of those who experience the disease despite receiving the vaccine. Long term can be thought of as beginning 1 year after the treatment and continuing for the lifetime of the individual.

Summary

In this chapter, we have looked at what each of the variables needed to complete a decision-making investigation attempts to measure. Probabilities, utilities, life expectancy, and costs are included in the assessment. Depending on the question being addressed and the type of investigation being conducted, the investigator may need to obtain the best available measurements of probabilities, utilities, life expectancies, and costs. These are called *base-case estimates*. When doubt exists about the accuracy of the base-case estimates, the investigator may need to make educated guesses of what are called *realistic high* and *realistic low values*. These provide a means of quantitatively incorporating uncertainty into the decision-making process.

In the next chapter we examine how the results are presented and look at how the realistic high and realistic low estimates can be used to incorporate uncertainty into the decision-making investigation.

REFERENCES

1. Hastie R, Dawes RM. *Rational Choice in an Uncertain World: The Psychology of Judgment and Decision Making*. Thousand Oaks, CA: Sage Publications; 2001.
2. Gold MR, Siegel JE, Russell LB, Weinstein MC. *Cost–Effectiveness in Health and Medicine*. New York, NY: Oxford University Press; 1996.
3. Petitti DB. *Meta–Analysis, Decision Analysis, and Cost–Effectiveness Analysis: Method for Quantitative Synthesis in Medicine*. 2nd ed. New York, NY: Oxford University Press; 2000.

[11.23] Unrelated costs include the cost of treating other diseases that occur unrelated to the disease being treated. Gold recommends that the costs of treating unrelated disease be included during the years of life that would have been lived without the intervention and either included or excluded for the additional years of life. In addition, Gold's recommendations allow either inclusion or exclusion of nonmedical future costs, such as food and shelter. We will assume that these are excluded, as is increasingly the practice in most cost–effectiveness analyses. If long-term nonhealth care costs are included, an otherwise successful intervention may be viewed as very expensive because it requires society to support the costs of daily living for the additional years of life. The exclusion of these costs implies a social decision to consider the value of a year outside the work force to be just as valuable as a year in the work force.

4. Greenberg RS, Daniels SR, Flanders WD, Eley JW, Boring JR. *Medical Epidemiology*. 4th ed. New York, NY: Lange Medical Books; 2005.

5. Guyatt G, Rennie D. *Users' Guides to the Medical Literature: A Manual for Evidence-Based Practice*. Chicago, IL: AMA Press; 2002.

6. Sox HC, Blatt MA, Higgins MC, Marton KI. *Medical Decision Making*. Boston, MA: Butterworth-Heinemann; 1988.

7. Levin HM, McEwan PJ. *Cost–Effectiveness Analysis: Methods and Applications*. 2nd ed. Thousand Oaks, CA: Sage Publications; 2001.

8. Van den Hout WB. The GAME estimate of reduced life expectancy. *Med Decis Making*. 2004;24:80–88.

---

thePoint ✳ Visit http://thePoint.lww.com for interactive Q&A, flaw-catching exercises, searchable eBook, and more!

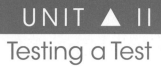

12 Decision and Cost-Effectiveness Analysis: M.A.A.R.I.E. Framework—Results, Interpretation, and Extrapolation

The results component of the M.A.A.R.I.E. framework for decision-making investigations asks us to address the issues of estimation, inference, and adjustment. The aim of estimation is to provide the best possible estimation of the strength of the relationship, that is a measure of the magnitude of the advantage of the best option compared to the conventional or standard option. Inference produces what we will call a *credibility interval* that is parallel to confidence intervals around the estimate in other types of investigations. Adjustment aims to take into account the differences between the timing of events using a process called discounting.

Let us look more closely at what we mean by estimation, inference, and adjustment in a decision-making investigation.(1,2)

RESULTS

Estimation

Estimation is a summary measurement that results from an investigation. It aims to summarize the magnitude of the advantage of the best intervention compared to the conventional or standard intervention. Each type of decision-making investigation produces one or more summary measurements. The measurement is different, however, if we are dealing with an expected-utility decision analysis, a quality-adjusted life years (QALY) decision analysis, a cost-and-effectiveness analysis, or a cost–utility analysis.

The differences between the summary measurements used in different decision-making investigations depend largely on the factors that are used to measure the outcomes. Probabilities alone may be used, or utilities and life expectancy may be incorporated. Cost may be used, or the investigation may focus exclusively on net effectiveness.

To see what we mean by these different estimates, let us return to our transthoracic laser coronaryplasty (TLC) and Cardiomagic example.

Figure 12.1 reproduces the previous decision tree for TLC and Cardiomagic incorporating probabilities and utilities of each final outcome. The summary measurement for this decision-making investigation is the difference in expected utility:

$$0.9912 - 0.9808 = 0.0104$$

This measurement may have little intuitive meaning in and of itself. However, what we will call a quality-adjusted number needed to treat can be calculated as 1 divided by this difference between the expected utilities. Here, the *quality-adjusted number needed to treat* equals the following:

$$1 \div 0.0104 \approx 96$$

This quality-adjusted number needed to treat tells us that on average, 96 individuals need to be treated with TLC instead of Cardiomagic to produce one additional life at full health.[12.1]

[12.1] For simplicity TLC and Cardiomagic are being compared. As we will see later it is important to compare each of these to the standard or conventional intervention. The quality-adjusted number needed to treat is being interpreted as the number of individuals who need to be treated with TLC as opposed to Cardiomagic to obtain one additional life at full health that would otherwise have resulted in an outcome with a utility of 0 (death) if treated with Cardiomagic. That is, how many individuals, who would have otherwise died, need to be treated to obtain the equivalent of one life saved at full health. As with all uses

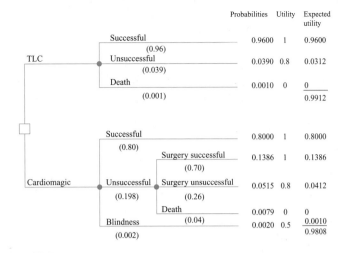

Figure 12.1 A decision tree incorporating probabilities and utilities for each outcome of TLC.

Now let us look at the summary measurement that can be used when a decision-making investigation produces results measured in QALYs. The data from the QALY decision analysis we discussed previously are presented in Table 12.1.

This data allow us to easily present the difference in QALYs per use by subtracting the 17.12 QALYs for Cardiomagic from the 17.44 QALYs for TLC:

$$17.44 - 17.12 = 0.32$$

TABLE 12.1	Quality-Adjusted Life Years (QALYs) for TLC and Cardiomagic			
	Probability	Utility	Life Expectancy	QALYs
TLC				
Successful	0.9600	1	18	17.28
Unsuccessful	0.0390	0.8	5	0.16
Death	0.0010	0	0	0
Total QALYs				17.44
Cardiomagic				
Successful	0.8000	1	18	14.40
Successful after surgery	0.1386	1	18	2.49
Unsuccessful after surgery	0.5150	0.8	5	0.21
Death after surgery	0.0079	0	0	0
Blindness	0.0020	0.5	18	0.02
Total QALYs				17.12

of expected utility, the meaning of the results assumes that we are willing to add together changes in utility from different individuals. Thus, we are assuming that preventing two cases of blindness, which provide two individuals an increase in utility from 0.5 to 1, is worth the same as providing full health at a utility of 1 compared with death at a utility of 0 for one individual.

Again, this may not have very much meaning in and of itself. In parallel to the measurement of expected utilities, we can calculate a quality-adjusted number needed to treat as follows:

$$1 \div 0.32 \approx 3$$

Thus, on average, an additional QALY results from treating approximately three patients with TLC instead of Cardiomagic. The quality-adjusted number needed to treat to produce an additional life saved or alternatively an addition QALY is thus useful summary measures for effectiveness. They tell us the number of individuals who need to receive the intervention of interest, as compared with the alternative, to produce one additional life saved or alternatively one additional life year at full health.

Cost-effectiveness Measures

The estimates for cost–utility analyses are presented in two ways that need to be understood and distinguished. Table 12.2 shows us the QALYs produced by TLC and Cardiomagic and also the costs of TLC and Cardiomagic. The table also shows this data for the conventional or standard treatment. These data allow us to calculate two types of summary measures. One is the *cost-effectiveness ratio*. The other is known as the *incremental cost-effectiveness ratio*.[12.2]

Let us examine the data for the decision using the three alternatives for single-vessel coronary artery disease (Table 12.2).

TABLE 12.2	Cost and QALYS of the TLC, Cardiomagic, and Conventional Treatment	
	Cost	**QALYs**
TLC	$116,600	17.44
Cardiomagic	$50,000	17.12
Conventional treatment	$20,000	15

Cost-effectiveness ratios
TLC, $116,600/17.44 = $6,686/QALY
Cardiomagic, $50,000/17.12 = $2,920/QALY
Conventional treatment, $20,000/15 = $1,333/QALY

The cost-effectiveness ratios for the decision alternatives for single-vessel coronary artery disease would be calculated as follows:

Cost-effectiveness ratio of TLC = $116,600 ÷ 17.44 QALYs = $6,686/QALY

Cost-effectiveness ratio of Cardiomagic = $50,000 ÷ 17.12 QALYs = $2,920/QALY

Cost-effectiveness ratios measure the average cost of an option divided by the average health outcome if that option is used. The comparison being used in a cost-effectiveness ratio is sometimes called the *do-nothing option*. The do-nothing option implies that there is an option that has no cost and produces no benefit. Thus, it might be called a zero-cost zero-effectiveness option. Cost-effectiveness ratios allow us to compare options for intervention for different diseases or conditions because all options are compared with the same do-nothing or zero-cost zero-effectiveness option.

Incremental cost-effectiveness ratios, as opposed to cost-effectiveness ratios, make what is often a more relevant comparison between two options. That is, they ask about the additional cost to obtain additional effectiveness for a particular disease or condition. Incremental cost-effectiveness ratios

---

[12.2] The special type of cost-effectiveness analysis called a cost-and-effectiveness study can also use cost-effectiveness and incremental cost-effectiveness ratios. However, for these studies, the cost-effectiveness ratio is cost per outcome, such as cost per life saved or cost per diagnosis made. The incremental cost-effectiveness ratio then measures the additional cost required to achieve an additional outcome such as a life saved or diagnosis made.

compare the option of interest with the conventional treatment, that is, the current standard treatment for a particular disease or condition. Thus, incremental cost-effectiveness ratios are the preferred comparison when we are asking about the best option to address one particular disease or condition.

Using the data from Table 12.2, let us look at the incremental cost-effectiveness ratios comparing TLC with conventional treatment and Cardiomagic compared with conventional treatment.

TLC versus conventional treatment

$$= \frac{\$116,600 - \$20,000}{17.44 \text{ QALYs} - 15 \text{ QALYs}} = \frac{\$96,600}{2.44 \text{ QALYs}} = \$39,590/\text{QALY}$$

Cardiomagic versus conventional treatment

$$= \frac{\$50,000 - \$20,000}{17.12 \text{ QALYs} - 15 \text{ QALYs}} = \frac{\$30,000}{2.12 \text{ QALYs}} = \$14,151/\text{QALY}$$

Notice that the incremental cost-effectiveness ratios are much greater than the cost-effectiveness ratios. This is the usual situation and reflects the different questions addressed by these two types of ratios. The cost-effectiveness ratio asks about the average cost of obtaining an outcome such as a QALY. This cost is really being compared with the do-nothing option that is assumed to have zero costs and zero effectiveness.[12.3]

Incremental cost-effectiveness ratios, on the other hand, are usually comparing a new intervention with the existing conventional intervention. To the extent that the conventional intervention already has a reasonable degree of effectiveness, it should not be surprising that there are substantial costs per additional unit of effectiveness (i.e., per QALY). Thus, it is important to recognize that the incremental cost-effectiveness ratio is asking about the additional cost per additional unit of effectiveness measured as QALYs.

Which ratio to use depends on the question being asked. Usually the question has to do with a choice between alternative treatments for a particular disease or condition. In this situation, the incremental cost-effectiveness ratio is the most informative. In fact, incremental cost-effectiveness ratios are now expected as part of a cost-effectiveness analysis comparing possible interventions for a single disease or condition. In general, comparing each new treatment to conventional treatment is the most helpful means of comparing different interventions for the same condition.

Inference: Sensitivity Analysis

In "Studying a Study," we showed how statistical significance testing and confidence intervals can be used to perform inference. A similar approach, called *sensitivity analysis* and credibility intervals are, used in decision-making investigations. Sensitivity analysis is a general term used to describe a series of methods for identifying factors in a decision-making investigation and determining the influence each factor has on the results of the investigation. The analyses we have looked at so far use measures that are called *base-case estimates*. Base-case estimates represent the best available data or the investigators' best guess at the true value for the factor. Sensitivity analyses are an effort to examine the consequences if a base-case estimate does not turn out to be accurate. Thus, investigators often try to define a realistic high value and a realistic low value that reflect the potential range of values. Together, we can think of these as parallel to the 95% confidence interval. This interval has been referred to as the *credibility interval*.

Sensitivity analyses are often classified as *one-way* or *multiple-way sensitivity analysis*. In one-way sensitivity analysis, one factor at a time is examined to determine whether varying its level within the credibility interval alters the conclusions of the investigation.

[12.3] The costs are compared with the do-nothing or zero-cost zero-effectiveness option, which is assumed to have zero cost and zero effectiveness even when that is not a realistic possibility. For instance, even when there is no intervention, there may be costs such as custodial care.

Let us look at how a one-way sensitivity analysis might be performed[12.4]:

Table 12.3 summarizes the results of a one-way sensitivity analysis that varies measures of the utility of blindness for the comparison of TLC and Cardiomagic. For this one-way sensitivity analysis, a high estimate and a low estimate are used in addition to the base-case estimate that was used in the original analysis. The high estimate is designed to reflect the upper end of what is felt to be a realistic range of possible values, whereas the low estimate is designed to reflect the lower end of this realistic range.

When looking at the results of a one-way sensitivity analysis, we are interested in determining whether the relationships between the decision options change when the high or the low estimate is substituted for the base-case estimate. If using the realistic high or realistic low estimate for

TABLE 12.3	Cardiomagic versus Conventional Therapy: One-Way Sensitivity Analysis for Utility of Blindness		
	Incremental Cost (Baseline)	Incremental QALYs	Incremental Cost-Effectiveness Ratio
Blindness utility 0.8 (high)	$30,000	2.13	$14,085
Blindness utility 0.5 (base-case)	$30,000	2.12	$14,151
Blindness utility 0.2 (low)	$30,000	2.11	$14,218

a factor such as cost, probability, or utility alters our preference for one option over another, then we say that the recommendation is sensitive to a particular factor. For instance, in constructing the decision tree for Cardiomagic, we used a base-case utility for blindness of 0.5. Now look at what happens in Table 12.3 if we alter the utility of blindness from a high of 0.8 to a low of 0.2. This change has very little impact on the expected utility, and the recommendation to use Cardiomagic is not affected. When a decision is not affected by changes in a factor within its realistic range, we say that the decision is not sensitive to the factor.

Table 12.4 shows a one-way sensitivity analysis for Cardiomagic and cost. Notice that the impact of the realistic high and realistic low cost estimates on the incremental cost-effectiveness ratio is substantial. However, even the use of the high estimate produces an incremental cost-effectiveness ratio of $28,302/QALY, which is well below the $39,590/QALY incremental cost-effectiveness ratio for TLC. Thus, despite the substantial change in cost per QALY, the conclusion that Cardiomagic is more cost effective than TLC is not sensitive to the estimates of cost.

It is important to look at key factors one at time and examine how their realistic high and low values may influence a recommendation. However, these one-way sensitivity analyses underestimate the uncertainty that exists because variation in more than one factor is at work at the

TABLE 12.4	Cardiomagic versus Conventional Therapy: One-Way Sensitivity Analysis for Costs		
	Incremental Cost	Incremental QALYs (Baseline)	Incremental Cost-Effectiveness Ratio
Cardiomagic cost high	$60,000	2.12	$28,302/QALY
Cardiomagic cost base-case	$30,000	2.12	$14,151/QALY
Cardiomagic cost low	$20,000	2.12	$9,434/QALY

[12.4] Note that the definition of sensitive to a factor used here is not the only possible use of the term. At times the term sensitive will be used when a substantial change occurs even thought it does not alter the recommendation. Other one-way sensitivity techniques are used for special purposes. One is *threshold analysis*, which varies key factors to determine the level of these factors that would alter the recommendation obtained from a particular decision-making investigation. Threshold analyses aim to determine the toss-up points or thresholds at which a different recommendation would be made.

same time in practice. Thus, it is often important for the investigators to perform a multiple-way sensitivity analysis, altering two or more factors simultaneously.

An extreme but commonly used and easy to understand form of multiple-way sensitivity analysis is called the *best case/worst case analysis*. Best case/worst case analysis reflects the investigators' attempt to create scenarios in which two or more key factors are favorable within a realistic range (best case) or unfavorable within a realistic range (worst case). These scenarios are not designed to reflect the very worst or very best possible outcomes, but rather the extremes of the realistic range.[12.5]

Table 12.5 shows how a best case/worst case analysis might look for the incremental cost-effectiveness ratios of TLC compared with conventional treatment. Two important factors, the probability of success and the cost, are initially set at the most favorable realistic estimates and then both are set at the least favorable realistic estimates.

When the probability of success and the cost for TLC are set at their most favorable realistic level (best case), the incremental cost-effectiveness ratio is $31,202/QALY. This best-case situation for TLC can then be compared with the base-case estimate for Cardiomagic. This

TABLE 12.5 Cost Effectiveness of TLC versus Conventional Treatment: Best Case/ Worse Case Analysis		
	Incremental Cost	Incremental Cost-Effectiveness Ratio
TLC best case success = 98%	$85,000	$31,202/QALY
TLC base case success = 96%	$96,600	$40,000/QALY
TLC worst case success = 90%	$120,000	–$500,000/QALY

best-case situation for TLC is still far greater than the $14,151/QALY base-case estimate for Cardiomagic. This provides convincing evidence that Cardiomagic is more cost effective than TLC, and this conclusion is not sensitive to the cost of TLC or its effectiveness within the realistic ranges.

When the probability of success and the cost of TLC are set at their least favorable realistic level (worst case), the incremental cost-effectiveness ratio is –$500,000. This negative number implies that, given these unfavorable assumptions, TLC is now less cost effective than conventional treatment. If these unfavorable assumptions are true, then by spending $500,000 on TLC, we are reducing the effectiveness by 1 QALY compared with using conventional treatment. Thus, our multiple-way sensitivity analysis has raised some degree of uncertainty as to whether TLC is actually a better treatment than conventional therapy.

Adjustment: Discounting

In general, adjustment is performed to take into account differences in alternatives that can affect the results. In decision-making investigations, the timing of events is a very important factor that needs to be taken into account as part of the adjustment. Timing of events is important for both decision analysis and cost-effectiveness analysis.

[12.5] The best case/worst case sensitivity analysis is often considered too demanding an approach because it is unlikely that uncertainties in multiple key variables will act in the same direction. Other forms of multiple-way sensitivity analyses are increasingly being used to calculate the confidence intervals or credibility intervals. Several complicated mathematical approaches are used to obtain these estimates. The best known is the *Monte Carlo Simulation*, which aims to establish credibility intervals by randomly selecting levels of each of the key variables using computer simulations. By performing a large number of these simulations, a distribution of results can be obtained and used to calculate a credibility interval.

To understand the impact of the timing of events, let us take another look at TLC. Recall that using the base-case estimate, TLC has been found to be more effective in treating single-vessel coronary artery disease compared with conventional treatment. It produces a substantially greater probability of favorable short-term outcomes despite its slight increase in adverse outcomes.

Short-term net effectiveness in comparison with conventional treatment still leaves open questions regarding TLC's impact on favorable outcomes in the long term, as well as possible long-term adverse outcomes. Assume that the following information is now available:

Mini-Study 12.1 ■ More than a decade after the widespread use of TLC began, it was recognized that late effects on the coronary artery made it more likely to close, producing a higher incidence of late myocardial infarction.

In most decision-making situations, not all events occur at the same time. The impacts of treatment may be immediate or delayed for many years. Even in the absence of an intervention, a disease may not have an impact until many years later. Note that people who experience the late effect on the coronary artery have still received the advantage of the favorable short-term outcome. That is, on average, they have lived longer.

The most common and accepted method for taking into account the consequences of the timing of events is *discounting*.[12.6] Discounting is a method for taking into account the fact that the benefits, harms, and costs that occur in the future are given less importance than those that occur immediately. The concept of discounting comes from economics and is most easily understood in terms of costs. However, it is important to recognize that discounting or taking into account the timing of events needs to be conducted for costs, benefits, and harms. An adverse outcome in the distant future is not as bad as an adverse outcome that occurs in the immediate future. Similarly, a favorable outcome in the distant future is not valued as highly as a favorable outcome that occurs in the immediate future. For instance, with Paresis A vaccine, the favorable outcome of prevention of paralysis does not necessarily occur immediately. A case of Paresis A prevented may occur several years in the future.

The concept of discounting can be understood by recognizing that most people prefer to receive $100 today rather than $100 a year from now. This is the situation even if the payoff a year from now takes inflation into account. That is, most people prefer $100 now to receiving $100 plus a guaranteed adjustment for inflation a year from now. As economists see it, if you receive $100 today, you generally can invest the money and, on average, receive a *real rate of return*. The real rate of return means that 1 year from now, you will have more than $100 even after the adjustment for inflation.

Looked at the other way, most people would prefer to pay $100 a year from now rather than today. A dollar paid in the future is not as costly as a dollar paid today. In fact, when performing discounting, the investigator is really calculating the amount of money that needs to be invested today to pay bills that are not due until a future time. The amount of money that needs to be invested today is called the *discounted present value* or *present value*. To calculate the discounted present value, the investigator needs to choose what is called a *discount rate*. Choosing a 3% annual

---

[12.6] The two basic approaches to taking into account the effects of timing are discounting and incorporating the timing of events into utilities. Most experts consider discounting of costs, favorable outcomes, and adverse outcomes to be the proper approach for decision analysis and also for cost-effectiveness analysis. In decision analysis, however, timing of events may at times be incorporated into utilities. Note that decision trees are structured to reflect the sequence of events, but they do not tell much about the time intervals between events. Long-term consequences are not necessarily distinguished from short-term consequences in a decision tree. Unless explicit discounting occurs, outcomes are usually dealt with as if they occur simultaneously. That is, a discount rate of 0% is used or the impact of timing is incorporated into the measurement of utilities.

discount rate implies that approximately $97 need to be put aside and invested today to ensure the availability of an inflation-adjusted $100 a year from now. If the discount rate is 5%, only about $95 needs to be put aside today to ensure the availability of an inflation-adjusted $100 a year from now.[12.7]

What is the proper discount rate? Economists generally agree that costs should be discounted to reflect the real rate of return, which is the rate that can be expected on average from investing money after taking into account the impact of inflation. There the agreement ceases because the real rate of return is neither constant nor predictable. However, the accepted range of discount rates is between 3% and 5%. A 3% discount rate is recommended when performing a sensitivity analysis. A second analysis to determine the consequences of using a 5% realistically high and a 1% realistically low discount rate can also be performed.

The discount rate for favorable and adverse effects should generally be the same as the discount rate used for costs. If different rates are used, the following situation can occur:

> **Mini-Study 12.2** ■ In discounting costs, favorable outcomes, and adverse outcomes for Paresis A vaccine, costs were discounted at 5%, but favorable outcomes were discounted at 3%. The authors concluded that since interventions that could be implemented in the future were much less expensive, it is desirable to wait to implement a Paresis A vaccine campaign.

Discounting costs at a greater discount rate than favorable outcomes always encourages delay. If costs are discounted at a greater rate than favorable outcomes, then every year, it looks desirable to wait until the next year because in future years, it will cost less to produce a favorable outcome. Thus, regardless of the discount rate that is used, it is important to discount cost, favorable outcomes, and adverse outcomes at the same discount rate. It is not enough just to discount costs. It is generally accepted that favorable and adverse outcomes also need to be discounted, and at the same discount rate as costs.

We have now examined the results that are produced through a decision-making investigation. Let us now turn our attention to the interpretation component of the M.A.A.R.I.E. framework.

INTERPRETATION (3,4)

Cost-Effectiveness Ratios

As with other types of investigations, interpretation is designed to evaluate the meaning of the results for the types of individuals who are included in the investigation. With decision-making investigations, no individual or group is actually included in the investigations. Rather, the investigator usually creates a model designed to simulate the situation facing particular types of individuals. Thus, the interpretation of a decision-making investigation should address the investigation's meaning for the types of individuals for which the investigation was designed.

Often, the most important and confusing interpretation in a decision-making investigation is the meaning of the cost-effectiveness ratios. Let us take a close look at how we interpret these ratios for the types of studies on single-vessel coronary artery disease and Paresis A vaccine that we have already examined. Since we are comparing interventions for two different conditions, we will use the cost-effectiveness ratios when making comparisons. That is, we will compare each of our options with the do-nothing or the zero cost–zero effectiveness option.

[12.7] Note that if the discount rate is 0%, then $100 needs to be put aside to ensure the availability of $100 a year from now. Thus, if discounting is not performed, the investigator is really assuming a discount rate of 0%.

As we have seen, the cost-effective ratios of the three options for treating single-vessel coronary artery disease are obtained as follows:

TLC: $116,600 ÷ 17.44 QALYs

Cardiomagic: $50,000 ÷ 17.12 QALYs

Conventional treatment: $20,000 ÷ 15 QALYs

We previously found that Paresis A vaccine reduced the cost by $2,000 per QALY compared with the do-nothing option—the only available alternative. Thus,

Paresis A vaccine: −$2,000 ÷ 1 QALY

To compare the Paresis A cost-effectiveness ratio with the TLC cost-effectiveness ratio, we need to calculate the cost of 17.44 QALYs when using Paresis A as follows:

Paresis A vaccine: −$34,888 to gain 17.44 QALYs

To examine the implications of these cost-effectiveness ratios, their components can be plotted on a cost–QALYs graph. Figure 12.2 is a cost–QALYs graph. Notice that it contains four areas, or quadrants, labeled A, B, C, and D. The zero point for the graph depends on the comparison being made. When we are addressing one condition such as single vessel coronary artery disease, the comparison would be the conventional or standard therapy. When we are comparing interventions for different conditions such as Paresis A and single vessel coronary artery disease we can compare the interventions to the do-nothing or zero cost-zero effectiveness option.

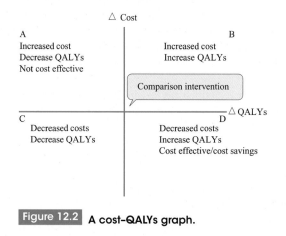

Figure 12.2 **A cost-QALYs graph.**

Figure 12.3 uses a cost–QALY graph to plot the cost-effectiveness ratios for the options to treat single vessel coronary artery disease and to prevent Paresis A.

Use of a cost–QALYs graph allows visual comparison between options for the same condition and/or different conditions. Each of the four quadrants has a different implication. Quadrant D, where Paresis A vaccine is located, is the ideal quadrant. Here, there is increased effectiveness as measured by QALYs and reduced cost as measured in dollars. The cost-effectiveness ratio in quadrant D is thus negative. When an option is located in quadrant D, it is cost-saving/effectiveness-increasing. This is a special situation in which we can unequivocally say that the results are cost-effective.

At times, this situation is called *cost savings*. Use of this term results in considerable confusion because cost savings can also result when the number of QALYs are reduced. This is the situation when the results are in quadrant C, in which there is a cost reduction accompanied by an effectiveness reduction as measured by reduced QALYs. Quadrant C is more accurately labeled cost-reducing/effectiveness-reducing.

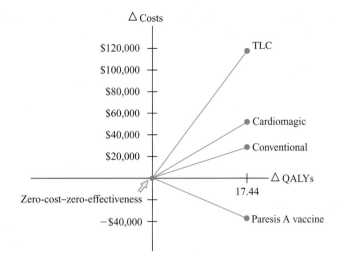

Figure 12.3 **Cost-QALYs graph depicting cost-effectiveness ratios.**
This graph allows comparison between options for the same condition
or for different conditions. Note that cost-effectiveness ratio rather than
incremental cost-effectiveness ratio is used here since interventions for
different conditions are being compared.

When interpreting decision options that fall into quadrant C, it is important to recognize that they may be labeled cost-effective if the decision-maker concludes that a relatively small reduction in QALYs is worth the substantial reduction in cost. At times, it may be reasonable to substantially reduce costs even though effectiveness is also reduced. However, calling this approach cost-effective obscures what is happening. It is better to label this cost-reducing/effectiveness-reducing and then to separately determine whether the reduction in cost justifies the reduction in effectiveness.

Quadrant A is also a clear-cut result. In this quadrant, the costs are increased and the effectiveness is decreased. Therefore, neither costs nor effectiveness supports using an option that falls in quadrant A, and such options should be labeled as not cost-effective.

Most alternatives being considered by QALY cost-effectiveness studies end up in quadrant B. These decision alternatives increase both cost and effectiveness. When an alternative is located in quadrant B, it is very important to determine the magnitude of the cost-effectiveness ratio and to be sure their meaning is clear.

When treatments are located in quadrant B, where both costs and effectiveness are increased, we are faced with the difficult questions of where to draw the line. When determining where to draw the line, it is important that we compare the options with conventional treatment, not with the do-nothing option. Thus, incremental cost-effectiveness ratios rather than cost-effective ratios should be used when deciding whether an intervention which increases cost as well as increasing effectiveness is considered cost effective.

Let us review the data we have obtained on incremental cost-effectiveness ratios for TLC and Cardiomagic compared with the conventional treatment:

Mini-Study 12.3 ■ The incremental cost-effectiveness ratios for TLC compared with conventional treatment is approximately $40,000 per QALY, and the incremental cost-effectiveness ratio for Cardiomagic compared with conventional treatment is approximately $14,000 per QALY. Should either or both of these options be considered cost-effective?

The answer depends on how cost-effectiveness is defined. Considerable controversy exists regarding the methods for interpreting these results and deciding which treatments should be labeled cost-effective. Various methods have been used to try to categorize the results of incremental cost-effectiveness ratios to be able to establish a level which is considered cost-effective. This has been very controversial because determining what dollar figure to use to draw the line requires placing a monetary value on a QALY. Take a look at Learn More 12.1 to better understand how a dollar figure is currently placed on a QALY.

LEARN MORE 12.1 ■ HOW MUCH IS A QALY WORTH? ■ An important and controversial question in cost-effectiveness analysis has been What is a QALY worth? There are several potential approaches to this question that have been attempted.

One method used in the past was to place a monetary value on a QALY was the *human capital approach*, which attempts to convert a QALY into a dollar value based on recipient's ability to contribute economically. This approach has been criticized because it only includes activities that result in financial payments and thus undervalues those who work without monetary payments, the retired, and low-wage groups.

Efforts have been made to use what economists call a *willingness-to-pay approach*. These approaches are attractive to economists but have been very difficult to implement. Past practices based on malpractice awards and legislative liability decisions have been used as evidence of a society's willingness to pay. In general, using malpractice awards result in placing a very high monetary value on a QALY, whereas using legislative reimbursement formula places a very low monetary value on a QALY.

A simple but useful approach is to use the per capita income, or the per capita gross domestic product (GDP) of the nation in which the investigation is conducted or to which the results will be applied. The question then become what can a country afford rather than what is a QALY worth?

Today, there is a general consensus that the question really is "What can a society afford?" and not "What is a QALY worth?" Often the per capita GDP is used as an approximation of what a society can afford to pay for a QALY. Therefore, acceptable and unacceptable ranges depend heavily on a society's economic wealth. The $14,000 figure is clearly within the per capita yearly income for North America and most of Europe and Japan. However, the $40,000/QALY may not be considered cost-effective even in many developed countries.

In addition, neither of these options would be considered cost-effective in a developing country with a per capita income of $3,000. However, in nations with low per capita incomes, the costs may also be substantially lower.

When a definitive value is set on a QALY, the investigation is really a cost–benefit analysis because equating a QALY with a set monetary figure allows all outcomes to be converted to dollars. Remember that the essential difference between cost-effectiveness analysis and cost–benefit analysis is that in cost-benefit analysis, outcomes and costs are both explicitly measured in monetary units.

In the United States, where the per capita gross domestic product is approaching $50,000 the following general approach is often used:

1. Incremental cost-effectiveness ratios of less than $50,000/QALY are generally considered cost-effective.

2. Incremental cost-effectiveness ratios of $50,000 to $100,000 are considered borderline cost-effective.

3. Incremental cost-effectiveness ratios of $100,000 or greater are generally considered not cost-effective.

This approach makes it clear that the approximately $14,000 incremental cost per QALY for Cardiomagic is considered cost-effective in the United States. The incremental cost of approximately $40,000 per QALY for TLC would also be considered cost-effective in the United States as long as conventional therapy is used as the comparison option.

However, if Cardiomagic becomes accepted as standard or conventional treatment, the use of TLC looks very different.

Let us calculate the incremental cost-effectiveness ratio comparing TLC with Cardiomagic:

$$\text{TLC versus Cardiomagic} = (\$116,600 - \$50,000)/(17.44 - 17.12 \text{ QALYs})$$
$$= \$66,600/0.32 \text{ QALYs} \approx \$208,000/\text{QALY}$$

This large incremental cost-effectiveness ratio tells us that to produce an additional QALY using TLC instead of Cardiomagic costs over $200,000 per QALY.

What are the implications when an intervention falls clearly outside the range of cost-effectiveness from the social perspective? First, it is important to note that when an intervention is clearly outside the cost-effectiveness range, it may still be more effective than the alternatives. In fact, TLC has been found to be slightly more effective than Cardiomagic, producing 17.44 QALYs per use compared with 17.12 QALYs for Cardiomagic. These additional QALYs, however, are very expensive to achieve.[12.8]

It is important to recognize that an intervention that has been declared not cost-effective from a social perspective may look quite different from an individual perspective. An individual who has the personal resources or adequate insurance coverage may well favor the use of TLC rather than Cardiomagic despite the extremely high cost per extra QALY.

Subgroups: Distributional Effects

We have already seen that cost-effectiveness analysis may be viewed as being biased in favor of the young over the old. In addition, we have seen that a bias exists in cost-effectiveness analysis toward the healthy as opposed to the permanently and severely disabled. In particular situations, there may be additional tendencies to favor one group over another. To understand these impacts, it is important to examine the results of a decision-making investigation to determine what types of individuals receive the favorable outcomes and what types experience the adverse outcomes. In addition, it is important to focus on the types of individuals who bear the financial costs. This is parallel to looking at subgroups.

The process of interpreting the results of a decision-making investigation is not limited to interpreting the summary measures such as incremental cost-effectiveness ratios. Summary measures, by definition, are averages. They are designed to summarize the average results. Average results do not tell the whole story for two fundamental reasons. First, the average does not in and of itself says much about what types of individuals experience the favorable outcomes and what types experience the adverse outcomes or must pay the additional costs. Examining the types of individuals who experience the favorable and adverse outcomes as well as the costs in decision-making investigations is known as examining the *distributional effects* of the intervention.

To illustrate the distributional effects, let us return to the Paresis A example and consider an aspect of the vaccine that we have not focused on previously. That is, which type of individual experienced the favorable and the adverse outcomes of the vaccine.

[12.8] The fact that a country cannot afford to generally provide everyone in need with an expensive service does not preclude a society from paying for its use under specific circumstances or for unique group(s) of patients. Ideally, these are justified as being subgroups who obtain substantial benefit thus lowering the incremental cost–effectiveness ratio. Several political, economic, and even research rationales may be made for heavily subsidizing a limited number of expensive services.

The favorable outcome of the Paresis A vaccine is the prevention of paralysis. The adverse outcome is the rare occurrence of a Paresis A-like illness among children of parents who have voluntarily had their children vaccinated.

It is unfortunate whenever anyone experiences the adverse outcomes of an intervention. However, when children (or their parents) voluntarily agree to accept the treatment after they are made aware of known adverse effects, they are accepting the adverse outcomes as part of the treatment. However, that is not the situation if the treatment is not accepted voluntarily. Imagine that the following new information is available on the impact of the Paresis A vaccine:

Mini-Study 12.4 ■ It has been found that the live attenuated virus contained in the Paresis A vaccine can spread to other children. Children exposed to their vaccinated peers are often protected, whereas a few children unknowingly exposed to vaccinated children may experience the Paresis A-like illness.

Thus, the impact of the adverse effects of the vaccine may fall on persons who never voluntarily agreed to receive the vaccine. Some may argue that submitting individuals to harm without their (or their parents') agreement is not an acceptable approach even if it results, on average, in improved outcomes at reduced costs. Regardless of how you view this controversy, it is important to recognize the distributional effects and at times take them into account when making decisions or recommendations based on decision making investigations.[12.9]

Meaning from other Perspectives

As we have seen, the initial analysis in a decision-making investigation should be performed from the social perspective. That is, we need to consider the harms, benefits, and costs regardless of who experiences the benefits or harms and regardless of who pays for the costs.

However, in addition to conducting a decision-making investigation from a social perspective, it may also be presented from the perspective of particular users of the investigation. These users may be insurance companies who pay the healthcare bills over the short run; government insurance systems that pay the healthcare bills over the longer run; or hospitals, health systems, or groups of professionals that receive payment for providing services.

When an analysis is conducted from a user perspective, it may not include all of the benefits, harms, and costs that should be considered from the social perspective. This can lead to potentially conflicting interpretations, as illustrated in the next example:

Mini-Study 12.5 ■ A decision-making investigation conducted from the social perspective found that TLC cost approximately $40,000/QALY and Cardiomagic cost approximately $14,000/QALY. The data were then examined from the perspective of a hospital system and an insurance company. The hospital system received payment for the TLC procedure and favored the use of TLC. The insurance company was not responsible for the cost of medications, and its findings strongly favored use of the medication Cardiomagic.

[12.9] Distributional effects often raise issues of social justice related to the impact on groups in society who have a lower socioeconomic status or are otherwise disadvantaged. Disproportionate negative impacts on groups who are already at a social disadvantage are often seen as violating principles of social justice.

In addition to the focus on reimbursement, providers of care are also concerned with their costs of providing services. Costs from the social perspective are very different from costs from a provider's perspective, as illustrated in the next example:

> **Mini-Study 12.6** ■ A reviewer of TLC, Cardiomagic, and the Paresis A vaccine literature looked at the relative costs and effectiveness from the social perspective. He concluded that for the same expenditure of funds, more QALYs could be obtained by providing all children with Paresis A vaccine and reducing the use of TLC. A hospital administrator whose hospital performed large number of TLC procedures argued in response that from the hospital's perspective, if TLC procedures were reduced in half, it would only serve to substantially increase the cost of performing the remaining TLC procedures.

The perspective of the insurance company can be understood by examining what they need to pay for as part of their health insurance policy. The provider or institutional perspective is reflected in the approach of the hospital administrator. From his perspective, costs are seen quite differently than from the social perspective. For instance, institutions have fixed costs, such as equipment, that remain regardless of how many TLC procedures they perform. The social and institutional perspectives may both be true as seen from different points of view.[12.10]

These examples indicate the limitations of cost-effectiveness analysis when conducted from specific user perspectives. Decision-making investigations are designed for the social perspective and should be interpreted primarily from the social perspective. That is, cost-effectiveness analysis is most useful for setting policies that apply to large numbers of institutions or a large population. Most users are interested primarily in their own reimbursements or costs. Thus, cost-effectiveness analysis may be presented from user perspectives, but the results should be interpreted with great caution.[12.11]

We have examined how the results of a decision-making investigation can be applied to the type of individuals included in the decision-making model. Finally, as with other types of investigations, we turn our attention to efforts to extrapolate the data.

EXTRAPOLATION (5,6)

In decision-making investigations, as in other types of studies, we need to consider the impact of extrapolation to similar populations, beyond the data, and to other populations. We first need to consider the impact of extrapolating the results to all individuals who are similar to those included in the investigation.

[12.10] Institutions may have personnel costs that cannot be reduced for lower volume because they need the equipment to be staffed regardless of volume of services. In addition, change itself involves economic (and psychological) costs. Institutions may have special concerns regarding the effect that the change will have on its reputation, cash flow, or other local effects. The social perspective views all costs and outcomes as averages for the future and does not take any of these factors into account. Thus, any one institution looking at a cost-effectiveness study will not necessarily agree that the conclusions drawn from the social perspective apply to them.

[12.11] Note that the government perspective and the social perspective are not the same. If a government provides insurance coverage, it may have a payer perspective. When comprehensive lifetime benefits are provided, including Social Security, that provide living expenses for the elderly, the tendency is even to go beyond the social perspective to try to include the additional living expenses for the additional years of life. Inclusion of these costs has been controversial, but they are not generally included from the social perspective. Payer perspectives may also be influenced by the special characteristics of the subgroup of individuals for whom they are responsible. Insurance companies that cover generally healthy individuals may look at recommendations quite differently than an insurance plan that covers the general population or individuals who have advanced disease.

To Similar Populations

Decision-making investigation may form the basis for the development of recommendations or guidelines for practice. Before decision-making investigations can serve this purpose, we need to examine their implications for the target population which should include individuals who are similar to the populations modeled the decision-making investigations.

Let us assume that a decision-making investigation has indicated that additional QALYs can be obtained at a cost that is considered cost-effective. If we want to extrapolate these results to a similar population in a practice setting, we need to consider the impact that will occur in practice.

First, it is important to address the meaning of effectiveness. The QALYs gained are not gained equally by all individuals who undergo the treatment. Some will experience a major positive outcome, some will experience no change, and some will experience only an adverse effect.

An appreciation of the impact of QALYs gained helps to avoid the following common but incorrect extrapolation of the results of a cost-effectiveness study:

Mini-Study 12.7 ■ A reviewer of the cost-effectiveness literature noted that the effectiveness of Cardiomagic was 17.12 QALYs per use compared with 15 QALYs per use for conventional therapy. The reviewer concluded that this was a quite small difference, especially because the impact occurs by adding years at the end of life.

The additional 2.1 QALYs gained per use are actually quite impressive. Few interventions provide this large an increase in QALYs. Cardiomagic is being used to treat single-vessel coronary artery disease, a condition that can be immediately fatal in middle-aged patients. For those who experience the benefit, the impact may be immediate and substantial. That is, when it is effective, it can be expected to prolong the life of younger individuals, as well as extend the longevity of the elderly. Thus, QALYs gained should not be viewed as added on only at the end of life.

In addition, to understand the impact of a decision-making study on a target population similar to the one included in the investigation, it is also important to appreciate the overall or *aggregate effects*. When extrapolating to a target population that has similar characteristics to the population used to construct or model the decision tree, the investigators are interested in the overall or aggregate effect. The aggregate effect will often depend on the size of the target population.

In decision analysis using QALYs, for instance, aggregate effectiveness may be reported as the total number of QALYs that would result if the intervention was applied to all individuals in a particular population who are similar to those included in the investigation.

Let us see the potential aggregate population impact by comparing the results of TLC and Paresis A vaccine in the next example:

Mini-Study 12.8 ■ A reviewer of the Cardiomagic and Paresis A vaccine cost-effectiveness literature noted that Cardiomagic provides on average 2.5 additional QALYs per use, whereas Paresis A vaccine provides far less than 1 QALY per use. Nevertheless, he noted that in the United States, using Cardiomagic for all patients with single-vessel coronary artery disease will provide 1.5 million QALYs compared with conventional treatment. Because of the large number of children who are susceptible to Paresis A and the large number of QALYs gained per case prevented, using the Paresis A vaccine for all children will provide 4 million QALYs. Therefore, he concluded that Paresis A vaccine is more effective than Cardiomagic.

Care must be taken when using measures of aggregate effectiveness to compare different types of interventions, such as Paresis A vaccine and treatment of single-vessel coronary artery disease, that are applied to two very different target populations. Cost-effectiveness ratios address the average impact of an intervention. Aggregate impact on a population addresses a different question than the cost-effectiveness ratios. Aggregate impact asks questions that depend on the particular composition and size of a target population. Aggregate impact does not compare directly one procedure or approach with another. Rather, it compares the impact of the procedure plus the characteristics and size of the target population. This approach may be useful at times for making population-based decisions, but it requires additional data and additional assumptions that are not part of the results of a cost-effectiveness analysis.

Beyond the Data

Extrapolation often requires that we extend the results to situations for which we do not have data. We have called this extrapolation beyond the data. An investigator may conduct this form of extrapolation using *linear extrapolation*. That is, the investigator may assume that more effort to implement an intervention will produce additional QALYs in direct proportion to the increased effort. This linear assumption may not hold true, especially when extending beyond the range of the data.

Cost, for instance, may not increase in a linear fashion as volume increases. The costs of increasing the scale or volume of services provided are referred to as *marginal costs*. Let us see what we mean by marginal costs in the following example[12.12]:

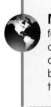

Mini-Study 12.9 ■ As Paresis A vaccine programs were implemented, it was found that the cost per vaccine delivered fell initially as the program grew and could more efficiently use personnel and publicize the program using mass media. However, as the program continued to expand, costs per vaccine delivered began to rise again as extra efforts were needed to identify and to obtain access to the most difficult-to-reach individuals.

Economists refer to *economies and diseconomies of scale*. The initial reduced cost per vaccine delivered is an example of an economy of scale, whereas the eventual increase in cost per vaccine delivered is an example of a diseconomy of scale.

To Other Populations

Extrapolation to populations with different characteristics can lead to very misleading results. Let us first look at the potential for problems when we extrapolate the results of a decision-making investigation to a new population, nation, or culture:

[12.12] The term *marginal costs* is sometimes equated with incremental costs. The two terms are not consistently used in the literature. However, it is important to distinguish between two very different concepts. Incremental cost addresses the question of the additional costs that occur when comparing one option with another under the conditions being modeled. Marginal cost relates to the changes in cost that occur when the conditions of practice are used rather than the conditions modeled in the investigation. Specifically, the conditions of practice often include a larger scale of operation that the one assumed in the decision-making investigation.

Mini-Study 12.10 ■ Paresis A vaccine was introduced into the rural areas of a developing country where a dependable source of electricity for refrigerating the vaccine could not always be assured. In this setting, the results of the intervention were very different in that the cost was considerably reduced, but so was the effectiveness. Once the problems with handling the vaccine were addressed, the intervention was found to cost only $1,500 per QALY. Unfortunately, this was considered more than the developing nation could afford to pay.

This example illustrates many of the problems with extrapolating from one population to another. The costs of labor and of delivering services may be much less in a developing country. However, if special training or equipment is needed for effectiveness, then effectiveness may also be reduced. Even if the cost-effectiveness ratios are substantially lower in a developing nation, the nation may not be able to afford the treatment. Thus, it is a very difficult task to extrapolate cost-effectiveness data and results from one society to another.

Extrapolation to groups with different characteristics can also produce misleading conclusions. For instance, imagine the following extrapolation of the TLC and Cardiomagic results:

Mini-Study 12.11 ■ The successful use of Cardiomagic for single-vessel coronary artery disease was so convincing that the results were widely extrapolated to recommend use of Cardiomagic for patients with severe coronary artery disease in two or more vessels. The favorable outcomes were not as great, and the adverse outcomes were greatly increased when Cardiomagic was applied to this new group of individuals.

It is not surprising that the outcomes will be different when an intervention is applied to groups with more severe or different types of disease. Therefore, just as in other types of investigations, it is very important in decision-making investigations to carefully examine the types of individuals who are included in the options being compared. Extrapolation to other groups carries assumptions that may not hold true among the new group of individuals to whom the results are extrapolated.

Finally, it is important to remember that cost-effectiveness investigations, like all studies, are conducted assuming a set of current alternatives and data. The alternatives may change rapidly, and unfortunately, cost-effectiveness analyses may sometimes be considered out-of-date by the time they are completed. The alternatives used in a decision-making investigation are often a simplification of the decision-making process used in clinical practice. Increasingly, efforts are being made to incorporate more realistic decision making into decision trees as discussed in Learn More 12.2.

LEARN MORE 12.2 ■ **IMPROVING DECISION ANALYSIS** ■ Decision analyses generally aim to compare two or a limited number of possible interventions. Generally, they act as if the choice to be made is to select one and only one intervention. In practice, it is often possible to select two or more interventions or to utilize one intervention followed by a second intervention if and when the first fails.

The development of prediction and decision rules increasingly forms the basis for more targeted efforts to tailor treatment to individuals based on their prognosis and their response to previous treatment(s). Thus, in theory, it is possible to create complex options that tailor the treatment to the individual and their responses to therapy.

(Continued)

Modeling these options using traditional decision analysis techniques creates extremely complicated decision trees with very large numbers of estimations that need to be made. To illustrate the basic issues, imagine the following:

Mini-Study 12.12 ■ An investigator looked at the possibility that both TLC and Cardiomagic can be used on a patient. The decision tree used a prediction and decision rule to determine which treatment should be given first. Then depending on the individual's outcome they were observed, treated, or given the other treatment.

This process rapidly creates a decision tree that is too large to fit on a printed page, although it can easily be handled by a computer. There are a very large number of probabilities and utilities that need to be considered. Nonetheless, this is the type of decision that we are faced with as our technology advances. Expect to see increasingly sophisticated computer techniques being applied to these types of decisions.

Despite the potential problems and difficulties in conducting decision-making investigations, it is important to recognize the contributions that these types of investigations make to clinical care and public health. The requirements to measure and express results quantitatively can improve communication. Decision-making investigations require the investigator to apply numbers to vague terms such as "rare" and "common," and "likely" and "unlikely." The need to explicitly define the decision-making process means that consequences must be defined and uncertainties recognized. Uncertainty always exists in decision-making. Formal decision-making investigations help us to measure and to determine the impact of uncertainty.

The decision-making literature is an important part of the movement toward evidence-based decision making in health care and public health. Decision-making investigations require the investigator to spell out in great detail the available evidence and the assumptions that have been made in filling the holes when evidence is not available. In decision-making investigations, the investigator must be able to respond to demands to show the evidence and justify the assumptions.

The forms of decision-making investigations that incorporate costs have added an entire new dimension to the health research literature. Previously, clinical and public health decision-making relied almost exclusively on issues of benefits and harm, that is, favorable and adverse outcomes. Technological advances in recent years have opened up so many therapeutic and preventive alternatives that no society can afford to do everything. Cost-effectiveness studies, despite their many limitations, often present the best available method for systematically choosing between the available options. For this reason, cost-effectiveness studies are now widely published in the health research.

Questions to Ask—Decision and Cost-Effectiveness Analysis

These questions to ask can be used as a checklist when reading decision analyzes and cost-effectiveness analyzes.

Method—Investigation's purpose and target population

1. **Study question and study type:** What is the study question and the type of decision-making investigation?
2. **Target population:** What is the target population to which the investigator wishes to apply the results?
3. **Perspective:** From what perspective is the investigation being conducted?

(Continued)

Questions to Ask—Decision and Cost-Effectiveness Analysis *(Continued)*

Assignment—Options and outcomes being investigated

1. **Options:** What options are being evaluated?
2. **Relevant options and realistic outcomes:** How are the options modeled? Are the options relevant to the study questions, and do they include realistic outcomes?
3. **Timing horizon:** How far into the future will the investigators look to determine outcomes?

Assessment—Measurement of outcomes

1. **Probabilities and utilities:** How are the probabilities and the utilities obtained, and is their measurement accurate and precise?
2. **Life expectancy:** Are life expectancies used and if so, were they appropriate to the study question?
3. **Costs:** How are the costs obtained, and do they accurately and precisely reflect the social perspective?

Results—Comparison of outcomes

1. **Estimation:** Is the summary measurement appropriately expressed, for example, QALYs, incremental cost-effectiveness etc.?
2. **Inference:** Is an appropriate sensitivity analysis conducted?
3. **Adjustment:** Is an appropriate method of discounting for present value used?

Interpretation—Conclusions for the target population

1. **Cost-effectiveness ratios:** Are the estimates such as cost-effectiveness ratios correctly interpreted?
2. **Subgroups:** Are the distributional effects on subgroups examined?
3. **Meaning from other perspectives:** What are the implications from perspectives other than the social perspective?

Extrapolation—Conclusions for other populations

1. **To similar populations:** Is the meaning for the average individual in the target population as well as the aggregate population impact addressed?
2. **Beyond the data:** If extrapolation beyond the data was conducted, is only a linear extrapolation used and are marginal effects of the scale of operation considered?
3. **To other populations:** If extrapolation to other populations is conducted, are differences from the target population of the investigation considered?

REFERENCES

1. Petitti DB. *Meta-Analysis, Decision Analysis, and Cost-Effectiveness Analysis: Method for Quantitative Synthesis in Medicine.* 2nd ed. New York, NY: Oxford University Press; 2000.
2. Gold MR, Siegel JE, Russell LB, Weinstein MC. *Cost-Effectiveness in Health and Medicine.* New York, NY: Oxford University Press; 1996.
3. Sox HC, Blatt MA, Higgins MC, Marton KI. *Medical Decision Making.* Boston, MA: Butterworth-Heinemann; 1988.
4. Greenberg RS, Daniels SR, Flanders WD, Eley JW, Boring JR. *Medical Epidemiology.* 4th ed. New York, NY: Lange Medical Books; 2005.

5. Guyatt G, Rennie D. *Users' Guides to the Medical Literature: A Manual for Evidence-Based Practice.* Chicago, IL: AMA Press; 2002.

6. Levin HM, McEwan PJ. *Cost-Effectiveness Analysis: Methods and Applications.* 2nd ed. Thousand Oaks, CA: Sage Publications; 2001.

---

the**Point** ✳ Visit http://thePoint.lww.com for interactive Q&A, flaw-catching exercises, searchable eBook, and more!

13 A Guide to the Guidelines

Most practitioners encounter evidence in their daily practice through the use of guidelines or recommendations. *Evidence-based guidelines* or *evidence-based recommendations* attempt to synthesize the evidence in order to provide a wide range of recommendations for making decisions. Recommendations for clinical practice are not new; they are as old as the teaching of the health professions. What is different about today's guidelines is the emphasis on evidence instead of authority or eminence. That is we have moved from eminence-based recommendations to evidence-based recommendations.

When reviewing an evidence-based recommendations or guideline, it is possible to use the M.A.A.R.I.E. framework to organize our approach and to help us identify the questions to ask. Figure 13.1 illustrates the application of the M.A.A.R.I.E. framework for reviewing guidelines.

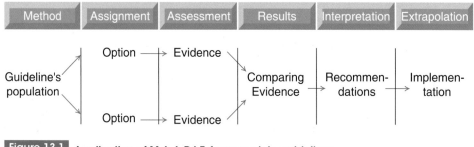

Figure 13.1 Application of M.A.A.R.I.E. framework to guidelines.

METHOD (1–3)

The Purpose of Guidelines

The movement to develop evidence-based guidelines was strongly motivated by the finding that clinicians in similar communities often have widely different practices for common and/or costly decisions. These decisions range from if and when to do surgery to whom to hospitalize. From these investigations, it was concluded that differences in practice not based on evidence result in unnecessary cost and unnecessary variations in quality. Only evidence could determine which practices were best, and only the development and acceptance of evidence-based guidelines could reduce these variations. These are the roots of the movement to develop evidence-based guidelines.

The original purposes for clinical guidelines were outlined by the Institute of Medicine as follows:

1. Assisting clinical decision making by patients and practitioners
2. Educating individuals or groups
3. Assessing and assuring the quality of care
4. Guiding allocation of resources for health care
5. Reducing the risk of liability for negligent care

Evidence-based guidelines were initially aimed at individual decision making by individual clinicians. Today, evidence-based guidelines have been developed for the full range of clinical activity, from prevention though palliation. Perhaps as a reflection of the success of the evidence-based guidelines movement, today guidelines are being applied not only for the care of individual patients by individual clinicians but also for institutional and population-based decision making. Institutional guidelines such as those for reducing the risk of anesthesia, preventing human immunodeficiency virus (HIV) infection after needle stick injury, or controlling tuberculosis in a hospital setting are now widely used.

Community guidelines have become central to public health efforts to improve population health. Community guidelines are increasingly bringing to bear the evidence for effective intervention, such as those to control tobacco use, lead paint exposure, and childhood obesity. Guidelines for responding to crises from bioterrorism to environmental contamination are now accepted as standard operating procedures.

Thus, we begin our examination of guidelines by asking about a guideline's goal. What is it aiming to achieve, and at what level—the individual patient or clinician, the institution, or the community? To illustrate key issues in development and implementation of evidence-based recommendations we will use colon cancer as an example. Let us imagine that we were examining the following type of guideline on colon cancer screening and prevention:

Mini-Study 13.1 ■ Colon cancer guidelines aim to establish indications and methods for screening those at average risk of colon cancer. They also aim to provide guidance for the use of aspirin for prevention of colon cancer.

This type of guideline is targeted at the individual clinical level when it addresses the goal of screening individual patients. When it addresses the issue of promotion of aspirin for prevention of colon cancer, it looks to the population or community level as well as the individual level. Both of these approaches have the goal of reducing the mortality rate from colon cancer, but they aim to intervene in different ways. Thus, the first question we need to ask when looking at a guideline is, What is its goal and how does the guideline hope to achieve it?

A Guideline's Target Population

It is key to understand the target population or the practice-based group for which the guideline is intended. Guidelines may be directed at narrowly defined groups or they may be directed at large numbers of individuals defined only by age or gender, as illustrated in the next example:

Mini-Study 13.2 ■ Guidelines for screening for colon cancer are developed for the average male or female 50 years and older with or without a family history of colon cancer. They are not designed to apply to those with diseases that predispose them to colon cancer, such as ulcerative colitis or familial polyposis.

This description gives us a clear understanding of the target population for the guideline. It indicates that the guideline is designed for screening, which implies that it is aimed at asymptomatic patients. The target group is those 50 years and older, and applies to both those with and without a family history of colon cancer. This is important because family history is a known risk factor for colon cancer, and the guideline might have excluded or treated this group separately.

In addition, the description indicates that the guideline does not apply to the much smaller group of individuals who are at increased risk because of predisposing diseases. It is important to appreciate from the beginning who is included and who is excluded. Guidelines, like investigations, usually have inclusion and exclusion criteria.

The Guideline's Perspective

The guideline movement has spawned an increasing number of "players" who are rapidly developing guidelines, often to serve specific or even proprietary agendas. The vast array of guidelines and guideline developers makes it useful to classify them to get a better idea of the perspectives of the authors. We might classify guideline developers as follows:

- Government agencies that seek qualified and broadly representative individuals for a committee or task force to independently develop evidence-based guidelines. In the United States, such agencies as the United States Preventive Services Task Force (USPSTF of the Agency for Healthcare Research and Quality [AHRQ]), the National Institutes of Health, and the Centers for Disease Control and Prevention have followed this approach.

- Professional societies such as the American College of Surgeons, the American College of Physicians, and many other clinically oriented professional societies.

- Nonprofit patient-oriented groups such as the American Heart Association and the American Cancer Society.

- For-profit and not-for-profit providers of care, including Kaiser-Permanente and national associations of health plans.[13.1]

Each of these organizations has its own approach, its own priorities, and at times its own biases. Thus, it is important to appreciate the authorship of the guideline so that the potential user can look for potential conflicts of interest that may subtly or not so subtly influence the way the guideline was developed or structured, as illustrated in the next example:

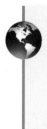

Mini-Study 13.3 ■ Recommendations for colon cancer screening were made by a government task force, a society of endoscopists, and a national consumer-oriented cancer society. The endoscopists recommendations stressed the use of colonoscopy, which allows examination of the entire colon. The consumer-oriented society stressed the use of occult blood testing and periodic sigmoidoscopy for patients who sought screening. The government task force recommended reaching as many patients as possible using various options for screening.

Even assuming the best of intentions, different groups will interpret the evidence differently. Those with experience with and interest in a technical procedure such as colonoscopy are often inclined to recommend its use. Those who represent consumers will often emphasize satisfying the desires of those who seek care and minimizing the harm or discomfort for those who do. Broadly representative groups may seek to reach large numbers of individuals, hoping to benefit as many as possible. Those seeking to reach large number of individuals may leave open as many options for implementation as possible to circumvent the most controversial of issues, such as which is the best method for screening.

There is no universally accepted approach to developing and presenting guidelines. Perhaps the most structured and rigorous approach in widespread use was developed by the United States Preventive Services Task Force (USPSTF). We will utilize their approach throughout this chapter.

Having defined the goal, the target population, and the perspective of guidelines, we will address the questions of assignment.

[13.1] For-profit corporations such as pharmaceutical companies rarely develop guidelines on their own because of their overt conflicts of interest. However, they may provide funding for other groups to develop guidelines. Thus, knowing the funding source supporting the guideline development is also important.

ASSIGNMENT (1,2,4)

The process of assignment addresses the options to consider; the types of evidence to include; and the decision making approach, that is deciding how to decide. Let us take a look at each of these three questions of assignment beginning by examining the selection of options to consider.

Options Being Considered

Guidelines should identify the options that are being evaluated as well as potential options that are being omitted, as illustrated in the following example:

Mini-Study 13.4 ■ A group of colon cancer screening guidelines compare sigmoidoscopy, colonoscopy, and virtual colonoscopy. They do not consider double-contrast barium enema or occult blood testing.

These guidelines are explicit about which methods they include for consideration and which ones they omit. Often the guidelines will only indicate which options are considered and leave to the reader the task of recognizing which options are omitted. It is important to recognize the omissions as well as the inclusions because exclusion implies that the omissions are not recommended.

Evidence—Structure and Types of Evidence to Include

The method of structuring the evidence can take several forms. As we have seen, decision making can be organized using a decision tree that defines the options, the decisions, and the outcomes of each decision, often including utilities of the outcomes as well as their probabilities. Use of a decision tree may at times guide the construction of a guideline. When that is the case, the decision tree should ideally appear in the guideline.

Often, however, other analytical frameworks and approaches are used. As we saw in our discussion of screening, the framework for evaluating a screening procedure ideally should require fulfilling four criteria: substantial morbidity and mortality, early detection improves outcome, screening is feasible, and screening is acceptable and efficient.

The evidence for evidence-based guidelines may be gathered and organized utilizing a systematic review, which as we have discussed may include a meta-analysis. Systematic review is an effort to collect and present all the relevant research evidence to address specific clinical or public health questions. As we have seen, systemic reviews may combine quantitative and qualitative methods, and often address a range of issues relevant to practice-based decision making. A meta-analysis may be used as part of a systematic review focused on a well-defined issue in which investigations are already available.

Thus, an article presenting an evidence-based guideline should indicate how the evidence is organized, as indicated in the following example:

Mini-Study 13.5 ■ A systematic review of cohort and randomized controlled trials of cancer screening was conducted to address questions of indications for screening, methods for screening, costs of screening, and frequency of screening, as well as patient acceptance. A meta-analysis was used to examine whether there were differences in the effectiveness of different screening methods.

As this example illustrates, methods of presenting the evidence may be combined. Systematic reviews are often the starting point for collecting and presenting the evidence. The evidence may then be structured to address key questions using methods such as meta-analysis.[13.2]

The types of evidence being included are usually organized into benefits, harms, and financial cost.[13.3] These broad categories are usually adequate to include a wide range of important considerations. Not all of these categories of evidence may be included. In additional other potentially relevant issues may or may not be included such as patient and provider acceptance as illustrated in the next example:

Mini-Study 13.6 ■ A guideline for colon cancer screening makes recommendations based upon on the net effectiveness—that is, the benefit minus the harm of the techniques. Issues of cost, patient acceptance, and provider reimbursement were not considered.

Thus the assignment process requires the investigator to define the categories of evidence that will be included and which will be excluded.

Decision Making Approach

In addition to deciding whether to take into account benefits, harms, and costs as well as other potential issues, it is also important to understand how they will be combined. Combining data is governed by the decision making approach being used. For instance imagine the following situation:

Mini-Study 13.7 ■ In evaluating the options for colon cancer screening, the potential methods were first evaluated for net effectiveness—that is, their benefits and harms were considered. For the two methods that demonstrated the greatest net effectiveness, cost was subsequently considered to determine which technique was recommended.

It is not unusual for developers of guidelines to separate issues of benefits and harms from those of costs. They may argue that there is no reason to consider costs unless an option reaches a certain level of net effectiveness. This approach may have the effect of excluding those options that have greatly reduced costs and modestly reduced effectiveness.

As we have seen, decision analysis and cost-effectiveness analysis are formal methods that can be used to combine considerations of benefits, harms, and costs. Decision analysis and cost-effectiveness analysis are built on decision criteria that we have called expected utility. That is, when we use an expected-utility approach, we seek to maximize the net effectiveness or the net benefits for the average person.

Maximizing expected utility is not the only possible decision making approach for combining benefits, harms and costs. Other approaches can include minimizing the harm or, maximizing the potential benefits as illustrated in the next example:

[13.2] There are several other methods for organizing and presenting data. Together, these have been called *analytical frameworks*. The Unites States Preventive Services Task Force, for example, has developed analytical frameworks for each of its areas of focus, that is, screening, immunization, counseling, and chemoprevention.

[13.3] Not all considerations in decision making relate directly to benefits, harms, and costs. Issues of ethics, for instance, may not directly relate to any of these outcomes. Guidelines can and should make as explicit as possible the types of evidence that are being considered.

Mini-Study 13.8 ■ Colon cancer screening by flexible sigmoidoscopy was considered as an option to be performed by primary care physicians. However, when using this option, if a biopsy is needed, a repeat examination and biopsy by a gastroenterologist is strongly recommended.

Here, the option for flexible sigmoidoscopy does not allow primary care physicians to perform a biopsy even if this, on average, would reduce the cost or even increase the benefit. The potential for greater harm through perforation, when the procedure is performed by those with less training and experience, is presumable paramount in recommending this option.[13.4]

Thus, the process of assignment may be summarized as the process of defining the options, organizing the evidence and deciding how to decide. Once this process is complete, we can go on to the assessment process.

ASSESSMENT (2,3,5)

The process of assessment in evidence-based recommendations requires us to look at the outcomes for each of the options being considered. The assessment process uses the decision making approach for making recommendations set forth in the assignment component. As part of the assessment process, we need to look at the sources of the data on outcomes; how the outcomes were measured; and how holes in the evidence were handled.

Sources of the Evidence on Outcomes

An evidence-based guideline should identify the specific sources of evidence on outcomes. In addition, it should provide specific information that will allow subsequent assessment of the quality of the evidence. Specifically, the types of investigations, the number of participants, and the specific outcomes measures being used are important. This can be illustrated as follows:

Mini-Study 13.9 ■ Evidence from a large randomized controlled trial has established the benefits and harms of screening for colon cancer. The trial demonstrated that fecal occult blood testing annually reduces the mortality from colon cancer for asymptomatic individuals 50 years and older regardless of their family history. Well-designed prospective cohort studies suggest that sigmoidoscopy every 3 to 5 years in addition to fecal occult blood testing further reduces mortality. A large randomized controlled trial demonstrated that virtual colonoscopy is approximately as effective as colonoscopy in detecting large but not small polyps.

As we will see, the types of investigations used to obtain the evidence on outcomes will become important issues when the guideline developers attempt to score the quality of the evidence.

Measurement of Outcomes

The measurement of outcomes may include benefits, harms, and costs. The definitions used to assess outcomes need to be made explicit as part of the assessment process as illustrated in the following example:

[13.4] Note that each of these methods implies that the options can be examined side by side. That is all the necessary information is available at the same time. Often, however, a decision needs to be made before all the necessary information is available on all the relevant options. In this situation the decision approach that has been called *satisficing* may be especially useful. *Satisficing* aims to achieve a good enough solution one that is acceptable to the decision maker.

Mini-Study 13.10 ■ Harms and benefits of screening for colon cancer were measured over the lifetime of the individual. Costs from a social perspective were taken into account only when options had approximately the same net effectiveness and also when considering the frequency of screening.

This guideline provides key information on how the measurements were conducted. It provides the time horizon for measurement, that is, the lifetime of the individuals. It also indicates how costs were calculated—that is, using a social perspective. Guidelines are expected to make available far more details. However, these details may not be readily available as part of a published article. Increasingly, however, these details should be available on a supplementary web site that accompanies a published article on guidelines.

Filling Holes in the Evidence

Evidence-based guidelines differ most dramatically from the traditional approach to recommendations in the way they treat expert opinion. In the traditional approach, experts informally reviewed the evidence and reached their own conclusions using their own approach. In evidence-based guidelines, quantitative evidence from well-conducted investigations is considered the most reliable form of evidence.

In evidence-based guidelines, expert opinion is itself considered a form of evidence. In terms of quality, however, expert opinion is regarded as the least dependable form of evidence. Thus, expert opinion is often used only when there are holes in the evidence that cannot be filled in by available investigations or other data.

Since expert opinion is itself considered a form of evidence, evidence-based guidelines often use a systematic process for collecting and incorporating expert opinion. Rather than selecting one particular expert, they may use a process designed to determine whether there is agreement among experts. If there is little or no agreement, guidelines may develop a realistic range of values based on expert opinion.

Two basic approaches to obtaining expert opinions have been called the *consensus conference* and the *Delphi approach.* The consensus conference approach, originated by the National Institutes of Health, aims to bring together face-to-face a broad range of experts to determine whether they can agree upon a predefined set of questions. Every effort is made to define those issues in which a group of experts can reach agreement. Using a consensus conference approach, when agreement is not possible, the range of realistic values might be defined.

In the Delphi approach, a representative group of experts is again included. However, in this approach, the participants never meet each other and their identities are not known to each other. The approach begins by having each participant address the questions posed, followed by formal feedback of all the responses to all of the participants. Each participant then may change their response or further justify their initial opinion. The process is continued until the participants have reached a consensus or made it clear that a range of opinions exist.

Let us see how these approaches to incorporating expert opinion might be used in the development of evidence-based guidelines, as in the following example:

 Mini-Study 13.11 ■ The evidence on colonoscopy's harms in practice were not available in the literature. A majority of an expert group using a Delphi approach believed that use of colonoscopy as an initial screening method would result in a probability of perforation of approximately 1 per 1,000 uses. Based on the Delphi approach, this best-guess estimate of the probability of perforation along with low- and high-realistic estimates were obtained.

Expert opinion here has been translated into what we previously called best guess plus realistic high and realistic low estimates. This example illustrates the degree to which developers of evidence-based recommendations regard expert opinion as a form of data that needs to be systematically collected and presented.

RESULTS (1,4)

The results component of evidence-based guidelines consists of the synthesis of the evidence upon which recommendations can be based. Thus, when looking at results, we will focus on the quality of the evidence, the methods for addressing uncertainties in the evidence, and the options that were eliminated on the basis of the evidence.

Scoring the Quality of the Evidence

The overall quality of the evidence can be judged using the following key criteria:

1. Study design and conduct of the investigations that produced the evidence
2. Relevance of the investigations to the target population
3. Coherence of the evidence supporting contributory cause and improvement in clinically important outcomes

We will refer to these criteria as study design and conduct, relevance, and coherence. Let us see what is meant by each of these criteria.

Study Design and Conduct

The developers of guidelines need to begin by assembling the available investigations related to potential recommendations. As with a meta-analysis, it is important that they undertake a complete search of the available evidence.

Developers of guidelines often evaluate the research evidence using a hierarchy of research types, starting with the highest quality type of study design as follows:

- Randomized controlled trials
- Prospective cohort studies
- Retrospective cohort studies and case-control studies

Lower quality study designs use what is called a *time series* or what we have called a before-and-after study. In a time series, there is no simultaneous control group. In a before-and-after study the study group after an intervention may be compared with the same group's outcomes before the intervention. One form of time series is exemplified by the introduction of penicillin in the 1940, in which the dramatic results compared with historical controls receiving the previous treatment, made clear the effectiveness of penicillin at least in the short run.

In evidence-based guidelines, the lowest quality of evidence is reserved for respected authorities, descriptive studies, case reports, and even the report of expert committees.

Meta-analyses are often evaluated based on the types of investigations included in the meta-analysis. Thus, a meta-analysis made up exclusively of randomized controlled trials may be considered the highest form of evidence.

It is important to recognize, however, that the type of study design alone does not ensure the quality of the investigation. Although prospective cohort studies by definition lack randomization, their size and the efforts to identify and adjust for confounding variables may make up for this inherent limitation. Likewise, the inherent tendencies for biases in retrospective cohort studies and case-control studies may be partially or fully overcome by good study design. Thus, the authors of guidelines need to consider both the design and conduct of the investigations that produce the evidence used in evidence-based guidelines. Table 13.1 outlines the system of categorizing study design and conduct that has been used by the USPSTF when grading the evidence.

TABLE 13.1	Hierarchy of Research Designs	
Category of Study Designs	Type of Study Design	Issues in Conduct of the Study
Category I	Evidence obtained from at least one properly randomized controlled trial	Statistical power, success of randomization, success of masking, completeness of follow-up
Category II-1	Evidence obtained from well-designed studies without randomization (prospective cohort studies)	Statistical power, comparability of study and control groups, completeness and length of follow-up, adjustment for potential confounding variables
Category II-2	Evidence obtained from well-designed retrospective cohort or case-control studies	Comparability of cases and controls, biases in assessment, completeness of assessment, adjustment for potential confounding, variables, potential for reverse causality
Category II-3	Evidence obtained from multiple time series with versus without the intervention, or dramatic results in uncontrolled experiments (such as the results of the introduction of penicillin treatment in the 1940s) could also be regarded as this type of evidence (dramatic changes in rates)	Quality of historical comparisons—short term before-and-after comparisons with clear-cut outcome measurements are more reliable
Category III	Opinions of respected authorities based on clinical experience, descriptive studies, and case reports, or reports of expert committees	Was a method used to establish a consensus of expert opinion—i.e., was it representative of expert experience?

Adapted from Agency for Healthcare Research and Quality. U.S. Preventive Services Task Force Guide to Clinical Preventive Services. Vol 1. AHRQ Publication No 02-500.

Thus, in developing evidence-based recommendations, the first step is to determine the degree to which the key studies have study design types high in the hierarchy of research designs and are well-conducted studies. The USPSTF refers to this evaluation as determining *aggregate internal validity*. Specifically, aggregate interval validity is the degree to which the studies provide valid evidence for the population and the setting in which it is conducted.

Relevance

In addition to evaluating the quality of the investigations, it is also important to evaluate their relevance. Relevance refers to the degree to which the intervention of interest has been investigated in groups or populations that are similar to the populations of interest—that is, the target population for whom the intervention is intended. The USPSTF calls the evaluation of relevance *aggregate external validity*.[13.5]

[13.5] The USPSTF is interested in the applications of preventive services to primary care. Thus, they define aggregate external validity as the extent to which the evidence is relevant and generalizable to the population and conditions of typical primary care practice.

Expert opinion may be needed to evaluate relevance. However, the process should begin by examining the evidence itself. To evaluate the relevance of an investigation, guideline developers need to ask such questions as, Are the types of patients studied and the methods used typical of the types of patients and methods that are encountered in typical clinical practice? For example, primary care practice if the intervention is designed for primary care. Table 13.2 summarizes the types of factors that can affect the relevance of an investigation and gives an example of each factor.

TABLE 13.2	Factors Affecting Relevance of the Evidence	
Factor	**Meaning**	**Example**
Patient relevance—biological analogy	Are there biological reasons to believe that the results obtained in a study will be different in another population?	Data on colon cancer might be extrapolated from men to women, but data on coronary artery disease might not be
Patient relevance— demographic, risk, and clinical differences	Were the populations studied different from the populations for which the intervention is intended in ways that may affect the results?	Studies on older, severely ill patients may not apply to younger, generally healthy individuals
Intervention relevance— relationship of the intervention to clinical practice	Was the intervention method used in the investigations similar to those routinely available or feasible in typical practice?	An investigation that used special equipment to monitor the patients, special incentive to increase adherence to treatment, or special methods to reduce or detect side effects may not be directly relevant to use in clinical practice
Intervention relevance— relationship of the investigations' setting to clinical practice	Were the special characteristics of the research settings likely to affect the results?	Were differences such as availability of consultants, 24-hour coverage, or increased attention as part of research likely to alter the outcome in the usual clinical setting?

Adapted from Agency for Healthcare Research and Quality. U.S. Preventive Services Task Force Guide to Clinical Preventive Services. Vol 1. AHRQ Publication No. 02-500.

Coherence

Finally, in addition to evaluating the study design and conduct and relevance of the evidence, it is important to ask what we will call coherence questions—does the evidence fit together? Coherent evidence requires that we ask

- Are there gaps in the evidence or does the evidence hold together as a convincing chain demonstrating efficacy or contributory cause?
- Has it been demonstrated that the intervention actually improves important health outcomes? That is, has effectiveness been demonstrated for outcomes that are important for the quality and/or length of life?

Thus high quality evidence should allow us to demonstrate effectiveness as well as efficacy. Ideally, we want to demonstrate that clinically important end points are improved and not just early surrogate end points unless these surrogate end point can be shown to correlate closely with important clinical end points.

Scoring the Quality of the Evidence

Guideline developers thus need to combine considerations of design and conduct with questions of relevance and coherence to produce an overall measurement of the quality of the evidence. A scoring system for the overall evidence has been used by the USPSTF. It classifies the overall quality of the evidence as

- Good
- Fair
- Poor

Table 13.3 outlines the definition of each category of quality and the meaning of the category. When these summary judgments regarding the quality of the evidence are used, the reader of the guidelines needs to appreciate the types of reviews and conclusions that should lie behind the final score. For instance, imagine the following conclusions about the quality of the evidence:

TABLE 13.3	Scoring the Overall Quality of the Evidence	
Evidence	**USPSTF Definition**	**Meaning**
Good quality	Evidence includes consistent results from well-designed, well-conducted studies in representative populations that directly assess effects on health outcomes	When considering the design and conduct of the investigations, the relevance of the studies, and the coherence of the evidence, a convincing case for effectiveness in practice can be made
Fair quality	Evidence is sufficient to determine effects on health outcomes, but the strength of the evidence is limited by the number, quality, or consistency of the individual studies, generalizability to routine practice, or indirect nature of the evidence on health outcomes	When considering the design and conduct of the investigations, the relevance of the studies, and the coherence of the evidence, there are no fatal flaws or holes in the evidence that invalidate a conclusion of effectiveness in practice
Poor quality	Evidence is insufficient to assess the effects on health outcomes because of limited number or power of studies, important flaws in their design or conduct, gaps in the chain of evidence, or lack of information on important health outcomes	When considering the design and conduct of the investigations, the relevance of the studies, and the coherence of the evidence, there are fatal flaws or holes in the evidence that invalidate a conclusion of effectiveness in practice

Adapted from Agency for Healthcare Research and Quality. U.S. Preventive Services Task Force Guide to Clinical Preventive Services. Vol 1. AHRQ Publication No 02-500.

Mini-Study 13.12 ■ All available evidence on the use of colonoscopy for screening for colon cancer was formally reviewed. The authors of the guidelines concluded that the quality of the evidence was good.

A conclusion of good evidence implies that a systematic effort was made to identify the evidence; the evidence was derived from high-quality study types; and the investigations were well conducted. It also implies that the studies' populations were relevant to the guidelines, and the evidence produced a coherent conclusion that the intervention improves clinically important outcomes. Thus, behind the increasingly common summary statement of good, fair, and poor quality lie a great deal of careful review plus, at times, considerable amounts of subjective judgment. A score of good evidence is often difficult to achieve. Identifying fatal flaws is often relatively straightforward. Thus a score of fair is often the default score.

Addressing Uncertainties

Because of the inherent limitation of the evidence and the need for subjective opinion when scoring the evidence, it is important that guideline developers make efforts to address the uncertainties that inevitably remain.

As we saw in our discussion of decision analysis and cost-effectiveness analysis, one method for addressing the remaining uncertainties is sensitivity analysis. At times, guidelines may be subjected to formal sensitivity analysis, especially when they are built upon decision trees or other formal quantitative decision models, as illustrated in the next example:

 Mini-Study 13.13 ■ Using a formal decision analysis the net effectiveness of virtual colonoscopy was not sensitive to whether or not the procedures were conducted every 5 or every 10 years. However, conducting virtual colonoscopy screening more frequently would substantially increase the costs.

More often, the remaining uncertainties are addressed subjectively, as illustrated in the next example:

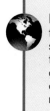 **Mini-Study 13.14** ■ The net effectiveness of colonoscopy as a screening technique for colon cancer is believed to be dependent on the availability of skilled colonoscopists who can rapidly and reliably examine the entire colon. Estimates of the number of currently available colonoscopists and the number that could be expected in the future based on current reimbursement rates led to the conclusion that colonoscopy was not an option that could be currently recommended for general use in screening.

Behind this type of result are a series of quantitative and subjective judgments that address the uncertainties regarding the usefulness of colonoscopy as a screening technique. This type of informal sensitivity analysis is often used to draw conclusions despite the uncertainties that remains.

Eliminating Options

The process of examining the results ends with an effort to determine whether any of the options being considered can be eliminated from further consideration. Eliminating options, like addressing uncertainties, may be done formally or informally.

The formal approach to elimination of options asks whether any of the options can be eliminated by what are called *dominance* and *extended dominance*. Let us see what we mean by dominance and extended dominance in the next example:

> **Mini-Study 13.15** ■ When cost and net effectiveness were considered, double-contrast barium enema every 3 to 5 years was more expensive and less effective than flexible sigmoidoscopy every 3 to 5 years. Thus, double-contrast barium enema was eliminated from further consideration. Sigmoidoscopy every year was eliminated because it was more expensive and had approximately the same effectiveness as sigmoidoscopy every 3 to 5 years plus fecal occult blood testing every year.

When one option is more effective and less expensive than another option, it is said to be dominant. The less-effective and more-expensive option is dominated by the more-effective and less-expensive option. Thus, the dominated option can be eliminated from further consideration, as illustrated in the example above for double-contrast barium enema.

Extended dominance usually implies that two options are approximately equally effective, but one option costs more to produce the same effect. The option that costs less is said to have extended dominance. Thus, in this example, sigmoidoscopy every 3 to 5 years has extended dominance over sigmoidoscopy every year, and yearly sigmoidoscopy can be eliminated from further consideration.[13.6]

In summary, the results component of the M.A.A.R.I.E. framework for guidelines looks at the quality of the evidence, the efforts to incorporate remaining uncertainty, and the elimination of options. The results component is the basis for producing the evidence-based guidelines. However, before making evidence-based recommendations the investigators need to go on to examine the components of interpretation and extrapolation.

INTERPRETATION (4,6,7)

Interpretation asks the investigator to go beyond scoring the quality of the evidence and requires scoring the magnitude of the impact. Once the magnitude of the impact has been scored it can be combined with the score for the quality of the recommendation to produce an overall grade for the strength of the recommendation. As we will see recommendations are graded as A,B,C,D, or I. Finally interpretation addresses the issues of perspective looking at how the interpretation of the recommendations may be affected by the perspective of the users of the recommendation.

Scoring the Impact of the Intervention

Recommendations require more than high quality evidence. They require conclusions about the magnitude of the impact on health outcomes. When the quality of the evidence is fair or good, then it is important to also make a judgment about the magnitude of the health benefit that can be expected for the average person for whom the service or intervention is recommended. Thus,

---

[13.6] This definition of extended dominance implies that net effectiveness is more important than cost as an initial criteria. Cost is only taken into account when the options have nearly equal net effectiveness. This reflect the approach often used in guideline development, although it is possible to envision an approach to extended dominance in which cost is considered first due to a fixed budget.

we need to ask not only does it work, but how well does it work? That is, does it have clinically important impact?

The magnitude of the impact may be classified in quantitative terms using measures such as odds ratios or relative risk, number needed to treat, lives saved, or quality-adjusted life years. Any of these measures may be used, depending on the circumstances.

These quantitative measures are used by the USPSTF and other guideline developers as the basis for scoring the magnitude of the impact as follows:

- substantial
- moderate
- small
- zero/negative

Unfortunately, there are no accepted rules for what fulfills each of these scores. Thus, there is a role for subjective judgments. To better understand this process, let us take a look at how an intervention might be classified as substantial.

The overall grade needs to take into account both the harm and the benefit to produce a score for the net effectiveness (benefit minus harm). However, in classifying the magnitude of the effect, it is often useful to separately score the magnitude of the benefit and the magnitude of the harm.

The benefit may be substantial from an individual perspective if it has a large impact on an infrequent condition that poses a major burden at the individual patient level. Phenylketonuria (PKU) screening of newborn infants is an example of this type of impact.

Alternatively, the benefit may be considered substantial if it has at least a small impact on a frequent condition in a large population. Reducing coronary artery disease by increasing physical activity may be an example of this type of impact.

The magnitude of harm may be substantial because it occurs frequently, such as the side effects of many medications. Alternatively, it may be substantial even when infrequent because of its life-threatening potential, such as anaphylaxis, aplastic anemia, or life-threatening arrhythmia.

In addition, when considering the harms of an intervention, the authors of the guideline need to define which harms are considered relevant. For instance, the USPSTF defines harms as including direct harm from the service, such as side effects and complications. It also takes into account what it calls the indirect harm, such as the consequences of increased follow-up testing and screening, psychological effects, and loss of insurability.

Scoring the magnitude of the impact of the intervention then requires the guideline authors to follow the basic steps we outlined in decision analysis. That is, they need to measure the benefits, measure the harms, and place a utility on the outcomes.

Thus, in making evidence-based recommendations, it is often important to incorporate utilities. But whose utility? The USPSTF uses utilities reflecting the "general values of most people." When there is little agreement on utilities, an average utility may be used.

Grading the Recommendations

Now we have seen the rather complicated steps that are needed to score the quality of the evidence and the impact of the intervention. Despite the complicated nature of the process, the net effectiveness may be presented using an overall grade of A, B, C, D, or I. Just as in many educational institutions, these overall grades reflect scores obtained along the way as well as well as a bit of subjective judgment. Like grades in courses, there is a category for incomplete, what is called "I" for insufficient. Table 13.4 indicates the grading categories used by the USPSTF. Notice that when the evidence it poor, the magnitude of the net effectiveness is always "I."

TABLE 13.4	Grading the Strength of the Recommendations			
Quality of the Evidence	Net Benefit Substantial	Net Benefit Moderate	Net Benefit Small	Net Benefit Zero/Negative
Good	A	B	C	D
Fair	B	B	C	D
Poor	I	I	I	I

System for grading evidence-based recommendations incorporating the scores on the quality of the evidence and the magnitude of the impact.

Adapted from Agency for Healthcare Research and Quality. *U.S. Preventive Services Task Force: Guide to Clinical Preventive Services.* Vol 1. Rockville, MD: Agency for Healthcare Research and Quality. AHRQ publication no 02-500.2001.

Thus, behind the grading of the recommendation is considerable evidence as well as judgment. Increasingly, recommendations are presented with these letter scores, as illustrated in the next example:

> **Mini-Study 13.16** ■ Recommendations for treatment of men and women with stage 2 colon cancer were based on evidence from well conducted randomized controlled trials on a representative sample of men and women with stage 2 colon cancer. The evidence demonstrated that men and women with stage 2 colon cancer who received the recommended treatment had twice the survival at 10 years compared to those that received the conventional treatment.

This recommendation would receive a grade of A. The evidence is obtained from well conducted randomized controlled trials which put it at the top of the hierarchy of study types. The evidence is relevant since it is obtained from a representative sample of the target population that is men and women with stage 2 colon cancer. Finally it is coherent since it measures a clinically important outcome that is survival. In addition to having a score of good quality evidence, the recommendation also has a magnitude of the impact score of substantial since the intervention has a large impact, doubling the long-term rate of survival. By combining the score of good for the quality of the evidence and the score of substantial for the magnitude of the impact using Table 13.4, the overall grade for the strength of the recommendations is A.

Table 13.5 outlines the meaning of the potential grades for the strength of the recommendations.

TABLE 13.5	Meaning of the Grades for the Strength of the Recommendations		
Levels of Recommendation	Action	Justification	Implications
A	USPSTF strongly recommends that clinicians routinely provide the service to eligible patients	Good evidence of substantial health benefit	This category represents an evidence-based recommendation to provide the service on a routine basis to all those for whom it is intended
B	USPSTF recommends that clinicians routinely provide the service to eligible patients	The quality of the evidence is good or fair, and the net benefit is at least moderate	In this category, a priority may be placed on A over B level services, considering constraints of time and resources, i.e., costs

(Continued)

TABLE 13.5	Meaning of the Grades for the Strength of the Recommendations *(continued)*		
Levels of Recommendation	**Action**	**Justification**	**Implications**
C	The USPSTF makes no recommendation for or against routine provision of the service	There is at least fair evidence, but the balance of benefits and harms is too close to justify a general recommendation	Clinicians may choose to offer the service on other grounds. For instance, an individual patient may be expected to gain greater benefit than the average patient observed in studies, or an individual patient's values or utilities are unusual enough to justify the service
D	The USPSTF recommends against routinely providing the service to asymptomatic patients	There is at least fair evidence that the service is ineffective (has zero net benefit) or that harms outweigh benefits	This category represents an evidence-based recommendation not to provide the service on a routine basis
I	The USPSTF concludes that the evidence is insufficient to recommend for or against routinely providing the service	The evidence is classified as poor or conflicting, and the balance of benefits and harms cannot be determined	This category implies that an evidence-based recommendation cannot be made, and decisions whether to provide the service must be made on grounds other than scientific evidence

USPSTF, U.S. Preventive Services Task Force.
Adapted from Agency for Healthcare Research and Quality. *U.S. Preventive Services Task Force: Guide to Clinical Preventive Services.* Vol 1. Rockville, MD: Agency for Healthcare Research and Quality. AHRQ publication no 02-500.

Classification of the recommendations is may be linked with specific implications for implementation. Recommendations may be classified as[13.7]

- Standards
- Guidance
- Alternatives

"Standards" imply that the intervention is intended for routine use when specific conditions are met; that is, it is expected that it will be implemented. Clinically, standards may be seen as indications. The implication is that a standard "must" be implemented.[13.8]

"Guidance" implies that the decision whether or not to use an intervention depends on the presence or absence of indications plus contraindications. The implication of guidance is that an intervention "should" be performed unless a contraindication is present.

[13.7] The term "guideline" is often used instead of guidance. Since "guideline" also refers to the overall set of recommendations, its use in this context may cause confusion. The term "option" is often used rather than "alternative." Because "option" is also used to indicate one particular intervention, it will not also be used to indicate that more than one option may be chosen.
[13.8] At times, standards may imply that an implementation must not be performed.

"Alternatives" imply that there is more than one potential intervention, none of which can be generally recommended over the others. The choice between interventions is made on the basis of individual provider and/or patient preference. Thus, the implication of alternatives is that the intervention "may" be used.

The following example demonstrates how standards, guidance, and alternatives can all be included in the same evidence-based guideline:[13.9]

> **Mini-Study 13.17** ■ Screening for colon cancer is indicated for all those 50 years and older. It should generally use a method that effectively screens both the proximal and distal colon and rectum. This may include yearly screening for fecal occult blood plus flexible sigmoidoscopy every 3 to 5 years, colonoscopy every 10 years, or virtual colonoscopy every 5 to 10 years.

This guideline incorporates standards, guidance, and alternatives. Screening is indicated for all men and women 50 years and older. This implies that screening "must" be offered. Guidance is provided, recommending that a method of screening "should" be used that effectively screens both the proximal and distal colon plus the rectum. The use of "should" implies that contraindications to a complete screening of the colon may exist. Finally, the guideline states three alternatives that "may" be used, implying that any of these methods fulfill the intent of the guideline.

Perspective of the Recommendations

Recommendations like other decision-making tools should generally take the social perspective. That is they should incorporate benefits, harms, and if included, costs regardless of who experiences the benefits, harm, or costs. Other perspectives such as that of an insurance system such as Medicare or a large health plan such as Kaiser-Permanente might also be used. When other perspectives are used, they need to be identified.

Evidence-based recommendations may also consider the distributional impacts of what they recommend. This may require special emphasis on vulnerable or high-risk groups to be sure that they do not experience potential harms or are included in the benefits.

To understand the perspective of the recommendations, it is also important to consider whether the recommendations focus on individuals, groups/institutions, or communities/the general public. The focus of recommendations may be on individual patients, but it may alternatively be on all hospitals with pediatric intensive care units or emergency departments in central cities. Recommendations may address the need for population-based services ranging from food processing to radon reduction.

The following screening recommendations demonstrate how recommendations might take a social perspective and focus the recommendations on multiple levels:

> **Mini-Study 13.18** ■ Recommendations for colon cancer screening emphasize the need to make screening widely available and to offer screening to all those older than 50 years without counterindications. Because of the low rate of acceptance of screening, clinicians are encouraged to offer multiple screening methods and make multiple requests over several years. Hospitals are encouraged to provide convenient and accessible services. Insurance companies are encouraged to provide all those insured with coverage for the procedures. Public information efforts should encourage colon cancer screening and should make special effort to reach groups with low rates of prior use of screening.

[13.9] Standards, guidance, and alternatives can be seen as having legal and financial implications. The implications of guidelines for malpractice and insurance coverage are still evolving and controversial. However, guidelines are increasingly being linked to insurance coverage and liability decisions.

By including all those older than 50 years, not just those who currently seek health care, the recommendations are taking a social perspective. These recommendations focus on the colon cancer screening of individuals including those at high risks due to low rates of prior screening. However, the focus of the recommendations is not limited to individual clinicians. Institutions such as hospitals and insurance companies are all part of the recommendations as are population-based efforts designed to inform the public. Learn More 13.1 explores the implications of taking a broader systems thinking approach to evidence-based recommendations.

LEARN MORE 13.1 ■ SYSTEMS THINKING AND EVIDENCE-BASED RECOMMENDATIONS ■ Evidence-based recommendations are designed to focus on one intervention at a time based on the best available research evidence. The research methods that inform evidence-based recommendations utilizes study designs that take into account, adjust for, or control for potential confounding variable. They adjust for these potential confounding variables in order to measure the impact of the one primary factor of interest sometime called the *main effect*. By looking at one factor at a time, evidence-based recommendations may miss the opportunity to take advantage of the interaction between risk factors or interventions as illustrated in the next example:

Mini-Study 13.19 ■ A chronic two pack per day cigarette smoker is trying to reduce his risk of lung cancer which you calculate as a relative risk of 10. The evidence-based recommendations focus on use of drugs and support systems to assist in cigarette cessation. There is no mention of testing his home for high radon levels which itself carries a relative risk of 5. When both long term cigarette smoking and high levels of radon exposure are present the risk of lung cancer is multiplied. Thus the relative risk of lung cancer is approximately 50. If high-dose radon exposure is removed, his relative risk of lung cancer would be close to 10 instead of 50.

Looking at one factor or intervention at a time has been called a *reductionist approach*. Looking at one intervention at a time prevent us from seeing the potential for interactions between risk factors or between treatments that can magnify the impact of the hazard or magnify the impact of interventions.

In addition to looking at one intervention at a time, evidence-based recommendations are largely focused on interventions at the individual level especially those that can be implemented in conjunction with a health care provider. Thus, evidence-based recommendations for cigarette smoking may miss the types of population-based interventions that have demonstrated effectiveness as illustrated in the next example.

Mini-Study 13.20 ■ Evidence-based recommendations focus on efforts to prevent individuals from starting cigarettes, assisting with smoking cessation efforts, screening for lung cancer, and treating lung cancer once it is diagnosed. They do not address issues at the population level such as the impact of cigarette taxes, restrictions on smoking in public places, or regulation of nicotine content of cigarettes despite the fact that these interventions have been shown to assist smokers who are trying to quit cigarette smoking.

Evidence-based recommendations are increasingly being seen as a subset of a broader approach to looking at problems known as *systems thinking*. Systems thinking looks at the full range of factors that cause disease and the full range of interventions that prevent, cure, and reduce disability.

Systems thinking can be looked at as a three-step process:

1. **Explanation:** Identifying the risk factors and interventions that influence the course of the disease or condition.
2. **Operation:** Describing the interactions between the risk factors and interventions looking for bottlenecks that can be addressed to

(Continued)

improve outcomes and leverage points that can be focused on to magnify the impact of interventions.

3. **Prediction:** Understanding the changes that are occurring over time to better understand what can be expected in the future.

Thus with cigarette smoking, system thinking might produce the following:

- **Explanation:** Cigarettes are an addiction that is best prevented rather than treated. Treatment needs to interrupt the cycle of addiction based on pharmacological and personal support systems that interrupt the addiction cycle.
- **Operation:** Individual behavioral characteristics, peer group actions, and population interventions all influence the process of starting cigarettes and the ease of cigarette cessation. Bottlenecks include continued high levels of nicotine in cigarettes. Leverage points include the opportunity to intervene in early pregnancy when women are especially motivated to stop smoking.
- **Prediction:** National efforts to focus on smoking during pregnancy and nicotine levels in tobacco are likely to prevent large number of individuals from starting and assist a substantial number in stopping. By 2020, we are likely to be left with a hard-core group of long-term smokers in whom screening for lung cancer and treatment of the disease will become even more important than they are now.

This type of systems thinking is increasingly being applied to health problems ranging from drug safety, to food safety, to complex problems such as cardiovascular disease, motor vehicle injuries, and HIV/AIDS.

We can look at systems thinking as an *integrative* approach as opposed to a reductionist approach. An integrative approach brings together evidence from a range of sources and uses evidence to examine a problem as a whole considering its clinical course from prevention to rehabilitation, as well as possible interventions from individual, to group, to population interventions.

Thus, in the future, expect to see evidence-based recommendations using a system approach that bring together diverse strategies and examines how to make changes at the systems level not just how to treat individuals.

The interpretation of the recommendations provides the basis for considering efforts to implement the recommendations in practice which is the focus of extrapolation, the final component of the M.A.A.R.I.E. framework.

EXTRAPOLATION (7,8)

Extrapolation of evidence-based recommendations or guidelines is the process of going beyond the conclusions drawn in the interpretation component to ask questions about the implications for practice. Implementation of guidelines in clinical or public health practice requires us to ask how guidelines should be implemented; for what populations the guideline should be used; and whether there is a process for updating or revising the guidelines.

Implementation in Target Population

Issues of implementation may include methods for organizing the delivery of services, promoting the services to those most in need, documenting efforts to offer the service etc.

The process of implementation of guidelines may be presented as an algorithm. Algorithms are usually constructed to provide a step-by-step decision-making process that is displayed as a graphical flowchart. Algorithms allow a visual display of the decision-making process recommended in a guideline. Algorithms may be quite complex. Regardless of the complexity, algorithms are constructed by using a set of rules much like the rules used in the construction of decision trees.

In algorithms,

■ an ellipse states or defines the decision to be made

■ six-sided figures incorporate questions that need to be answered

■ boxes indicate an action that needs to be taken

By tradition, algorithms begin at the top and move down, indicating the ordering of the process.

As illustrated in Figure 13.2 algorithms usually pose an issue such as, Should this patient be screened for colon cancer? They then ask specific question to determine whether a particular individual is a candidate for screening. This algorithm could be extended to decide between the potential forms of screening and what to do if the patient decides not to have a screening test.[13.10]

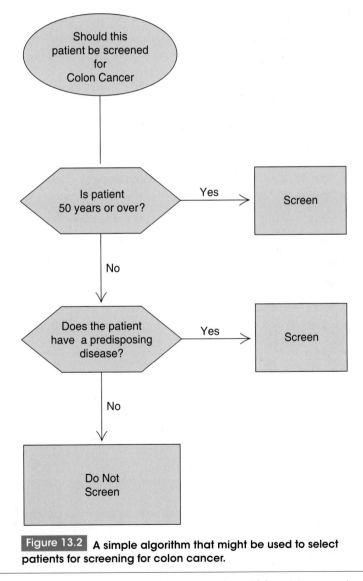

Figure 13.2 **A simple algorithm that might be used to select patients for screening for colon cancer.**

[13.10] Algorithms are often used to allow delegation of implementation to those with less training or experience. Algorithms are also used to clarify the underlying thinking process built into guidelines, identify possibilities that are not addressed by guidelines, or to teach the approach included in guidelines. Algorithms are only one method for implementation of guidelines.

Methods for implementation also include issues that occur before or after the issues addressed by algorithms. For instance, how should patients be sought for screening or how should the decision be documented. Let us take a look at these types of issues in the next hypothetical example:

Mini-Study 13.21 ■ Priority in screening programs for average-risk individuals should be on widely covering the population with at least one screening intervention rather than repeatedly screening the same individuals. Thus, a reminder system should be implemented to identify and remind all those 50 years and older who have not received a recommended colon cancer screening test to make an appointment.

Algorithms usually address what to do when confronted with an individual patient. This implementation issue goes further. It addresses what should be done to identify patients and offer them screening. This type of implementation issue implies that organized health care delivery systems carry a responsibility that extends beyond a responsibility for those who present for care. This broadened responsibility may be incorporated into the methods for implementation.

At the other end of the process are issues of implementation related to documentation of what has or has not been done, as illustrated in the following hypothetical example:

Mini-Study 13.22 ■ Patients who are seen in primary care practice for other purposes should be advised to undergo a screening procedure at approximately age 50. Documentation that this advice was provided should be included in the patient's medical record. Those who indicate they do not wish to undergo screening should be asked to sign a release, indicating that they have understood the recommendation and do not wish to undergo screening.

Thus, the processes for implementing guidelines go beyond the guidelines themselves. They ask us to extrapolate guidelines into practice. When extrapolating into practice, we need to recognize that it is possible to extend the recommendations to those who were not included in the initial target population. Thus, we need to examine the extent to which guidelines are extended beyond the target population.

Implementation Beyond the Target Population

When actually implementing a guideline, as with extrapolation of investigations, it is important to consider whether the guideline is being extrapolated beyond the target population. This may occur when a recommendation is extended to those at lower risk, perhaps younger or healthier patients, or to other countries or regions that have different prevalence or severity of a disease, as illustrated in the next example:

Mini-Study 13.23 ■ The colon cancer screening guideline on the use of colonoscopy developed for the United States are also recommended for other developed countries with a high-mortality rate from colon cancer, but were not recommended for less-developed countries and for populations with lower mortality rates from colon cancer.

This type of extrapolation is intentionally cautious. It is going beyond the data but recognizing the dangers of extrapolating conclusions between societies with very different distributions of disease and resources. A recommendation for widespread use of colon cancer screening using colonoscopy would have required a long list of questionable assumptions.

Presentation, Review, and Revision (6-9)

Evidence-based recommendations are now in widespread use. The AHRQ maintains a comprehensive Clearinghouse web site of the growing number of evidence-based recommendations now available. (9) The Guidelines Clearinghouse allows side-by-side comparison of two or more guidelines that address the same basic issues.

The 2010 U.S. health reform legislation utilized the A-B-C-D-I grading system and helped ensure coverage for clinical preventive services that receive a grade of A or B by the USPSTF.

The growing acceptance of evidence-based guidelines increasingly calls for standardized method for presenting guidelines. The Conference on Guideline Standardization (COGS) developed a list of expected information that needs to be included in guidelines. (6) The COGS list is summarized in Table 13.6.

TABLE 13.6	Conference on Guideline Standardization—List of Expected Information
Topic	**Description**
1. Overview material	A structured abstract that includes the guideline's release date, status (original, revised, updated), and print and electronic sources
2. Focus	Primary disease/condition and intervention/service/technology that the guideline addresses. Indicate any alternative preventive, diagnostic, or therapeutic interventions that were considered during development
3. Goal	The goal that following the guideline is expected to achieve, including the rationale for development of a guideline on this topic
4. Users/setting	The intended users of the guideline (e.g., provider types, patients) and the settings in which the guideline is intended to be used
5. Target population	The patient population eligible for guideline recommendations and list any exclusion criteria
6. Developer	The organization(s) responsible for guideline development and the names/credentials/potential conflicts of interest of individuals involved in the guideline's development
7. Funding source/sponsor	The funding source/sponsor and describe its role in developing, and/or reporting the guideline. Disclose potential conflict of interest
8. Evidence collection	The methods used to search the scientific literature, including the range of dates and databases searched, and criteria applied to filter the retrieved evidence
9. Recommendation grading criteria	The criteria used to rate the quality of evidence that supports the recommendations and the system for describing the strength of the recommendations. Recommendation strength communicates the importance of adherence to a recommendation and is based on both the quality of the evidence and the magnitude of anticipated benefits or harms

(Continued)

TABLE 13.6	Conference on Guideline Standardization—List of Expected Information *(Continued)*
Topic	**Description**
10. Method for synthesizing evidence	How evidence was used to create recommendations, e.g., evidence tables, meta–analysis, decision analysis
11. Prerelease review	How the guideline developer reviewed and/or tested the guidelines before release
12. Update plan	Whether or not there is a plan to update the guideline and, if applicable, an expiration date for this version of the guideline
13. Definitions	Unfamiliar terms and those critical to correct application of the guideline that might be subject to misinterpretation
14. Recommendations and rationale	Recommended action precisely and the specific circumstances under which to perform it. Justify each recommendation by describing the linkage between the recommendation and its supporting evidence. Indicate the quality of evidence and the recommendation strength, based on the criteria described in topic 9
15. Potential benefits and harms	Anticipated benefits and potential risks associated with implementation of guideline recommendations
16. Patient preferences	The role of patient preferences when a recommendation involves a substantial element of personal choice or values
17. Algorithm	When appropriate a graphical description of the stages and decisions in clinical care described by the guideline
18. Implementation considerations	Anticipated barriers to application of the recommendations. Provide reference to any auxiliary documents for providers or patients that are intended to facilitate implementation. Suggest review criteria for measuring changes in care when the guideline is implemented

Adopted from Yale Center for Medical Informatics. COGS: the conference on guideline standardization. http://gem.med.yale.edu/cogs/statement.do. Accessed August 6, 2011.

As we have seen, the development of guidelines usually requires assumptions for which there is little or no data. In addition, uncertainty is often addressed by a subjective process such as the use of expert opinion. As time passes, evidence may be available that addresses these uncertainties and assumptions. In addition, new options may be available that have increased benefits or decreased harms or costs. Thus, it is important when examining a guideline to determine its publication date.

Guidelines should include a process and timetable for revision, as illustrated in the next example:

Mini-Study 13.24 ■ Review of this guideline should occur after adequate evidence is available to assess the benefits, harms, and costs of virtual colonoscopy. The evidence of effectiveness of colonoscopy every 10 years compared with sigmoidoscopy every 3 to 5 years plus fecal occult blood testing every year should be reviewed in 3 years to determine whether use of these methods continues to be recommended. A comprehensive review of the guidelines should be conducted in 5 years.

The rapid pace of change that is going on in health and health care requires that most guidelines be formally reviewed either when specific data is available or on a set timetable. When a guideline is out-of-date, the reader of the guideline needs to be very cautious in accepting its conclusions.

As we have seen, guidelines have become a key method for integrating evidence into practice. The use of the M.A.A.R.I.E. framework can help us organize our approach to reviewing guidelines and help us identify their uses and limitations.

Questions to Ask—A Guide To The Guidelines

The following questions to ask can serve as a checklist when reading evidence-based guidelines.

Method—Guideline's purpose and target population

1. **Purpose:** What is the purpose of the guidelines?
2. **Target population:** What is the target population for whom the guidelines are intended?
3. **Perspective:** What is the perspective of the authors of the guideline?

Assignment—Options, structuring the evidence, and decision criteria

1. **Options:** What options are being considered?
2. **Evidence—structure and types of evidence to include:** How is the evidence gathered and organized and what types of evidence are included? e.g. benefits, harms, costs?
3. **Decision making approach:** How will the types of evidence be combined to make decisions or recommendations?

Assessment—Presenting the evidence on outcomes

1. **Sources of evidence:** What sources of evidence are used to measure the outcomes?
2. **Measurement of outcomes:** How are the outcomes measured?
3. **Filling holes in the evidence:** How are holes in the evidence addressed? For example, expert opinion, consensus, conference, Delphi method etc.

Results—Synthesizing the evidence

1. **Scoring the quality of the evidence:** Is a scoring system used to score the quality of the evidence?
2. **Addressing uncertainties:** How are remaining uncertainties addressed? For example, sensitivity analysis, subjective judgment, etc.
3. **Eliminating options:** What approach is used to eliminate options?

Interpretation—Making recommendations

1. **Scoring the magnitude of the impact:** Is a scoring system used to score the magnitude of the impact of the intervention?
2. **Grading the strength of the recommendation:** Combining scores for the quality of the evidence and the magnitude of the impact, what grade can be given to the strength of the recommendations?
3. **Perspective of the recommendations:** Are the recommendations made from the social perspective and/or other perspectives and are they focused on individuals, institutions, and/or communities?

Extrapolation—Implementation

1. **Implementation in target population:** Do the recommendations include methods for implementation in the target population?
2. **Implementation beyond the target population:** Are recommendations made for implementation beyond the target population?
3. **Presentation, review, and revision:** Are the recommendations presented using a standardized approach? Is there a timetable for revision of the guidelines?

REFERENCES

1. Harris RP, Helfand M, Woolf SH, et al; Methods Work Group, Third US Preventive Services Task Force. Current methods of the US preventive services task force: a review of the process. *Am J Prev Med.* 2001;20(suppl 3):21–35.

2. Institute of Medicine. *Guidelines for Clinical Practice: From Development to Use.* Washington, DC: National Academies Press; 1992.

3. Centers for Disease Control and Prevention. The community guide: what works to promote health. http://www.thecommunityguide.org/index.html. Accessed August 5, 2011.

4. Agency for Healthcare Research and Quality. *U.S. Preventive Services Task Force Guide to Clinical Preventive Services.* Vol 1. AHRQ Publication No 02-500.

5. Fink A, Kosecoff J, Chassin M, Brook RH. Consensus methods: characteristics and guidelines for use. *Am J Public Health.* 1984;74(9):979–983.

6. Institute of Medicine. *Clinical Practice Guidelines We Can Trust.* Washington, DC: National Academies Press; 2011.

7. Yale Center for Medical Informatics. COGS: the conference on guideline standardization. http://gem.med.yale.edu/cogs/statement.do. Accessed August 6, 2011.

8. Margolis CZ, Cretin S, eds. *Implementing Clinical Practice Guidelines.* Chicago, IL: Health Infosource; 1999.

9. Agency for Healthcare Research and Quality. *National Guideline Clearinghouse.* www.guideline.gov. Accessed August 6, 2011.

thePoint ✳ Visit http://thePoint.lww.com for interactive Q&A, flaw-catching exercises, searchable eBook, and more!

14 Translating Evidence into Practice

Putting evidence into practice is perhaps the most challenging and important job facing us whether we are clinicians trying to improve the quality of medical care, public health practitioners trying to improve population health, or health researchers using evidence to design the next investigation. Regardless of how we use research evidence, there are a series of questions that we need to ask:

- How can research evidence be made as applicable as possible to practice?
- How can we go from evidence to implementation?
- What can we do when the evidence is not enough?

In this final chapter, we will take a look at these three questions to see how we can successfully translate evidence into practice.

MAKING EVIDENCE APPLICABLE TO PRACTICE

The first step in translating evidence into practice is to find the evidence. Various tools are now available to help you search the literature and find the evidence as discussed in Learn More 14.1.

> **LEARN MORE 14.1 ■ SEARCHING FOR THE EVIDENCE (1)** ■ Key to a successful search for evidence is defining the question(s) that you want to address. The mnemonic P.I.C.O. has been found to be useful in structuring questions for literature searches. P.I.C.O. stands for
>
> **P:** Patient population—For which group do you need information? For example, postmenopausal women
>
> **I:** Intervention (or Exposure)—What risk or intervention is of interest? For example, estrogen replacement therapy
>
> **C:** Comparison—With what intervention are you comparing the intervention of interest? For example, no estrogen replacement
>
> **O:** Outcomes—What is the impact of the intervention? For example, impact on incidence of osteoporosis, breast cancer, and/or endometrial cancer
>
> The P.I.C.O. components provide a basis for focusing a search of the health research literature. Evidence is published in a wide variety of sources including original research articles, meta-analyses and systematic reviews, practice guideline, and of course books. In addition, evidence is increasingly accessible from sources that are not published in standard reference sources such as doctoral dissertations, government and private reports, and conference presentations. The term *gray literature* is increasingly used to describe information, usually research and technical information, found outside the formally published literature but increasingly accessible through Internet sources.
> The process of searching the literature to ensure access to the most relevant and highest quality evidence is itself a challenge. Tool for searching over 5,000 journals in the health research literature have been developed by the National Library of Medicine (NLM). The NLM has developed sophisticated methods, using what are called Medical Subject Headings or *MeSH* terms, for accessing the literature through PUBMED and other databases. Understanding how to efficiently and effectively use these search methods

(Continued)

is an important skill. (2) The National Library of Medicine provides a range of tutorials. Several libraries in academic health centers also provide excellent introductory and advanced materials and tutorials to assist you in searching the literature. (3,4)

Increasingly, complete versions of high quality journals are available to individuals without charge. Many high quality journals now provide free access to full articles beginning 6 months after publication.

TRANSLATIONAL RESEARCH

Once you have found the available evidence, you need to ask about whether it is applicable to practice. We will begin by looking at ways that research evidence is being improved in an effort to make research evidence more applicable to practice. This effort has been summarized using the term *translational research*. (5) Figure 14.1 displays a model for the three steps in translational research that have been called T-1, T-2, and T-3.

The types of research that we have discussed up to this time have been called *translational research 1 or T-1* research. T-1 research generally looks at how basic sciences advances can be translated into clinical care under the ideal conditions of research investigations. T-1 research is the step within translational research of moving from basic science understandings to demonstration of efficacy of interventions; that is, Does it work under the ideal conditions of investigations?

T-2 translational research can be seen as the step within translational research of moving from the efficacy to the effectiveness of interventions. We will take a look at new types of randomized controlled trials that are attempting to improve our understanding of what works and what is most effective in practice.

T-3 translational research may be seen as the final step within translational research of addressing the implementation and evaluation of interventions in health care and public health delivery and their impact on groups and populations. As we will discuss, new and more comprehensive efforts to evaluate the success of interventions not just in isolation but as part of systems are key to T-3 research.

Both T-2 and T-3 research require that we expand our focus for research from traditional randomized controlled trials conducted under ideal clinical conditions designed to simulate a laboratory to the real-world conditions of clinical and population health practice. As Dr. Lawrence Green has written, (6) "If we want more evidence-based practice we need more practice-based evidence."

Translational Research 2

The goal of translational research 2 (T-2) has been described as deciding on "the right treatment for the right patient in the right way at the right time." (7) Much of T-2 research is not new. As we have seen in our discussion of safety, postmarket research is moving rapidly to incorporate data from clinical practice, relying heavily on newer types of cohort studies and selective use of case-control studies.

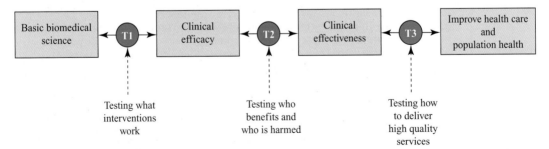

Figure 14.1 **Framework for translational research.** Adopted from Dougherty D, Conway PH. The "3T's" road map to transforming US health care: the "how" of high quality care. *JAMA*. 2008;299:2319–2321.

In addition to expanded use of cohort studies and case-control studies, T-2 research is stimulating new types of randomized controlled trials, which have become part of an effort known as *comparative effectiveness research.*

In particular, T-2 research is rapidly incorporating two new types of randomized controlled trials that have been called *equivalence trials*[14.1] and *pragmatic trials.* Let us take a look at each of these types of randomized controlled trials.

Equivalence trials are an increasingly important type of randomized controlled trials that are being used as part of comparative effectiveness research. (8) These types of randomized controlled trials are conducted when a new drug or other intervention has apparent advantages over an established intervention in terms of cost, and ease of use by patients or clinicians, or has fewer adverse effects etc. The study or alternative hypothesis of an equivalence or trial is that the new treatment is equivalent to the established or conventional treatment. In contrast to these types of studies, the traditional type of randomized controlled trial is referred to as a *superiority trial*, and the study hypothesis states that the new treatment is superior to the established or conventional treatment.

Let us look at a hypothetical equivalence trial to see some of the differences between these trials and the traditional randomized controlled trial or superiority trial:

Mini-Study 14.1 ■ An equivalence trial examines the impact of a new method for treating a specific type of myocardial infarction, which has been shown to have a 6% 1-year mortality rate given conventional treatment. A new treatment is found to be less invasive and cheaper. The investigation defines equivalence as between 5% and 7% mortality or one percent higher or lower than the conventional treatment. The randomized controlled trial includes 20,000 patients in the conventional treatment group and 20,000 in the new treatment group. The Investigational Review Board (IRB) carefully examines the measures of assessment and requires careful monitoring of the trial. The investigation is analyzed using an as-treated analysis rather than an intention-to-treat method. The observed mortality with the new methods is 6.2% compared with 6% for the conventional treatment. The 95% confidence interval for the new treatment's mortality rate is 6.8% to 5.6%. The investigators concluded that the methods are equivalent since the the 95% confidence interval around the efficacy of new method is within the predefined equivalence range.

First notice that the sample size required is much larger than we would expect from the usual superiority type randomized controlled trial. This is the situation because we are dealing with a very small hypothesized difference between the study group and the control group outcomes, and this results in a very large sample size. In fact, the required sample size is literally off the chart that we previously used to estimate the needed sample size for superiority type randomized controlled trials.

Second, extra attention needs to be given to the conduct of these studies since misclassification or bias in the assignment or assessment component often favors a smaller observed difference between the current and the new treatment. Thus, with equivalence trials, poor study design or poor implementation may produce results supporting equivalence. Thus, IRBs need to give extra attention to the element of study design and study implementation.

Third, use of as-treated or per-protocol analysis rather than intention-to-treat analysis is often recommended in these studies. Intention-to-treat analysis often results in smaller differences

---

[14.1] Equivalence trials are often called *noninferiority trials.* Technically, equivalence trials and noninferiority trials are distinguished from each other by the fact that an equivalence trial aims to establish that two interventions are equivalent, a whereas noninferiority trial aims to establish that a new intervention is not inferior, that is, not worse than an established intervention. Equivalence trial use two-tailed statistical significance tests since their alternative hypothesis allows for either treatment to be better than the other. Noninferiority trials use one-tailed statistical significance tests since they assume that the existing treatment is superior. This distinction makes little difference since two-tailed 95% confidence intervals rather than statistical significance tests are recommended for use in both types of studies. Equivalence and noninferiority trials will therefore be used as synonyms.

between the treatment groups, which in this situation would favor the conclusion of equivalence. The use of as-treated or per-protocol analysis makes it more difficult to establish equivalence.[14.2]

Now let us take a look at the second new type of randomized controlled trial called *pragmatic trials* that is increasingly being used a part of T-2.

Pragmatic Trials

Pragmatic trials are an increasingly important form of randomized clinical trials. The aim of pragmatic trials is to investigate two or more alternative interventions in the actual conditions of clinical practice. Thus, pragmatic trials can also be called *effectiveness trials*. A pragmatic trial differs from both superiority and equivalence trials in that pragmatic trials are not conducted under the strictly maintained conditions of traditional randomized controlled trials but rather aim to reflect the conditions of clinical or public health practice.

Let us look at the following simulated pragmatic trials to examine how it differs from other types of randomized controlled trials that we have discussed:

> **Mini-Study 14.2** ■ Children aged 6 to 12 with a history of recurrent episodes of asthma were recruited to participate in a pragmatic trial if they were members of a large health plan. No other inclusion or exclusion criteria were utilized. Each child was randomized to begin treatment with one of two commonly used approaches. The parents of each child were informed of the treatment assignment. Follow-up monitoring was at the discretion of the clinicians and the families. Outcomes were measured during a 5-year period and included patient satisfaction, adverse events, and cost measures as well as objective measures of lung function, growth, and levels of physical activity.

Notice that this pragmatic trial differs in a large number of ways from other types of randomized clinical trials.

- The entry criteria are very broad. This allows the pragmatic trial to be as representative as possible of the types of patients seen in clinical practice.
- No masking or blinding is performed. Since masking or blinding is not a part of clinical practice, removing masking or blinding makes the pragmatic trial more reflective of clinical practice, but it also may result in biases in assessment of the outcomes.
- Follow-up occurs at the discretion of the clinician and the family. Once again leaving follow-up to the clinician and the family makes the trial more reflective of clinical practice, but raises the possibility of bias in assessment.
- Outcome measures are longer term and more diverse including not only traditional short-term measures of efficacy but also longer-term benefits and harms as well as costs. Therefore, pragmatic trials can address longer-term issues of effectiveness and safety as well as cost issues. Thus, the outcomes of pragmatic trials may be useful for addressing long-term policy issues.

Table 14.1 summarizes these key differences between pragmatic trials and traditional randomized controlled trials. (9)

[14.2] In addition, the results of an equivalence or noninferiority trial are reported somewhat differently from a superiority trial. The results of an equivalence or noninferiority trial are reported as the observed study and control groups outcomes plus the 95% confidence interval of the study group outcome. If the 95% confidence interval of the study group outcome falls within the predefined equivalence range, in this case a 5% to 7% difference or a 1% increase or decrease in the mortality in the new treatment compared to the conventional treatment, then the new or study treatment is considered equivalent or noninferior to the conventional control treatment. (8)

TABLE 14.1	Key Differences between Traditional Superiority Randomized Controlled Trials and Effectiveness or Pragmatic Trials	
Question	**Efficacy—Can the Intervention Work?**	**Effectiveness—Does the Intervention Work When Used in Normal Practice?**
Setting	Well-resourced, "ideal" setting	Normal practice
Participants	Highly selected. Poorly adherent participants and those with conditions that might dilute the effect are often excluded	Little or no selection beyond the clinical indication of interest
Intervention	Strictly enforced and adherence is monitored closely	Applied flexibly as it would be in normal practice
Outcomes	Often short-term surrogates or process measures	Directly relevant to participants, funders, communities, and health care practitioners
Relevance to practice	Indirect—little effort made to match design of trial to decision making needs of those in usual setting in which intervention will be implemented	Direct—trial is designed to meet needs of those making decisions about treatment options in setting in which intervention will be implemented

Adapted from a table presented at the 2008 Society for Clinical Trials meeting by Marion Campbell, University of Aberdeen. Zwarenstein M, Treweek S, Gagnier JJ, et al. Improving the reporting of pragmatic trials: an extension of the CONSORT statement. *BMJ*. 2008;337:a2390. doi:10.1136/bmj.a2390.

Translational Research 3

Translational research 3 (T-3) has been described as follows: "T-3 activities address the 'how' of health care delivery so that evidence-based treatment, prevention, and other interventions are delivered reliably to all patients in all settings of care and improve the health of individuals and populations." (4) T-3 research may be seen as the final step within translational research of addressing the implementation and evaluation of interventions in health care and public health delivery and their impact on groups and populations. New and more comprehensive efforts to evaluate the success of interventions not just in isolation but as part of systems are key to T-3 research.

T-3 research builds upon earlier stages of translational research. In addition, it utilizes but going beyond traditional methods of evaluation. Traditionally, evaluation research has often focused on *before-and-after studies*, which are a special type of population comparison. Let us take a look at traditional forms of evaluation research. Then we will take a look at how traditional evaluation research is becoming modernized and becoming an important part of T-3 research. The following scenario outlines an important use of before-and-after studies:

> **Mini-Study 14.3** ■ Well-conducted randomized controlled trials of folic acid administration to women intending to get pregnant demonstrated a substantial and statistically significant reduction in spina bifida and other neural tube defects. Supplementation in pill form was recommended and adopted as national policy for all women of childbearing age. Before-and-after studies indicated little or no change in the average level of serum folic acid among women of childbearing age and no change in the national incidence of neurotube defects.

For many years, this type of evaluation study has served as the mainstay of investigation of the broader impact of interventions. In this situation, the before-and-after study was important to recognize the lack of a population impact of voluntary supplementation. This led to legally enforced food supplementation with folic acid, which was followed by an elevation of serum folic acid among women of childbearing age, as well as a substantial reduction in the incidence of neurotube defects.

Despite the continued importance of before-and-after studies, T-3 research requires increasingly sophisticated methods of evaluation that address the impacts of interventions on specific groups and populations including providing a better understanding of the strengths and limitation of interventions and how different interventions can work together as part of a system.

T-3 research is not generally based on randomized controlled trials. Increasingly, it relies on a coordinated set of quantitative and qualitative research designed to understand and improve the process of implementation.

A recent framework for evaluation research has been called the *RE-AIM framework*. (10) RE-AIM is a mnemonic that includes

- **R**each—How well the intervention can reach its target audience
- **E**ffectiveness—How benefits and harms, that is, net-effectiveness of the intervention when it succeeds in reaching its target audience
- **A**doption—Acceptance of the implementation among its target audience and other audiences
- **I**mplementation—How extensively an intervention is actually implemented among its target audience and other audiences
- **M**aintenance—Longer-term ability of the intervention to have long-term impacts on a problem as part of a system

The following scenario illustrates how evaluation research as part of T-3 might proceed:

> **Mini-Study 14.4** ■ An evaluation of interventions designed to have an impact on the national problem of neurotube defects looked at currently feasible interventions. These included food supplementation with folic acid, folic acid supplementation for women considering pregnancy, and screening for neurotube defects before the 20th week of pregnancy with subsequent observation, abortion, or selective use of intrauterine surgery. Benefits and harms were assessed taking into account the relative importance of different outcomes. The research found that together these approaches were able to reach a large percentage of women of childbearing age, had benefits that far exceed the harms, were widely accepted by patients and clinicians, and were likely to be implemented by clinicians and institutions. Policy changes in insurance coverage and U.S. Food and Drug Administration (FDA) food supplementation requirements facilitated the use of all these interventions as part of a system.

This scenario includes each of the components of the RE-AIM framework. The investigators have defined the reach of the interventions as extending to all women, all pregnant women as well as all women of childbearing age. Harms and benefits as well as the relative importance of different outcomes were taken into account in evaluating net-effectiveness. The acceptance of the interventions by the target audience was considered as well as its implementation by clinicians and institutions. Finally, the maintenance of the interventions as part of a system took into account the necessary policy changes including insurance coverage and FDA food supplementation regulations.

Many of these components such as acceptance of the interventions and the impact of insurance changes require qualitative research methods that take an in-depth look at a particular issue by gathering data from a small number of carefully chosen individuals. This type of comprehensive evaluation as part of T-3 research is in its early stage of development. Expect to see considerable attention, controversy, and change as this type of research matures and becomes an important part of translational research.

We have now looked at the types of investigations that are increasingly being used to help us translate evidence into practice. Let us now explore how we can go from evidence to implementation. To do this, we will explore additional factors beyond the evidence that influence decision making. We will start by examining ways that evidence is presented and framed that can produce misleading conclusions.

FROM EVIDENCE TO IMPLEMENTATION

Presenting and Framing the Evidence

Putting the research evidence into practice requires that we understand the ways that evidence is perceived. Perceptions depend heavily on how information is presented. To better appreciate the importance of how evidence is presented and perceived, let us look at what are known as *framing effects*. (11) Framing effects are ways that evidence is presented that can and often do alter the way it is perceived.

Two basic types of presentation issues have been shown to impact the choices we make.

1. Positive versus negative presentation
2. The order of the presentation

Let us look at a series of choices for you to make to better understand how these framing effects can influence how information is perceived:

> **Mini-Study 14.5** ■ You are confronted with a life-threatening disease. The following two options are offered to you. Which one of the options would you select?
>
> **Option #1:** A treatment that results in a 90% chance that you will be alive in 5 years.
> **Option #2:** A treatment that has a 2% chance of death each year for the next 5 years.

Even though these two options have the same outcome as measured using a decision analysis approach, many individuals prefer option #1 since it presents the data as a positive outcome focused on survival rather than option #2's negative outcome focusing on death. Presenting evidence in a positive light as in option #1 presents the outcome as a gain, whereas presenting evidence in a negative light as in option #2 presents the outcome as a loss. A fundamental principle of decision-making psychology stresses that losses loom larger than gains. (12) Everything else being equal, individuals prefer an option that is framed as a gain over one that is framed as a loss.[14.3]

Often it is best to present evidence both ways to ensure that the recipients have the opportunity to see the evidence from both a positive and a negative perspective.

[14.3] The fact that individuals generally prefer options framed as gains over those framed as losses means that many if not most individuals can have their decision making or their attitudes manipulated by the way that a decision or events are framed or perceived. These manipulations, in large part, focus on influencing the way individuals see their current situation that is the status quo. In decision-making language, these efforts are said to alter an individual's *reference point*. For instance, when individuals see their previous decisions as part of their current commitment to a course of therapy, they may see their past decisions as what is called *sunk costs*. Having put considerable effort into a treatment or other decision, they cannot quit now. The practice or "hanging crepe" or preparing the family for the worst by exaggerating the severity of the status quo may be another example of an effort to alter the reference point. Alternatively, individuals may feel or be convinced that their status quo should be seen in the light of the good health they experienced in the past and other options are viewed in light of their potential to return an individual to full health. When individuals view the status quo using the reference point of their previous state of good health, they may see the current status quo as a loss rather than returning to their previous state of health as a gain.

Individuals often find it easiest to compare two options at a time deciding which is best by performing a "side-by-side" comparison. When there are more than two options, it is common to select two of the most promising options and decide which of these two options is preferred. Other options are then compared one at a time with the currently preferred options to see whether the current preference remains the best or whether it needs to be replaced by another option. To be sure of the final preference, the process of comparing two options at a time continues to allow us to compare the preferred option with all other close calls. This approach may be used quite successfully for instance when choosing the best vision correction.

Often this approach works well. However, it also has the potential to be manipulated by the order in which the options are presented especially when we don't get a second chance to confirm our choice. For instance, decision making may be structured much like an election with a primary with a large number of candidates followed by a general election with only two candidates. As with election primaries, the final choice may greatly depend on how the primaries are structured. For instance, imagine the following example:

Mini-Study 14.6 ■ Imagine that you are deciding on observation versus surgery versus medicine as a treatment. Your preferences for these three options can be expressed as follows:

- Observation is better than surgery
- Surgery is better than medicine
- Medicine is better than observation

In the following comparisons, the decision is made based on your preferences as described above.

Approach #1
First decide on observation versus surgery—observation wins
Now decide on observation versus medicine—you prefer medicine

Approach #2
First decide on medicine versus surgery—surgery wins
Now decide on surgery versus observation—you prefer observation

Approach #3
First decide on observation versus medicine—medicine wins
Now decide on surgery versus medicine—you prefer surgery

Notice that when a decision is structured as a two-option choice, your final preference can be manipulated by the order in which the options are presented. Ideally when presenting multiple options, they can be laid out side by side comparing their advantages and disadvantages. This approach may help prevent the framing effect that can be unconsciously or consciously produced by those who determine the order of presentation of the options.

In decision analysis, the issues of positive versus negative presentation and the order of the presentation of the options do not come up. The data are presented using numbers and are neither a negative nor a positive presentation. In addition, all the options are addressed simultaneously, so there is no order of presentation.

In addition to framing effects that influence all or most of us, the ways that data are perceived can be influenced by individual attitudes. Understanding the impact of individual attitudes can go a long way to help us understand how evidence is utilized in practice.

Individual Attitudes and Decision-making Approaches

Research studies whether they are case-control, cohort, or randomized controlled trials, aim to estimate the average outcome for a study group compared with a control group. These outcomes tell us the proportion of the patients who receive net benefit from treatment compared with a comparison or control group.

Even when evidence-based guidelines appear to be targeted at the type of individual patient who you have before you, you may find that the recommended action is not acceptable to a particular patient. Let us take a look at a number of ways that individual's attitudes and approaches to decision making may produce a decision that appears to conflicts with the evidence. We will use the mnemonic D.R.U.G. to summarize these features of individual decision making. D.R.U.G. stands for discounting, risk-taking attitudes, uncertainty, and goals.[14.4]

Discounting

As we have discussed as part of decision analysis and cost-effectiveness analysis, most people would prefer to receive $100 today rather than the same amount 1 year from now. This is true even if you are protected against inflation (and deflation). Not only is a dollar generally worth more today than next year, but so are the benefits of health. In general, we would rather pay off a $100 debt in 1 year rather than today, and we would rather delay bad outcomes or harms if we can. As we have seen, this process of taking the timing of events into account is called discounting.

When formally synthesizing quantitative evidence, it is assumed that the discount rate used for benefits, harms, and cost is the same. The use of different discount rates artificially either encourages or discourages the use of a particular intervention. For instance, if we place a higher discount rate on benefits than we do on harms and costs, we will encourage the immediate use of interventions with immediate benefits and discourage the use of ones with delayed benefits.

Evidence-based studies and recommendations generally assume a 3% to 5% discount rate per year. A 5% discount rate implies that a benefit received, a harm suffered, or a cost paid 1 year from now has only 95% of the value compared to one that occurs in the immediate future.

Despite the fact that evidence-based studies use a relatively low discount rate and require the use of the same discount rate for benefits, harms, and costs, clinicians and patients may not agree with these rules. Let us see how this might happen, and the implications:

> **Mini-Study 14.7** ■ Imagine that you have a choice between two interventions. Option A is given now, that is, at the beginning of year #1. Option B is given at the beginning of year #2. The interventions are identical except for the timing of the deaths and the occurrence of side effects that only occurs with Option B. These options are displayed below.
>
> **Option A**
>
> Year #1   Year #2
>
> 20% death   0% death
>
> |-----------------------------------|-----------------------------------|
>   ↑
>   *Treat*

(Continued)

[14.4] Many of these decision-making attitudes and approaches are applicable to population decision making as well as individual decision making. For instance, societies as a whole as well as politicians interested in reelection often see the harms and benefits that occur in the immediate future as more important than those that occur at a later time.

Option B

Year #1	Year #2
0% death from	22% death

```
|-------------------------------------- |------------------------------------------ |
↑
Treat
```

Did you select Option B? Many if not most people do. Selecting Option B implies that your discount rate is at least 10% perhaps far more. That is, you place a greater value on benefits that occur immediately and less value on harms that occur in the future compared with the discount rate used in evidence-based studies. The discount rate for those who choose option B is at least 10% since the choice of Option B implies that you are willing to increase your probability of death from 20% to at least 22% if death can be delayed a year. Many people are willing to tolerate higher risks of death in the second year perhaps 24% or 26% or even higher indicating that they are using a discount rate of 20% to 30% or even higher. This is a far higher discount rate than the one that is incorporated into decision analyses, cost-effectiveness analyses, and evidence-based recommendations.

This tendency to value the immediate future far more than time in the longer-term future varies from person to person. However, it is very common for those with severe illnesses who anticipate a limited life span to view small gains in life span as extremely important. These gains may be of great importance since they allow an individual to settle their affairs, say their last words to those they love, or merely have time to reflect. Thus, we can expect those with severe illness to make choices that often are not consistent with evidence-based recommendations especially when there are trade-off between current benefits and future harms.

Discounting may influence decision making in healthy individuals as well. Adolescents are notorious for being willing to trade current benefits for future harms and heavily discounting the importance of future harms. When individuals heavily discount future harms, efforts to influence their decisions often need to be on short-term benefits and harms. For instance, if the long-term harms of cigarettes have little impact on an individual, emphasis can also be placed on immediate gains and short-term harms such as increased exercise ability, personal hygiene, or the harms during pregnancy.

The use of high discount rates for future events is a common and important part of individual decision making. At times, high rates of discounting can distort the decision-making process. Thus, we need to recognize when patients and policy makers are placing great importance on the present and try to feed back that information as part of the decision-making process.

Risk-Taking Attitudes

Decision analysis and evidence-based recommendations make the assumption that individuals are *risk neutral*. That is, when confronted with two equal expected utilities, that is, probability times utility, of harms and benefits, they will consider the situation a "toss-up." In fact, in practice, few toss up situations are perceived to exist. We generally tend to favor one option or another when confronted with options of equal expected utility as defined by decision analysis. Let look at the ways that individuals may express their risk-taking attitudes in the following scenarios:

Mini-Study 14.8 ▪ You are required to choose between two alternatives in situation A and also in situation B.

Situation A. Assume you have a serious disease that has resulted in a utility for the quality of health of 0.8 compared with your previous state of disease-free health (i.e., 1). Imagine that you are offered the following pair of options, but you can select only one of the two. Which of the following two alternatives do you prefer?

    #1. Select a treatment with the following possible outcomes:
- 50% chance of raising the quality of your health from 0.8 to 1 and
- 50% chance of an outcome that reduces the quality of your health from 0.8 to 0.6

    #2. Refuse the treatment and accept a quality of your health of 0.8.

Situation B. Assume that you have a serious disease that has resulted in a utility for the quality of health of 0.2 compared with your previous state of full health (i.e., 1). Imagine that you are offered the following pair of options, but can select only one of the two. Which of the following two alternatives do you prefer?

    #1. Select a treatment with the following possible outcomes:
- 10% chance of an outcome that raises the quality of your health from 0.2 to 1 and
- 90% chance of an outcome that reduces the quality of your health from 0.2 to 0.11

    #2. Refuse the treatment and accept a quality of your health of 0.2

Figures 14.2 and 14.3 display these decisions using decision trees.

    Did you choose #2 in situation A and #1 in situation B? Most, but not all, people do. To understand this exercise, you need to appreciate that in terms of the evidence, as defined by expected utility, option #1 and option #2 are identical or nearly identical in both scenario A and scenario B situation. That is, it is a "toss–up" between these two options when only probabilities and utilities are included, as demonstrated in Figures 14.2 and 14.3. Thus, the evidence does not argue for one option over the other. The choice really depends on your risk-taking attitude.

    What does it mean to choose option #2 in situation A and option #1 in situation B? In situation A, we begin with a utility of 0.8. For many people, this is a tolerable situation and they do not want to take any chances that they may be reduced to a lower, intolerable utility. Thus, they want to guarantee continuation at a tolerable level of health. This can be called the *guarantee effect*.

    In situation B, we begin with a utility of 0.2. For many people, this is an intolerable situation. These people are usually willing to take their chances of getting even worse in the hopes of a

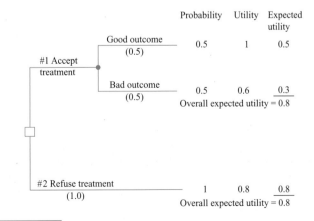

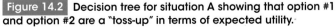

Figure 14.2 Decision tree for situation A showing that option #1 and option #2 are a "toss-up" in terms of expected utility.

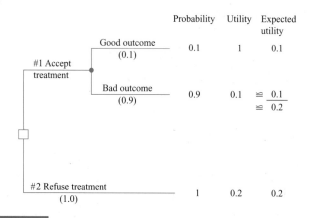

Figure 14.3 Decision tree for situation B should that option #1 and option #2 are approximately a "toss-up" in terms of expected utility.

major improvement in their health. When the quality of life is bad enough, most people are willing to take their chances and "go for it." This risk-taking behavior can be called the *long-shot effect*.

Thus, both risk-seeking and risk-avoiding choices are common, defensible, and reasonably predictable in specific types of situations. Risk-seeking choices are particularly prominent among the severely ill, whereas risk-avoiding choices are particularly common among the healthy or asymptomatic. Thus, it is important to recognize that recommendations that carry even a low probability of death or serious harm may be rejected by patients in generally good health. An option that carries a substantial probability of death or serious harm may be sought out by those who are seriously ill.

A minority of individuals prefers option #1 in both situations A and B. These individuals choose to take a risk even when confronted with a situation in which most people are risk-avoiders. These individuals have at times been termed *risk-takers*. Alternatively, a minority of individuals prefer option #2 in both situations A and B. These individuals choose to avoid risk even when confronted with a situation in which most people would be risk-seekers. These individuals have at times been termed *risk-avoiders*.

We need to recognize that most recommendations are made on the assumption of risk-neutrality, and decision-makers, whether clinicians or patients, often are not risk-neutral when they make decisions. (13) Therefore, it is not surprising that even the most carefully constructed evidence-based recommendations may not always make intuitive sense to patients and clinicians.[14.5]

Uncertainty

In most situations, people try to avoid uncertainty. Everything else being equal, most of us prefer situations with greater certainty. In fact, we often frame issues so that it appears that certainty exists even when it does not. This process is so common that it has a term to describe it, *pseudocertainty*. Pseudocertainty implies that an outcome is certain or guaranteed once a series of conditions have been fulfilled. The following scenario illustrates the concept of pseudocertainty:

Mini-Study 14.9 ■ A patient has been diagnosed with a disease and has an undiagnosed life-threatening complication. There is a 50% chance that the complication is A and a 50% chance that the complication is B. The treatment is 100% successful and has no adverse effects if the complication is A. It has no effect on complication B. The patient is given two choices:

#1. Treat the complication without making a diagnosis

#2. Diagnose the complication and treat the complication only if it is complication A

[14.5] A small number of individuals will choose option #1 in scenario A and option #2 in scenario B. These choices may be harder to explain. They usually relate to the interpretation of the meaning of a particular utility.

Overall, the two treatments provide an equal chance of cure, that is, 50% in both situations. Nonetheless, most patients and most clinicians favor choice #2. Choice #1 appears to offer certainty or 100% chance of cure. Notice, however, that this is pseudocertainty since the guarantee of cure depends on the patient having complication A not complication B. Thus, we are not dealing with true certainty but rather certainty contingent on uncertainty that is on pseudocertainty.

Even though we tend to favor situations of certainty, we are often faced with a great deal of uncertainty. Probabilities are themselves an expression of uncertainty. Often we cannot even rely on having precise or exact probabilities. Let us take a look at how we may react when exact probabilities are not available in the next scenario:

> **Mini-Study 14.10** ■ Imagine that you have just been diagnosed with a serious disease. Which of the following two options would you select?
>
> **#1.** Select a treatment with the following possible outcomes:
> - 50% chance of raising the quality of your health to 1 and
> - 50% chance of reducing the quality of your health to 0.6.
>
> **#2.** Select a treatment with the following possible outcomes:
> - Somewhere between a 40% and a 60% chance of raising the quality of your health to 1 and
> - Somewhere between a 40% and a 60% chance of reducing the quality of your health to 0.6.

On this question, people are often divided between option #1 and option #2. Option #1 has the advantage of greater certainty. Option #2 provides additional uncertainty since in addition to probabilities, there is uncertainty about the probabilities. Option #2 represents a realistic situation in decision making, which may be called the *uncertainty of uncertainty*. In this situation, patients are often looking for certainty in the form of recommendations that they can trust. Thus, when a treatment is recommended, they may read into option #2 "… for me the chances are better than average" or they may hear "… in my hands you can expect to do better than average."

Thus, the mere existence of uncertainty has a complicated impact on individual decision making. Some people look favorably on uncertainty, whereas others see it in a negative light.

Goals

Individuals may disagree with the evidence-based recommendations because they may reject the basic goals of evidence-based recommendations which are built on principles of expected utility. Remember that the goal of expected utility as used in decision analysis is to maximize the expected utility, that is, to maximize the average net benefit. A Nobel prize was won for the development of an alternative decision-making principle known as *satisficing*. (7) Satisficing implies that the aim of decision making is to achieve a good enough solution. Satisficing may occur because individuals place value not only on the outcome of care but also on the process of care.[14.6]

Often an important goal of patients is to maximize the process even at the expense of an optimal outcome. For instance, individuals view the ability to have control over the process as important in-and-of-itself regardless of the eventual outcome. We often consider hazards that we perceive as in our control as less threatening than ones that we perceive as out of our control. Fatal

---

[14.6] Satisficing may also occur because decision makers cannot make a decision with all of their options arrayed in front of them. As with job or apartment seeking, we often need to make decisions on the basis of only the known options that are available at one point in time. This type of situation may also occur in health care.

automobile collisions, for instance, are often seen as less likely than fatal airplane crashes, despite the fact that statistics show that commercial air travel is far safer than travel by automobile. Providing patients with control over their treatment choices and methods for implementation often results in reduced perceptions of the probability of harm and increased perceptions of the probability of benefits.

In addition, the process of decision making can influence how we regard the outcomes as illustrated in the following choice:

> **Mini-Study 14.11** ■ Which of the following situations do you prefer #1 or #2
>
> **#1.** You are being treated with drug A. You consider switching to drug B, but decide against it. Later you find out that you would most likely have had a better outcome if you switched to drug B.
>
> **#2.** You are being treated with drug B. You are offered the choice of drug A and decide to switch to drug A. Later you find out that you would most likely have had a better outcome if you stayed with drug B.

These two options produce the same outcomes, yet they may be perceived as quite different by most patients and by most clinicians. Option #1 may be considered an *error of omission*. That is, failure to act has produced the less than optimal outcome. Option #2 can be viewed as an *error of commission*. That is, action has produced the less than optimal outcome. From the perspective of the outcome as well as the ethics of decision making, these two options can be viewed as the same. A decision analysis would not recognize any difference.

However, many patients, clinicians, and at time the legal system do regard these as different. The way we view these options may be affected by our attitudes toward regret and responsibility. Individuals vary greatly in their "action orientation"; some see taking action or "doing something" as a positive, whereas others favor reflection as a positive.

Thus, the process of getting there and not just the results themselves can greatly influence the choices that are made by individuals. Decision analysis does not take the process of getting there into account. A good outcome is the same whether it occurs as the result of a preventive intervention or after many months of intensive care.

Finally, understanding the process of translating evidence into practice requires that we ask our third question: What do we do when evidence is not enough?

WHEN EVIDENCE IS NOT ENOUGH

From the earliest days of health research, it has been apparent that evidence in-and-of-itself is often inadequate to change minds and to change behavior. For instance, the classic works of Semmelweis that convincingly demonstrated that puerperal fever could be dramatically reduced by antiseptic hand washing were never accepted by his contemporaries. Perhaps it was the lack of an adequate "scientific" explanation or the implication of wrongdoing on the part of physicians. Once the germ theory of disease provided an explanation for Semmelweis' finding, antiseptic hand washing was institutionalized as one of the foundations of modern medicine and public health.

These barriers to change are still very much with us. It is discouraging to find that well-developed evidence-based recommendations are often not put into practice. Successful implementation of evidence-based recommendations often requires an organizational and systems approach in addition to education at the individual level. The types of approaches that are increasingly effective in implementing evidence-based guidelines are discussed in Learn More 14.2.

LEARN MORE 14.2 ■ IMPLEMENTING EVIDENCE-BASED RECOMMENDATIONS (9)■ Successful efforts to put evidence into practice have focused largely on the factors that facilitate implementation of evidence-based recommendations. Figure 14.4 displays what has been called the *push–pull* model.

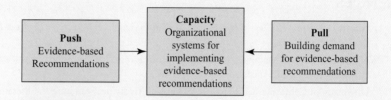

Figure 14.4 **Push–pull approach to successful implementation of evidence-based guidelines.** (Adapted from Curry SJ. Organizational intervention to encourage guideline implementation. *Chest.* 2000;118:40S–46S. [Figure 2].)

Push implies that the development of high quality evidence-based guidelines as described in Chapter 13 is a prerequisite for successful implementation, but are not enough in-and-of themselves to guarantee success. Pull implies the need for demand for implementation from professional and accrediting organizations, purchasers of health care, and acceptance of evidence-based recommendation by patients. Finally, the push and pull factors need to be reinforced by local organizational factors or capacity including health information systems, measurement of clinical outcomes, and peer acceptance.

Putting evidence into practice is now taking center stage in health care. Expect to see multiple simultaneous efforts designed to both push and pull the process.

As we have seen, translating evidence into practice is a complicated process that we are just beginning to understand and include as part of evidence-based research. New types of research such as equivalence research and pragmatic trials are being increasingly used to move beyond efficacy to effectiveness as part of T-2 research. In addition, evaluation research is becoming a vehicle for T-3 research and its efforts to understand how to successfully implement interventions in practice at the individual and population levels.

Acceptance of evidence-based guidelines by clinicians and at time by patients requires an understanding of the implementation process, that is, how evidence is perceived and incorporated into decision making. We need to appreciate that individuals perceive evidence and incorporate it into decision making in different ways than the ones we have encountered in decision analysis, cost-effectiveness analysis, and the development of evidence-based recommendations. The mnemonic DRUG may be used to summarize these differences. Individuals often heavily discount for events in the immediate future; they often are risk-takers or risk-avoiders in specific situation; they may see uncertainty as positive or alternatively as negative; and finally their goal may be a satisfactory outcome or an acceptable process rather than one that maximizes the expected utility of the outcome.

Finally, evidence is often not enough. We need to appreciate how evidence is or is not integrated into practice. This requires us to appreciate the organizational and systems factors that influence the acceptance of evidence-based recommendations. The elements that push and the elements that pull need to work in the same direction to successfully put evidence into practice.

Understanding the evidence obtained through research is an essential starting point for decision making, but it is not the end of the road. There is still an art as well as a science to decision making. Good practitioners need to combine the art and the science to help patients make decisions that they can live with.

REFERENCES

1. Guyatt G, Rennie D. *Users' Guides to the Medical Literature: A Manual for Evidence-Based Practice*. Chicago, IL: AMA Press; 2002.

2. National Library of Medicine. Medical subject headings (MeSH®). http://www.nlm.nih.gov/pubs/factsheets/mesh.html. Accessed August 7, 2011.

3. University of California San Francisco School of Medicine. Searching the literature for evidence-based medicine. http://missinglink.ucsf.edu/lm/EBM_litsearch/. Accessed August 7, 2011.

4. University of North Carolina Health Sciences Library. Searching the medical literature for the best evidence. http://www.hsl.unc.edu/Services/Tutorials/EBM_searching/pages/intro.htm. Accessed August 7, 2011.

5. Dougherty D, Conway PH. The "3T's" road map to transforming US health care: the "how" of high quality care. *JAMA*. 2008;299:2319–2321.

6. Green L. Guidelines and categories for classifying participatory research project in health. http://www.lgreen.net/guidelines.html. Page 1. Accessed July 20, 2011.

7. Slutsky JR. Moving closer to a rapid-learning health care system. *Health Aff (Millwood)*. 2007;26(2):w122–w124.

8. Piaggio G, Elbourne DR, Altman DG, Pocock SJ, Evans SJ; CONSORT Group. Reporting of non-inferiority and equivalence randomized trials: an extension of the CONSORT statement. *JAMA*. 2006;295(10):1152–1160.

9. Zwarenstein M, Treweek S, Gagnier JJ, et al. Improving the reporting of pragmatic trials: an extension of the CONSORT statement. *BMJ*. 2008;337:a2390. doi:10.1136/bmj.a2390.

10. National Cancer Institute. Implementation science: integrating science, practice, and policy. http://cancercontrol.cancer.gov/IS/reaim/. Accessed July 20, 2011.

11. Hastie R, Dawes RM. *Rational Choice in an Uncertain World: The Psychology of Judgment and Decision Making*. Thousand Oaks, CA: Sage Publications; 2001.

12. Tversky A, Kahneman D. Judgment under uncertainty: heuristics and biases. *Science*. 1974;185:1124–1131.

13. Curry SJ. Organizational intervention to encourage guideline implementation. *Chest*. 2000;118:40S–46S.

thePoint ✳ Visit http://thePoint.lww.com for interactive Q&A, flaw-catching exercises, searchable eBook, and more!

GLOSSARY

A

Accuracy Without systematic error or bias; on average the results approximate those of the phenomenon under study.

Actuarial Survival The actuarial survival is an estimate of life expectancy based on a cohort or longitudinal life table. The 5-year actuarial survival estimates the probability of surviving 5 years, and may be calculated even when there are only a limited number of individuals actually followed for 5 years.

Adjustment Techniques used after the collection of data to take into account or control for the effect of known or potential confounding variables and interactions. (*Synonym:* control for, take into account, standardize)

Adverse events An undesirable outcome often used in relationship to interventions including drugs and vaccines. As opposed to the term adverse effects or side effects adverse events do not imply a cause and effect relationship.

Affected by Time An increase in the duration of observation results in a greater probability of observing the outcome, and individuals are observed for different lengths of time.

Aggregate Impact The overall impact of an intervention on the entire population of individuals to whom it is directed.

Aggregate External Validity As used by the United States Preventive Services Task Force, the extent to which the evidence is relevant and generalizable to the population and conditions of typical primary care practice.

Aggregate Internal Validity As used by the United States Preventive Services Task Force, the degree to which the studies used to support an evidence-based recommendation provide valid evidence for the populations and the settings in which they were conducted.

Algorithm An explicit, often graphic presentation of the steps to be taken in making a decision such as diagnosis or treatment. May be used to present evidence-based guidelines or recommendations using a standardized graphical approach.

Allocation Concealment In a randomized controlled trial, the inability of the individual making the assignment to predict the group to which the next individual will be assigned.

Allocation Ratio In a randomized controlled trial the proportion of participants intended for each study and control group.

Alternative Hypothesis The statement of the hypothesis that is an alternative to the null hypothesis. In statistical significance testing, the choices are between the null hypothesis and an alternative hypothesis. The alternative hypothesis states that a difference or association exists. (*Synonym:* Study hypothesis)

Analysis of Covariance (ANCOVA) Statistical procedures for analysis of data that contain a continuous dependent variable and a mixture of nominal and continuous independent variables.

Analysis of Variance (ANOVA) Statistical procedures for analysis of data that contain a continuous dependent variable and more than one nominal independent variable.

Analytical Study All types of investigations that include a comparison group within the investigation itself (e.g., population comparison, case-control, cohort, and randomized controlled trials).

Analytical Frameworks A structure for thinking through and presenting the information relevant to a problem such as the development of evidence-based recommendations

Appropriate Measurement A measurement that addresses the question that an investigation intends to study, i.e., one that is appropriate for the study question.

Artifactual Differences or Changes Differences or changes in measures of occurrence that result from the ability, effort or definition of the disease or condition. without changes in the underlying rates. (*Synonym:* spurious, artificial differences or changes in rates)

Assessment The component of the M.A.A.R.I.E. framework in which the outcome or endpoint of the study and control groups are measured.

Assessment Bias A generic term referring to any type of bias in the process of measuring outcome. Recall, report, and instrument errors are specific types. (synonym: observation bias)

Assignment The component of the M.A.A.R.I.E. framework in which individuals become part of a study group or control group.

Association The strength of a relationship in one sample (or population) compared to another. Exist when the relationship is statistically significant.

As Treated Analysis A method for data analysis in a randomized controlled trial in which individual outcomes are analyzed based upon the actual treatment received. (*Synonym:* per protocol analysis)

At-Risk Population The population that is represented in the denominator of most rates— that is, those who are at risk of developing the event being measured in the numerator.

Attributable Risk Percentage The percentage of the risk, among those with the risk factor, that is associated with exposure to the risk factor. If a cause-and-effect relationship exists, It is the percentage of a disease that can potentially be eliminated among those with the risk factor if the impact of the risk factor is completely and immediately eliminated. (*Synonym:* attributable risk [exposed], etiological fraction [exposed], percentage risk reduction, protective efficacy)

Averaging Out The process of obtaining overall expected utilities for a decision tree by adding together the expected utilities of each of the potential outcomes included in the decision tree.

B

Base-Case Estimate The estimate used in a decision-making investigation that reflects the investigators' best available or best-guess estimate of the relevant value of a particular variable. High and low estimates reflect the extremes of the realistic range of values around this estimate.

Bayes' Theorem A mathematical formula that can be used to calculate posttest probabilities (or odds) based on pretest probabilities (or odds) and the sensitivity and specificity of a test.

Bayesian An approach to statistics that takes into account the preexisting probability (or odds) of a disease or a study hypothesis when analyzing and interpreting the data in the investigation.

Before-and-after study A special type of population comparison in which an outcome is measured in the same population before an after an intervention (see: population comparison)

Berksonian Bias A type of selection bias that may result from utilization of controls who are hospitalized at the same time as and place as the cases.

Bias A measurement that produces results which depart from the true values in a consistent direction. (*Synonym:* systematic error)

Biological Plausibility An ancillary, adjunct, or supportive criteria of cause-and-effect which implies that the relationship is consistent with a known biological mechanism.

Bivariable Analysis Statistical analysis in which there is one dependent variable and one independent variable.

Blind Assessment The evaluation of the outcome for participants in an investigation without the individual who makes the evaluation knowing whether the subjects were in the study group or the control group. (*Synonym:* masked assessment)

Blind Assignment Occurs when individuals are assigned to a study group and a control group without the investigator or the subjects being aware of the group to which they are assigned. When both investigator and subjects are "blinded" or "masked," the study is sometimes referred to as a double-blind study. (*Synonym:* masked assignment)

Broad Validation As used in prediction and decision rules, implies that the type of database used for validation differs substantially from the type of database used for derivation and initial validation of the prediction and decision rule.

C

Calibration An measure used in prediction and decision rules that measures performance of a prediction and decision rule by comparing its performance on participants whose characteristics are substantially above and substantial below the average value for all those included in the data.

Carry-Over Effect A phenomenon that may occur in a cross-over study when the initial therapy continues to have an effect after it is no longer being administered. What is know as a wash-out period is often used to minimize the potential for this effect.

Case-Based Case-Control Study A type of case-control study in which the control are selected from the same institution, such as a hospital, as the controls.

Case-cohort study A special type of case-control study in which the controls are sampled from the entire population thereby including the cases as potential controls.

Case-Control Study A study that begins by identifying individuals with a disease (cases) and individuals without a disease (controls). The cases and controls are identified without knowledge of an individual's exposure or nonexposure to factors being investigated. (*Synonym:* retrospective study)

Case Fatality The number of deaths due to a particular disease divided by the number of individuals diagnosed with the disease at the beginning of the time interval. It estimates the probability of eventually dying from the disease.

Case Finding Identification of an individual usually with a communicable disease with the intention of locating and treating their contacts.

Case-mix A term used to describe the types of patients that are included in a population especially to describe a population's range of patient prognoses (See: Case-Mix Bias)

Case-Mix Bias A form of selection bias that may be created when treatments are selected by clinicians to fit characteristics of individual patients resulting in different prognoses among those receiving different treatments.

Censored Data Occurs when collection of data is terminated at a particular point in time and the event of interest has not occurred but it is not known whether or not the outcome subsequently occurred or would have occurred. May be due to loss to follow-up, death from another cause or termination of the investigation.

Chain of causation   Occurs when factor A increases the probability of developing factor B and factor B increases the probability of developing factor C. When the relationship between factor A and factor C is being investigated factor B should not be treated as a confounding variable.

Chance Node   A circle in a decision tree that indicates that once a decision is made, there are two or more outcomes that may occur by a chance process.

Chi-Square Test   A statistical significance test that can be used to calculate a *P* value for a nominal independent and a nominal dependent variable.

Chi-Square Test for Trend   A statistical significance test that is used for a nominal dependent variable and a continuous independent variable.

Classification error   An error in categorizing an individual to study or control groups or to the presence or absence of the study outcome. This error can be either directional indicating the presence of a bias or non directional suggesting the impact of chance.

Clinical equipoise   A principle of research ethics implying that there is sufficient controversy within the expert health community about the preferred treatment to justify a randomized controlled trial.

Clinical sensibility   A term used in prediction and decision rules to refer to the practical barriers to use of these rules in clinical practice.

Clusters   Occcurence of an unexpected number of rare events in the a small geographic area or over a short period of time.

Coefficient of Determination   The square of a correlation coefficient. This statistic when appropriately used indicates the proportion of the variation in one variable (the dependent variable) that is explained by knowing the value of one or more other variables (the independent variables). The independent and dependent variable can be reversed without affecting the results. (See: correlation coefficient)

Cohort   A group of individuals who share a common exposure, experience, or characteristic. (*See:* cohort study, cohort effect)

Cohort Effect   A change in rates that can be explained by the common experience or characteristic of a group of individuals that cannot be expected to continue. This effect implies that current rates should not be directly extrapolated into the future.

Cohort Study   A study that begins by identifying individuals with and without a factor being investigated. These factors are identified without knowledge of which individuals have or will develop the outcome. These studies may be prospective or retrospective.

Collinearity   Sharing of information among independent variables. In a regression method this effect poses an issue of which independent variables to include in a regression equation. When two or more independent variables that are themselves associated are included as variables in a multivariable regression it leads to a reduced strength of the relationship for each of the associated independent variables. (*Synonym:* multicollinearity)

Comparative Effective research   A term describing investigations that compare two or more interventions both of which have undergone investigations establishing efficacy. This type of research may be seen as a component of translational research 2 or T-2.

Compassionate Use   An exemption to the FDA procedures that allows a drug to be used under specific non-investigational circumstances prior to its formal approval.

Concurrent Cohort Study   A cohort study in which an individual's group assignment is determined at the time that the study begins, and the study group and control group participants are followed forward in time to determine if the disease occur. (*Synonym:* prospective cohort study)

Confidence Interval (95%)   In statistical terms, the interval of numerical values within which one can be 95% confident that the value being estimated in the larger population lies. (*Synonym:* interval estimate)

Confidence Limits   The upper and lower extremes of the confidence interval.

Confounding Variable   A variable that is distributed differently in the study group and control group and that affects the outcome being assessed. In addition, this type of variable may not be part of the chain of causation. It may be due to chance or bias. (*Synonym:* confounder See: chain of causation)

Consensus Conference   As used here, a process for determining the presence or absence of a consensus by using face-to-face structured communication among a representative group of experts.

Continuous Data   A type of data with an unlimited number of equally spaced potential values (e.g., diastolic blood pressure, cholesterol).

Contributory Cause   Definitively established when all three of the following have been established: (a) the existence of an association between the cause and the effect at the level of the individual; (b) the "cause" precedes the "effect" in time; and (c) altering the "cause" alters the probability of occurrence of the "effect".

Control Group   A group of subjects used for comparison with a study group. Ideally, this group is identical to the study group except that it does not possess the characteristic or has not had the exposure under investigation.

Convenience Sample   A subset from a population that is assembled because of the ease of collecting data without considering the degree to which the sample is randomly selected or representative of the population of interest.

Conventional Care   The current level of intervention accepted as routine or standard care. (*Synonyms:* standard care, state-of-the-art care)

Correlation A statistic which may be used for studying the strength of an association between two variables, each of which has been sampled using a representative or naturalistic method from a population of interest.

Correlation Analysis A class of statistical procedures that is used to estimate the strength of the relationship between a continuous dependent variable and a continuous independent variable when both the dependent variable and the independent variable are selected by representative or naturalistic sampling.

Correlation Coefficient An estimate of the strength of the association between a dependent variable and an independent variable when both are obtained using naturalistic sampling. (e.g., Pearson's and Spearman's correlation coefficients.)

Cost-and-Effectiveness Studies As used here, the type of decision analysis study that compares the cost of achieving a common unit of effectiveness, such as a life saved or a diagnosis made.

Cost-Benefit Analysis The type of decision-making investigation that converts effectiveness as well as cost into monetary terms. Benefit in this type of analysis refers to net effectiveness, that is, the favorable minus the unfavorable outcomes.

Cost-Consequence Analysis A type of cost-effectiveness analysis in which harms, benefits, and costs are measured or described but not directly combined or compared.

Cost-Effective Describes the situation when one of the following has been demonstrated: an increase in net-effectiveness is considered worth the increase in cost; or a decreased net-effectiveness is considered worth the substantial reduction in costs; or there is reduced cost plus increased net-effectiveness.

Cost-Effectiveness Analysis A general term for the type of decision-making investigation in which costs are considered as well as harms and benefits.

Cost-Effectiveness Ratios The average cost per QALY obtained. The comparison alternative is not usually specified in which case it is the do-nothing or hypothetical zero cost–zero effectiveness alternative.

Cost-QALY Graph A graph that includes cost on the y-axis and QALY on the x-axis, and includes four quadrants with different interpretations related to cost-effectiveness.

Cost Savings A generic term implying that a reduction in cost may be accompanied by a reduction or an increase in effectiveness.

Cost-Utility Analysis The type of cost-effectiveness analysis that measures and combines benefits, harms, and costs, taking into account the probabilities and the utilities. These investigations often use QALYs as the measure of effectiveness and thus may be called cost-effectiveness analysis using QALYs. (*Synonym:* QALY cost-effectiveness study)

Cox Proportional Hazards Regression A statistical procedure for a nominal dependent variable and a mixture of nominal and continuous independent variables that can be used when the dependent variable is affected by time. (*Synonym:* Cox regression)

Credibility Intervals A term used in decision-making investigations to present the results in a form that parallels confidence intervals. The Monte Carlo method may be used to generate this intervals by performing large numbers of simulation's using the investigation's own decision-making model.

Cross-Over Study A type of paired design in which the same individual receives a study and subsequently a control therapy (or visa versa), and an outcome is assessed for each therapy.

Cross-Sectional Study A study that identifies individuals with and without the condition or disease under study and the characteristic or exposure of interest at the same point in time.

Cumulative Survival The estimate of survival derived for a life-table analysis calculated by combining the probabilities from each time interval.

D

Decision Analysis As used in decision-making investigations, refers to the type of investigations in which benefits and harms are included but not costs. Often used generically to refer to all quantitative decision-making.

Decison Maker A generic term designed to leave open the identify of the individual or institution that is actually making the decision. Can be patients, clinicians, health insurance companies etc.

Decision-Making Model A diagram or written description of the steps involved in each of the alternatives being considered in a decision-making investigation. A decision tree is a commonly used method.

Decision Node A square in a decision tree that indicates that a choice needs to be made. (*Synonym:* choice node)

Decision and Prediction Rule A prediction score that is converted into a test and used as the basis for making decisions. (*Synonym:* clinical prediction rule, clinical decision rule)

Decision and Prediction rule validation The process of determining whether use of decision rule to guide decision making improves outcome compared to the current method of decision making.

Decision Tree A graphic display of the decision alternatives, including the choices that need to be made and the chance events that occur.

Declining Exponential Approximation of Life Expectancy (DEALE) A specialized life-expectancy measure which combines survival derived for a longitudinal life table plus life expectancy based on age and other demographic factors derived from a cross-sectional life table.

Delphi Method A formal method for reaching group agreement in which the participants do not communicate directly with each other.

Determinant– A factor which is related to a disease or other condition but more remotely than a contributory cause or risk factor. Have been called "causes of causes".

Deductive reasoning A form of reasoning that begins with general principles or theories and derives specific conclusions or hypotheses.

Dependent Variable Generally, the outcome variable of interest in any type of research study. The outcome or end-point that one intends to explain or predict.

Derivation Cohort A subset of individuals from an existing database that is used to develop an initial prediction and decision rule.

Descriptive Study An investigation that provides data on one group of individuals and does not include a comparison group, at least within the investigation itself. Includes case series, time series and historical control studies.

Diagnostic Ability A term used here to indicate that the measurement of a test's performance includes a weighting of false positives compared to false negatives in addition to the discriminant ability.

Diagnostic Test A test conducted in the presence of symptoms compatible with a specific disease with the intention of identifying the presence of disease.

Difference A measure of the strength of a relationship that is obtained by subtracting a measurement in one sample (or population) from that of another sample (or population).

Direct Cause A contributory cause that is the most directly known cause of a disease (e.g., hepatitis B virus is the direct cause of hepatitis B infection, and contaminated needles are an indirect cause). The direct cause is dependent on the current state of knowledge and may change as more immediate mechanisms are discovered.

Disability Adjusted Life Years (DALY) A disease- or condition-specific measure of the number of life years lost from death and disability per population unit (such as per 1,000 population) compared to a current population with the longest life expectancy and no disabilities.

Discordant Pairs In a paired case-control study, the pairs of subjects in which the study and control members of the pair differ in their exposure or nonexposure to the potential risk factor.

Discounted Present Value The amount of money that needs to be invested today to pay a bill of a particular size at a particular time in the future. (*Synonym:* present value)

Discounting A method used in decision-making investigations to take into account the reduced importance of benefits, harms, and/or costs that occur at a later period of time compared to those that occur immediately.

Discrete Data Data with a limited number of categories or potential values. This type of data may be further classified as either nominal or ordinal data.

Discriminant Ability A measure of test performance that assumes that a false positive and a false negative are of equal importance. May be measured by the area under a ROC curve. (*Synonym:* area under ROC curve)

Diseconomies of Scale Increases in unit costs that accompany increases in the scale of production or implementation.

Dispersion Spread of data around a measure of central tendency, such as a mean or average.

Distribution Frequencies or relative frequencies of all observed values of a characteristic. Can be described graphically or mathematically.

Distributional Effects A term used in decision-making investigations that indicates that the average results do not take into account the distributions of the adverse and favorable outcomes among subgroups with different characteristics.

Dominance The situation when an alternative can be eliminated since it is inferior regardless of the utilities.

Do-Nothing Approach The hypothetical comparison alternative in calculation of cost-effectiveness ratios in which there is presumed to be zero cost and zero effectiveness.

Dose-Response Relationship This type of relationship is present if changes in levels of an exposure are associated with changes in the frequency of the outcome in a consistent direction. This type of relationship is an ancillary or supportive criterion for contributory cause.

Dread Effect A decision making bias in which the emotional impact of the outcomes biases the perception of its frequency

E

Ecological Fallacy The type of error that can occur when the existence of a group association is used to imply the existence of an individual association that does not exist at the individual level. (*Synonym:* population fallacy)

Economies of Scale Refers to reductions in unit cost that accompany increases in the scale of production or implementation.

Effect An outcome that is brought about, at least in part, by an etiological factor known as the cause.

Effect of Observation A type of assessment bias that results when the process of measuring an outcome alters the outcome being measured.

Effect Size A summary measure of the magnitude of the difference or association found in the sample. May not imply a cause and effect relationship.

Effectiveness The extent to which a intervention produces a beneficial impact when implemented under the usual conditions of clinical care for a particular group of patients.

Efficacy The extent to which a treatment produces a beneficial effect when assessed under the ideal conditions of an investigation.

Eligibility Criteria The combined set of inclusion and exclusion criteria that define those who are eligible for participation in an investigation (*Synonym:* entry criteria)

Equivalence Trial A type of randomized controlled trial designed to determine whether two or more interventions are equivalent in terms of outcome as contrasted to the traditional superiority trial (*See:* Non-inferiority trial)

Error of Commission An error or less than optimal outcomes that occur after an action is taken by a decision maker

Error of Omission A error or less than optimal outcome that occurs after an action is not taken by a decision maker.

Estimate A value calculated from sample observations that are used to approximate a corresponding population value or parameter. (*Synonym:* point estimate)

Event An episode or diagnosis of the condition or disease that appears in the numerator of a rate or proportion.

Evidence-Based Recommendations Structured set of recommended actions for clinical or public health practice indicating specific conditions for utilizing or not utilizing interventions. Based on evidence from the research literature combined with decision-maker preferences and expert opinion. (*Synonym:* evidence-based guideline, practice guidelines).

Exclusion Criteria Conditions which preclude entrance of candidates into an investigation even if they meet the inclusion criteria.

Expected Utility The results of multiplying the probability times the utility of a particular outcome. (*Synonym:* quality-adjusted probability)

Expected-Utility Decision Analysis The type of decision analysis that considers probabilities and utilities but does not explicitly incorporate life expectancy.

Exploratory Meta-analysis A meta-analysis in which there is not a specific hypothesis, and all potentially relevant investigations are included.

External Validity How well the conclusions can be applied to individuals, groups or populations not included in an investigation. When used for prediction and decision rules implies using additional databases beyond the database that was used for initial derivation and validation to establish the internal validity of the prediction and decision rule.

Extrapolation Conclusions drawn about the meaning of an investigation for those not included in the investigation. (*Synonym:* generalizability, external validity)

F

Factorial Design A method increasing used in randomized controlled trials to examine more than one intervention at a time. Most commonly two interventions are investigated each with two levels producing four possible groups.

Fail-Safe N The number of studies which must be omitted from a meta-analysis before the results would no longer be statistically significant. These additional studies are assumed to be of the same average size as the included studies and have, on average, an effect size of 0 for differences or 1 for ratios.

False Negative An individual whose result on a test is negative but who has the disease or condition as determined by the reference standard.

False Negative Rate The proportion of all negatives that are false negative. This rate is the complement of the predictive value of a negative i.e. the proportion of all negatives that are true negatives.

False Positive An individual whose result on a test is positive but who does not have the disease or condition as determined by the reference standard.

Final Outcome An outcome that occurs at the completion of a decision option. This outcome is displayed at the right end of a decision tree.

Fixed Costs Costs which do not vary with modest increases or decreases in the volume of services provided. Space and personnel costs are considered examples.

Fixed-Effect Model A type of statistical significance test that assumes that subgroups all come from the same large population. In meta-analysis, its use implies that there is homogeneity across the investigations.

Folding Back the Decision Tree A process in which probabilities are multiplied together to obtain a probability of a particular outcome known as a path probability. Calculations of path probabilities assume that the probability of each of the outcomes that occur along the path is independent of the other probabilities along the same path.

Forest Plot A graphical method which among its uses is the display of results of a meta-analysis including the effect size and confidence interval of each of the investigations included in the meta-analysis.

Framing Effect A decision making term that implies that the way evidence is presented or structured can influence the way it is perceived.

Frequentist An approach to statistics that as opposed to the Bayesian approach does not take into account the pre-existing probability. This approach is incorporated into traditional statistical significance testing and leads to an alternative interpretation of confidence intervals.

Funnel Diagram   A graphical method for evaluating whether publication bias is likely to be present in a meta-analysis.

G

Gaussian Distribution   A distribution of data assumed in many statistical procedures. This distribution is a symmetrical, continuous, bell-shaped curve with its mean value corresponding to the highest point on the curve. (*Synonym:* normal distribution)

Global Measures   Measurements that can only be made at the population level and do not have meaning at the individual level such as the national level of gross domestic product (GDP)

Gray Literature   Information, usually research and technical information, found outside the formally published literature but increasingly accessible through Internet sources.

Group Association   The situation in which a characteristic and a disease both occur more frequently in one group of individuals compared with another. Does not necessarily imply that individuals with the characteristic are the same ones who have the disease. (*Synonym:* population association, ecological association, ecological correlation)

Group Matching   A matching procedure used during assignment in an investigation that selects study and control individuals in such a way that the groups have a nearly equal distribution of a particular variable or variables. (*Synonym:* frequency matching)

Group Randomized Trials   A special type of randomized controlled trial in which the unit of randomization is groups such as hospitals, schools or communities instead of individuals (*Synonyms:* cluster randomized trials, community randomized trials)

Guideline   Indicates a recommendation for (or against) an intervention except under specified exceptions.

H

Hazard ratio   A measure of the strength of a relationship that is produced by a Cox proportional hazards regression and may be interpreted as a relative risk adjusted for multiple confounding variables.

Health Adjusted Life Expectancy (HALE)   A summary measurement that includes a measure of the quality of health, measured on a scale of 0 to 1, that is multiplied by the life expectancy.

Heuristic   A rule of thumb or method used in nonquantitative or subjective decision-making that generally uses only a portion of the potentially available data and thus simplifies the decision-making process.

Historical Control   A control group from an earlier period of time that is used to compare outcomes with a study group actually included in an investigation.

Homogeneous   When used in the context of a meta-analysis, refers to investigations which can be combined into a single meta-analysis because the study characteristics being examined do not substantially affect the outcome.

Homoscedasticity   An assumption of statistical methods for a continuous dependent variable implying equal variance of the dependent variable values in the population for each value of the independent variable(s). (*Synonym:* assumption of equal variance)

Human Capital   An approach to converting effectiveness to monetary terms that uses the recipient's ability to contribute to the economy.

Hypothesis-Driven Meta-analysis   A meta-analysis in which a specific hypothesis is used as the basis for inclusion or exclusion of investigations.

I

Incidence-prevalence Bias   A bias that occurs in cross-sectional study due to the fact that cross-sectional studies detect existing cases based on prevalence which is affected by the duration of the disease rather than new or incident cases which are not affected by the duration of the disease.

Incidence Rate   The rate at which new cases of disease occur per unit of time. Often calculated as the number of individuals who develop the disease over a period of time divided by the total person-years of observation.

Inclusion Criteria   Conditions which must be met by all potential candidates for entrance into an investigation.

Incremental Cost-effectiveness Ratio   The cost of obtaining one additional QALY using an alternative intervention compared with the use of the conventional intervention.

Independence   In testing is present when the results of one test does not affect the probability of obtaining the same results from a second test.

Independent Variable   Variable being measured to estimate the corresponding measurement of the dependent variable in any type of research study.

Index Test   The test of interest that is being evaluation by comparison with the reference standard or gold standard test.

Inductive reasoning   A method of reasoning that may be used to generate hypotheses by starting with specific situations and generalizing to a hypothesis? (*See:*deductive reasoning)

Inference In statistical terminology, is the logical process that occurs during statistical significance testing in which conclusions concerning a population are obtained based on data from a random sample of the same population. (*See:* statistical significance test)

Influence Diagram A graphical method for displaying decision making which displays the factors that affect a decision or outcome and their interactions.

Information Bias A systematic error introduced by the process of obtaining the investigation's measurement of outcome. (*Synonym: assessment bias*) (*See:* recall bias, reporting bias)

Informed consent Voluntary agreement to participate in an investigation given by an eligible individual or their legal proxy after approval of the content of the statement by an Institutional Review Board.

Integrative Approach An approach to evidence that aims to examine multiple factors and their interactions such as used in systems approaches (*synonym:* holistic*)

Intention to Treat A method for data analysis in a randomized controlled trial in which individual outcomes are analyzed according to the group to which they have been randomized even if they never received the treatment to which they were assigned. (*See:* As Treated)

Interaction Occurs when the probability of an outcome resulting from the presence of one variable is altered by the level of a second variable. May produce results which are less than or more than additive. (*Synonym:* effect modification, synergy)

Interim Analysis An analysis of the data that occurs during the course of an investigation

Internal validity A term used to address issues of assessment of the outcome as well as interpretation of the data for those included in the investigation.

Interobserver variability Variation in measurement by different individuals (*Synonym:* Inter-rater reliability)

Interpretation The drawing of conclusions about the meaning of any differences found between the study group and the control group for those included in the investigation. (*See:* internal validity)

Interpolation The process of filling in data values between points that are actually measured usually using a straight line to connect the observed data points.

Intervention A term that applies to a wide range of preventive, therapeutic, rehabilitative and palliative approaches

Intraobserver Variation Variation in measurements by the same person at different times.(*Synonym:* Test-retest reliability)

K

Kaplan-Meier Life Table A graphical display of survival data from a randomized controlled trial or a cohort study. Does not adjust for multiple confounding variables

Kappa A measure of agreement between two measurement that takes into account chance agreement. (*Synonym:*Kappa statistic)

Koch's Postulates A set of difficult to fulfill criteria developed for demonstrating cause-and-effect for communicable diseases. (see Modern Koch's Postulates).

L

Lead-Time Bias Overestimation of survival time due to earlier diagnosis of disease. Actual time of death does not change when this bias is present despite the earlier time of diagnosis.

Length Bias The tendency of a screening test to more frequently detect individuals with a slowly progressive disease compared with individuals with a rapidly progressive disease.

Life Expectancy The average number of years of remaining life from a particular age based on the probabilities of death in each age group in one particular year.

Life Table (Cohort or Longitudinal) A method for organizing data that allows examination of the experience of one or more groups of individuals over time when some individuals are followed for longer periods of time than others. (*See:* Kaplan-Meier life tables)

Life Table (Cross-Sectional or Current) A data technique that uses mortality data from one year's experience and applies the data to a stationary population to calculate life expectancies. (See: survival analysis)

Likelihood Ratio of a Negative Test A ratio of the probability of a negative test if the disease is present to the probability of a negative test if the disease is absent.

Likelihood Ratio of a Positive Test A ratio of the probability of a positive test if the disease is present to the probability of a positive test if the disease is absent.

Linear Extrapolation A form of extrapolation that assumes, often incorrectly, that levels of a variable beyond the range of the data included in an investigation will continue to operate in the same manner that they operate in the investigation. (*Synonym:* straight line extrapolation*)

Log-Rank Test A statistical significance test that is used in life-table analysis (*Synonym:* Mantel-Haenszel test)

Logistic Regression A multivariable method used when there is a nominal dependent variable and a nominal and continuous independent variable that are not affected by time.(*Synonym:* Multiple Logistic Regression Analysis)

M

Main Effect Refers to the relationship between the independent variable and the dependent variable that reflect the relationship stated in the study hypothesis.

Mann–Whitney Test A statistical significance test that is used for an ordinal dependent variable and a nominal independent variable.

Marginal Cost The impact on costs of greatly increasing the scale of operation of an intervention so that economies of scale and diseconomies of scale may impact the costs. Should be distinguished from incremental cost, which relates to the cost of one additional unit.

Markov Analysis A method of analysis used in decision-making investigations to take into account recurrent events such as recurrence of previous disease or development of a second episode of disease.

Matching An assignment procedure in which study and control groups are chosen to ensure that a particular variable is the same or similar in each group. Pairing is a special type in which an individual from the study group and from the control group are analyzed together.

McNemar's Test A statistical significance test for paired data when there is one nominal dependent variable and one nominal independent variable.

Mean Sum of the measurements divided by the number of measurements being added together. The "center of gravity" of a distribution of observations. A special type of average in which all values are given the same weight. (*Synonyms*: arithmetic mean, average)

Median The mid-point of a distribution where half the data values occur above and half occur below.

MeSH Headings Medical subject heading developed by the National Library of Medicine to search the peer reviewed health research literature

Meta-analysis A series of quantitative methods for systematically combining data from more than one investigation to draw quantitative conclusions which could not be drawn solely on the basis of the single investigations. (*See*: systematic review)

Method As used in the M.A,A.R.I.E. framework, the first component that addresses issues of hypothesis, study population, and sample size.

Modern Koch's Postulates A term used to refer to a modification of Koch's postulates for establishing causation for communicable diseases. Require epidemiological association, isolation, and transmission to establish causation for a pathogen. (*See*: Koch's Postulates)

Mode The point of greatest frequency in a graphic display of data

Monte Carlo Simulation A method used for sensitivity analysis in cost-effectiveness analysis and other applications that repeatedly samples the same population to derive a large number of samples whose distribution can be used to calculate point estimates and confidence or credibility ranges.

Mortality Rate A measure of the incidence of death. This rate is calculated as the number of deaths over a period of time divided by the number in the at-risk population at the beginning of the time interval.

Multivariable Analysis A statistical analysis in which there is one dependent variable and more than one independent variable.(see multivariate analysis).

Multivariate Analysis A statistical analysis in which there is more than one dependent variable. Commonly but incorrectly used as a synonym for multivariable analysis.

Mutually Exclusive Categories fulfill this definition if any one individual can be included in only one category.

N

Narrow Validation As used in prediction and decision rules, implies that the database used for validation is similar to the one used for derivation and initial validation of the prediction and decision rule.

Natural Experiment A special type of cohort study often used to provide evidence that altering the "cause" alters the "effect". The study and control groups' outcomes are compared with their own outcomes before and after a change is observed in the exposure of the study group.

Naturalistic Sample A special type of representative sample in which observations are obtained from a population in such a way that the sample distribution of independent variable values as well as dependent variable values is representative of their distribution in the population. (*See:* representative sample)

Necessary Cause A characteristic fulfills this definition if its presence is required to produce or cause the disease.

Nested case-control study A case-control study conducted using data originally obtained as part of a cohort study or randomized controlled trial.

Net-effectiveness The benefits minus the harms. In the context of decision analysis this is used as the measure of effectiveness.

N-of-1 Trial An investigation of a single individual suspected of having an adverse event resulting from an intervention. The investigator determines whether removal of the intervention reverse the adverse event and if so whether reuse of the intervention again produces the adverse event.

Nominal Data A type of data with named categories. May have more than two categories that cannot be ordered (e.g., race, eye color). May have only two categories i.e. dichotomous data, that can be ordered one above another (e.g., dead/alive). (see nominal variable)

Nominal variable A variable with two possible categories. The number of variables required to represent nominal data is equal to the number of potential categories of the nominal data minus one.

Nondifferential misclassification- Classification error that is the result of chance. The consequences of this type of misclassification error are to reduce the magnitude of the association below that which would be found in the absence of misclassification due to chance.

Noninferiority Trial   A type of randomized controlled trial similar to an equivalence trial designed to establish that the study treatment is not inferior to the control treatment. (*See:* equivalence trial)

Null Hypothesis   The assertion that no association or difference exists in the larger population from which the study samples are obtained

Number Needed to Treat   The number of patients, similar to the study patients, who need to be treated to obtain one fewer bad outcome or one more good outcome compared to the control group treatment.

Number-Prevented-in-the-Population   The potential number of cases of a disease or condition that may be prevented in a population of a particular size over a defined period of time. Calculated as the population attributable risk, times the incidence of disease times the population size.

O

Observational Study   An investigation in which the assignment is conducted by observing the subjects who meet the inclusion and exclusion criteria.

Observed Assignment   Refers to the method of assignment of individuals to study and control groups in observational studies where the investigator does not intervene to perform the assignment.

Odds   A ratio in which the numerator contains the number of times an event occurs and the denominator contains the number of times the event does not occur.

Odds Form of Bayes' Theorem   The formula for Bayes' theorem that indicates that the posttest odds of disease is equal to the pretest odds times the likelihood ratio.

Odds Ratio   A ratio measuring the strength of an association applicable to all types of studies employing nominal data but is required for case-control studies.

Off-label Prescribing   This type of prescribing occurs when an approved drug is used for indications or at dosages or duration other than those for which it is approved by the FDA.

One-Tailed Test   A statistical significance test in which deviations from the null hypothesis in only one direction are considered. Its use implies that the investigator does not consider a true deviation in the opposite direction from the study hypothesis to be possible.

Open label   Refers to an investigation usually of a therapeutic or preventive agent, in which there is no attempt to blind either the participants or the investigators.

Option   One alternative intervention being compared in a decision-making investigation. May also be used in practice guidelines to indicate that the evidence does not

support a clear recommendation or that inadequate data are available to make a recommendation.

Ordinal Data   A type of data with a limited number of categories and with an inherent ordering of the categories from lowest to highest. Says nothing about the spacing between categories (e.g., Stage 1, 2, 3, and 4 cancer).

Outcome   The phenomenon being measured in the assessment process of an investigation. In case-control studies, it is a prior characteristic; in concurrent cohort studies and randomized controlled trials, it is a future event which occurs subsequent to the assignment. (*Synonym:* endpoint)

Outcome Studies   A generic term which refers to investigations of the results of interventions regardless of the type of investigation used.

Outcomes Profile   The type of decision analysis that measures the benefits and harms but does not directly compare them. (*Synonym:* balance sheet)

Outliers   An investigation included in a meta-analysis or a subject in an investigation whose results are substantially different from the vast majority of studies or subjects, suggesting a need to examine the situation to determine why such an extreme result has occurred.

Over Adjustment   The error that occurs when investigators conduct an adjustment procedure using a variable that is in the chain of causation

Over Matching   The error which occurs when investigators attempt to study a factor closely related to a characteristic used to match or pair the study and control groups.

P

Paired test   A statistical significance test used when an individual from the study group is paired with an individual from the control group to prevent a confounding variable. (*Synonym:* matched test)

P Value   The probability of obtaining data at least as extreme as the data obtained in the investigation's sample if the null hypothesis is true.

Pairing   A special form of matching in which each study individual is paired with a control group individual and their outcomes are compared. (*See:* matching)

Parameter   A value that summarizes the distribution of data in of a large population such as the mean and the standard error.

Path Probability   The probability of a final outcome in a decision-making investigation. Calculated by multiplying the probabilities of each of the outcomes that follow chance nodes and that lead to a final outcome.

Pearson's Correlation Coefficient   The correlation coefficient that may be used when the dependent variable and the independent variable are both continuous and both have been obtained using a method of representative sampling i.e. naturalistic sampling.

Person-Years Equivalent to one person observed for a period of 1 year. Can be used as a measure of total observation time in the denominator of a rate.

Perspective In decision-making investigations, asks what factors should be consider when measuring the impact of the benefits, harms, and costs from a particular point of view. (*See:* social perspective, user perspective)

Phases I, II, III, IV The phases of pre-approval and post approval testing of drugs and vaccines on humans used by the U.S. Food and Drug Administration.

Phi A measure of agreement that unlike Kappa can be used when the measure of agreement is very high or very low by chance alone (*see:* Kappa)

Placebo A biologically inert substance or procedure that may under certain conditions be used by individuals assigned to a control group in a randomized controlled trial.

Placebo Effect The impact on outcome of an intervention that results from an indiviudal's belief that they are receiving effective treatment.

Plateau Effect A flat portion of a life-table or time-to-event curve at the right hand end of the curve that may reflect the fact that very few individuals remain in the investigation rather than indicating cure.

Population In statistics, one attempts to draw conclusions about a large group by obtaining a representative sample made up of individuals from this large group.

Population-Attributable Risk Percentage The percentage of the risk in a community, including individuals with and without a risk factor, that is associated with exposure to a risk factor. Does not necessarily imply a cause-and-effect relationship. (*Synonym:* attributable fraction [population], attributable proportion [population], etiological fraction [population])

Population Based Case-Control Study A type of case-control study in which both the cases and the controls aim to be a representative sample of a larger source population from which both the cases and control are obtained.

Population Comparison A research study designed to compare populations or one population over time (*Synonym:* ecological study**)**

Positive-if-Both-Positive As used here, a screening strategy in which a second test is administered to all those who have a positive result on the initial test. The results may be labeled positive only if both tests are positive. (*Synonyms:* serial testing, consecutive testing)

Positive-if-One-Positive As used here, a screening strategy in which two or more tests are initially administered to all individuals and the screening is labeled as positive if one or more tests produce positive results. *(Synonyms:* parallel testing, simultaneous testing),

Post hoc analysis A term used to describe an analysis of data, usually on subgroups, in which a hypothesis for the analysis was not put forth prior to collecting the data. (*See:* pre hoc analysis)

Post Market As used to describe the FDA processes, refers to research and monitoring efforts after FDA approval

Pragmatic Trial A randomized controlled trial for effectiveness comparing two or more interventions using populatio and setting consistent with the use of the intervention in practice. (*Synonym:* effectiveness trial)

Precise Without random error, without variability from measurement to measurement of the same phenomenon. (*Synonyms:* reproducibility, reliability)

Prediction A special form of extrapolation in which the investigator extrapolates to a future point in time. May also refer to efforts to develop a prognosis for one particular individual.

Prediction and Decision Rule The end result of developing a prediction score and setting cut-off lines that allow its use as a test to recommend actions. (*Synonym:* clinical decision rule).

Prediction Score A score derived from a prediction formulae that may be used as the basis for estimating prognosis or may be converted to a test for making decisions. (*Synonym:* prediction rule)

Predictive Value of a Negative Test The proportion of individuals with a negative test who do not have the condition or disease as measured by the reference standard.

Predictive Value of a Positive Test The proportion of individuals with a positive test who actually have the condition or disease as measured by the reference standard.

Pre hoc analysis A term used to describe an analysis of the data, usually on subgroups, in which a hypothesis for the analysis was put forth prior to collecting the data. (*See* post hoc analysis)

Premarket As used to describe the FDA process refers to phases 1,2, and 3 prior to FDA approval.

Pretest Probability The probability of disease before the results of a test are known. (*Synonym:* prior probability)

Prevalence The proportion of persons with a particular disease or condition at a point in time. Can also be interpreted as the probability that an individual selected at random from the population of interest will be someone who has the disease or condition. (*Synonym:* point prevalence)

Primary Endpoint The outcome measurement in a study which is used to calculate the sample's size. It should be a frequently occurring and biologically important endpoint though it may not be a clinically important endpoint. (*See:* secondary endpoint)

Probability A proportion in which the numerator contains the number of times an event occurs and the denominator includes the number of times an event occurs plus the number of times it does not occur.

Prognosis Prediction of outcome for an individual.

Propensity Score A special type of prediction score that can be used to measure the prognosis of individuals for purposes of adjustment for prognosis as part of research investigations.

Proportion   A fraction in which the numerator contains a subset of the individuals contained in the denominator.

Protocol Deviant   An individual in a randomized controlled trial whose treatment differs from that which the person would have received if the treatment had followed the rules contained in the investigation's protocol.

Proximal Cause   A legal term that implies an examination of the time sequence of cause-and-effect to determine the element in the constellation of causal factors that was most closely related in time to the outcome.

Pruning the Decision Tree   The process of reducing the complexity of a decision tree by combining outcomes and removing potential outcomes which are considered extremely rare or inconsequential.

Pseudocertainty   An impression of certainty in decision making created by framing a decision as certain once a series of conditions have been fulfilled.

Publication Bias   The tendency to not publish small studies that do not demonstrate a statistically significant difference between groups.

Purposive Sample   A set of observations obtained from a population in such a way that the sample's distribution of independent variable values is determined by the researcher and not necessarily representative of their distribution in the population.

Push-pull model   A model describing the systems, organizations and individual factors needed for successful implementation of evidence-based recommendation in health care.

Q

Q-statistic   A statistical significance test that has been used in meta-analysis. This statistical significance test has low statistical power for rejecting the null hypothesis of homogenity

Qualitative studies   As used here, research conducted without an intention of including a sample size designed to provide adequate statistical power to conduct statistical significance tests.

QALY Decision Analysis   The form of decision analysis that uses QALYs as the outcome measure.

Quality Adjusted Life Years (QALYs)   A measure which incorporates probabilities, utilities, and life expectancies. Is the equivalent of one additional year of life at full health for one person compared to death.

Quality-Adjusted Number Needed to Treat   As used here, a summary measurement that can be derived from an expected utility decision analysis. Measures the number of individuals, on average, who need to receive the better alternative in order to obtain one additional good outcome or one few bad outcomes.

R

Random Effects Model   A type of statistical significance test that does not assume that subgroups all come from the same large population. In meta-analysis, implies that there is heterogeneity across the investigations.

Random Error   Error which is due to the workings of chance, which can either operate in the direction of the study hypothesis or in the opposite direction.

Random Sampling   A method of obtaining a sample that ensures that each individual in the larger population has a known, but not necessarily equal, probability of being selected for the sample.

Randomization   A method of assignment in which individuals have a known, but not necessarily equal, probability of being assigned to a particular study group or control group. (*Synonym:* random assignment)

Randomization by blocks   Randomization that is accomplished using groups of individuals, perhaps from the same site, who have given their consent to participate and who are then randomized to study or control groups using a predefined allocation ratio.

Randomized Controlled Trial   An investigation in which the investigator assigns individuals to study and control groups using a process known as randomization. (*Synonym:* randomized clinical trial, experimental study)

Range   The difference between the highest and lowest data values in a population or sample.

Rate   Commonly used to indicate any measure of disease or outcome occurrence. From a statistical point of view, are those measures of disease occurrence that include a numerator which is a subset of the denominator and includes a unit of time. (e.g., incidence rate). (*Synonym:* true rate)

Rate Ratio   A ratio of rates often obtained from a population comparison. Should be distinguished from a relative risk and an odds ratio which imply that the data relates the outcomes to individual characteristics.

Ratio   A fraction in which the numerator is not necessarily a subset of the denominator, as opposed to a proportion.

RE-AIM framework   A framework for evaluation research as part of T-3 research that addresses questions of reach (R), effectiveness (E), adoption (A), implementation (I) and maintenance (M).

Real Differences or Changes   Differences or changes in the measurement of occurrence which reflect differences or changes in the phenomenon under study as opposed to artifactual changes.

Real Rate of Return   The rate of return that is used when discounting. It is designed to take into account the fact that money invested rather than spent is expected to increase in value above and beyond inflation.

Recall Bias   An assessment bias that occurs when individuals in one study or control group are more likely to remember past events than individuals in the other group.

Receiver-Operator Characteristics (ROC) Curve   A method used to quantitate the discriminant ability of a test based on the area under the curve. Can also assist in identifying an optimal cutoff line for a positive and a negative test.

Reductionist Approach An approach to evidence which aims to examine one factor of interest at a time as opposed to an integrative approach that looks at the impact of multiple factors at the same time.

Reference Case In decision-making investigations, it is the accepted method for presenting the data using the social perspective, best guess, or baseline estimates for variables, a 3% discount rate, and a series of other generally accepted assumptions.

Reference Interval The interval of test results which reflects the variation among those who are free of the disease. (*Synonym:* range of normal)

Reference Sample Group The sample used to represent the population of individuals who are believed to be free of the disease. (*Synonym:* disease-free group)

Reference Point In decision making refers to the status quo or alternative points of reference such as past health status that may be used by individuals to compare the potential outcomes of an intervention.

Reference Standard The criterion used to unequivocally define the presence and absence of the condition or disease under study. (*Synonym:* gold standard)

Regression Analysis A generic term describing any statistical method in which an outcome or dependent variable is related to one or more independent variables.

Regression to the Mean A statistical principle based on the fact that unusual events are unlikely to recur. By chance alone, measurements subsequent to an unusual measurement are likely to be closer to the mean. Subsequent measures may also return to the average due to social forces other than chance.

Relative Risk A ratio of the probability of developing the outcome in a specified period of time if the risk factor is present divided by the probability of developing the outcome in that same period of time if the risk factor is not present. The numerator and the denominator may be reversed.

Replacement Mortality At older ages reduction in death rates from one particular cause may result in increased rates from other causes.

Reportable Diseases Diseases or conditions that are expected to be reported by clinicians and laboratories to a governmental organization, often the local health department. (*Synonym:* notifiable disease)

Reporting Bias An assessment bias that occurs when individuals in one study or control group are more likely to report past events than individuals in the other group. Is especially likely to occur when one group is under disproportionate pressure to report confidential information

Representative sample A subset of a larger population that is obtained or drawn using a chance process and therefore resembles the large population.

Results The component of the M.A.A.R.I.E. that compares the outcome of the study and control groups. Includes issues of estimation, inference, and adjustment.

Retrospective Cohort Study A cohort study in which an individual's group assignment is determined before the investigator is aware of the outcome even though the outcome has already occurred. Uses a previously collected database. (*Synonym:* nonconcurrent cohort study, database research)

Reverse Causality The situation in which the apparent "effect" is actually the "cause."

Risk The probability of an event occurring during a specified period of time. The the numerator contains the number of individuals who develop the disease during the time period; the denominator contains the number of disease-free persons at the beginning of the time period. Is also used as a synonym for the probability of harm (*Synonym:* cumulative probability)

Risk Avoider In decision making an individual who decides on the status quo rather than an active intervention when the expected utility of the two options are the same

Risk Factor As commonly used, a generic term in which a factor that has been shown to be associated with an increased probability of developing a condition or disease. In this book, implies that at least an association has been established at the individual level. (*Synonym:* risk indicator) (*See* risk marker and risk predictor)

Risk Marker As used in this book a type of risk factor which is associated with an outcome at the individual level but it has not been establishes that the "cause" precedes the "effect".

Risk-Neutral The choice of alternatives is governed by expected utility and is not influenced by the tendency to either choose a risk-seeking or a risk-avoiding alternative

Risk Predictor As used in this book a type of risk factor that implies that an association at the individual level has been established and that the "cause' precedes the "effect" has been established. It does not imply that a contributory cause has been established.

Risk Taker In decision making an individual who decides on an active intervention rather than accepting the status quo when the expected utility of the two options are the same

Robust The assumptions of a statistical procedure can be violated without substantial effects on its conclusions.

Rule-of-Three The number of individuals who must be observed to be 95% confident of observing at least one case of an adverse effect. This number is three times the denominator of the true probability of occurrence of the adverse effect.

Run-In Period Pre randomization observation of patients usually designed to ensure that they are appropriate candidates for entrance into a randomized controlled trial, especially with regard to their adherence to therapy.

S

Sample   A subset of a larger population obtained for investigation to draw conclusions or make estimates about the larger population.

Sampling Error   An error introduced by chance differences between the estimate obtained in a sample and the true value in the larger population from which the sample was drawn.

Satisficing   A decision-making approach in which the goal is not to maximize expected utility but to maximize the chances of achieving a satisfactory solution.

Screening Test   Test conducted on an individual who is asymptomatic for a particular disease as part of a testing strategy to diagnose that particular disease.

Secondary Endpoint   An endpoint which is of clinical interest and importance, such as death, but which occurs too infrequently to use to calculate the sample's size.

Selection Bias   A bias in assignment that occurs when the study and control groups are chosen so that they differ from each other by one or more factors that affect the outcome of the study. A type of confounding variable that results from study design rather than chance (See: confounding variable)

Self-Selection Bias   A bias related to the assignment process in screening that may occur when volunteers are used in an investigation. The bias results from differences between volunteers and the larger population of interest, i.e., the target population.

Sensitivity   The proportion of those with the disease or condition, as measured by the reference standard, who are positive by the test being studied. (*Synonym:* positive-in-disease)

Sensitivity Analysis   A method used in decision-making investigations that alters one or more factors from their best guess or baseline estimates and examines the impact on the results. (*See*: Monte Carlo simulation)

Sequential Analyses   Methods of analysis that seek to determine whether an investigation should continue. Sequential analysis methods may permit an investigation to be terminated or stopped at an earlier time. (*See*: stopping rules)

Simpson's paradox   The unusual situation in which 2 sets of data that indicate a consistent outcome reverse direction when combined.

Social Perspective   The perspective that takes into account all health-related benefits, harms, and costs regardless of who experiences these outcomes or who pays these costs. Is considered the appropriate perspective for decision-making investigations.

Source Population   In a case-control study both the cases and the controls aim to be representative of this larger population.

Spearman's Correlation Coefficient   A correlation coefficient that can be obtained from a bivariable analysis when the dependent variable and the independent variable are both ordinal and are obtained through naturalistic sampling.

Specificity   The proportion of those without the disease or condition, as measured by the reference standard or gold standard, who are negative by the test being studied. (*Synonym:* negative-in-health)

Spectrum Bias   A bias in testing in which the participants do not reflect the spectrum of disease in the target population, such as excluding those with other diseases of the same organ system that may produce false negative or false positive results.

Spontaneous Reporting System   A voluntary FDA system for reporting adverse events associated with the use of drugs.

Standard Deviation   A commonly used measure of the spread or dispersion of data which measures how widely dispersed the values are around the mean.

Standardization (of a rate)   An effort to take into account or adjust for the effects of the distribution of a factor such as age or gender on the observed rates. (*See:* adjustment, standardized mortality ratio)

Standardized Mortality Ratio (SMR)   A ratio in which the numerator contains the observed number of deaths and the denominator contains the number of deaths that would be expected based on a comparison population. Implies that indirect standardization has been used to control for confounding variables.

Stationary Population   A population often defined as 100,000 birth that experiences no entry or exit from the population except for birth or death. Often used as the population for cross-sectional life table and life expectancy calculations.

Statistic   A value calculated from sample data that is used to estimate a value or parameter in the larger population from which the sample was obtained.

Statistical Power   The ability of an investigation to demonstrate statistical significance when a true association or difference of a specified strength exists in the population being sampled. Equals 1 minus the Type II error. (*Synonyms:* power, resolving power)

Statistical Significance Test   A statistical technique for determining the probability that the data observed in a sample, or more extreme data, could occur by chance if there is no true difference or association in the larger population (i.e., if the null hypothesis is true). (*Synonym:* inference, hypothesis testing)

Stopping Rules   Ethics procedures established as part of the investigation's protocol to conduct interim analyses at predetermined time(s) and stop the investigation if predetermine criteria have been met. (See: sequential analysis)

Stratification   A process used to control for confounding variables by making separate estimates for groups of individuals for each level of the confounding variable.

Stratum When data are stratified or divided into groups using a characteristic such as age, each group is known as a stratum.

Student's *t* Test A statistical test used for one continuous dependent variable and one nominal independent variable.

Study Group In a cohort study or randomized controlled trial, a group of individuals who possess the characteristics or who are exposed to the factors under study. In case-control studies, a group of individuals who have developed the disease or condition being investigated.

Study Hypothesis An assertion that an association or difference exists between two or more variables in the population sampled.

Study Population The population of individuals from which samples are obtained for inclusion in an investigation. (*Synonym:* study's population)

Subgroup Analysis Examination of the relationship between variables in smaller groups such as gender or age groups, obtained from the original study and control groups.

Subjective Probabilities Probabilities that are obtained based on perceived probabilities.

Sufficient Cause A characteristic fulfills this definition if its presence in and of itself will produce or cause the disease.

Summary Measure A measurement such as a relative risk or odds ratio designed to summarize the data obtained in an investigation.

Sunk cost In decision making refers to previous commitments made to a course of action that influence the way that a current decision is viewed. Financial costs may or may not be involved.

Superiority trial A term describing the traditional type of randomized controlled trial designed to compare a new intervention to a control group intervention with the hypothesis that the new intervention is superior to the control group intervention.

Supportive Criteria When contributory cause cannot be definitively established, additional criteria can be used to develop a judgment regarding the existence of a contributory cause. These include strength of association, dose-response relationship, consistency of the relationship, and biological plausibility. (*Synonym:* adjunct, ancillary criteria)

Surrogate Outcome The use of substitute measurements such as test results instead of an important clinical outcome to assess the outcomes of an investigation. In order to be an appropriate measure of outcome, these measurements must be strongly associated with an important clinical outcome. (*Synonym:* surrogate endpoint)

Survey A method of data collection in which data is collected from a sample of a population

Systematic literature search Formal approach to identifying all existing studies regardless of the type of study or whether or not they were published in the peer review literature

Systematic Review An evaluation of research that addresses a focused question using methods designed to reduce the possibility of bias. May use qualitative as well as quantitative methods. (*See:* meta-analysis)

Systems Approach An approach to problem solving that looks at the multiple influences on a problem and the interactions of these influences, identifies bottlenecks and leverage points, and looks for changes over time

T

Target Population The group of individuals to whom one wishes to apply the results of an investigation. May be different from the study population from which the sample used in an investigation is obtained.

Temporal Trend Long-term real changes in rates (*Synonym:* secular trend)

Test-Based Confidence Interval Confidence interval derived using the same data and same basic process as that used to perform a statistical significance test on a particular set of data.

Testing A generic term that implies the collection of information to assist in decision making such as diagnosis, screening, and prediction and decision rules.

Time dependent variable A dependent variable whose measurement is affected by the duration of observation fulfills this definition.

Time Horizon The follow-up period of time used to determine which potential outcomes that occur in the future will be included in a model for a decision-making investigation. (*Synonym:* analysis horizon)

Time-to-event curve A general term for a curve or plot displaying the data from a longitudinal or cohort life table.

Transformation A formulae applied to each observation in a dataset to covert the data to a distribution that fulfills the assumptions of a statistical method, such as the assumption of Gaussian distribution.

Translational research A generic term used to refer to the steps in moving from basic science advances to their use to improve outcomes of individual patients and entire populations.

Translational research 1 (T-1) The step within translational research of moving from basic science understandings to demonstration of efficacy of interventions under investigational conditions.

Translational research 2 (T-2) The step within translational research of moving from the efficacy to the effectiveness of interventions and developing evidence-based guidelines.

Translational research 3 (T-3) The final step within translation research of addressing the implementation and evaluation of interventions in health care and public health delivery and their impact on populations.

True Negative An individual who does not have the disease or condition, as measured by the reference or gold standard, and has a negative test result.

True Positive An individual who has the disease or condition, as measured by the reference or gold standard, and has a positive test result.

Two-Tailed Test A characteristic of a statistical significance test in which deviations from the null hypothesis in either the direction of the study hypothesis or in the opposite direction are considered possible.

Type I Error An error that occurs when data demonstrate a statistically significant result when no true association or difference exists in the larger population. The alpha level is the size of the this error which will be tolerated.

Type II Error An error that occurs when the sample's observations fail to demonstrate statistical significance when a true association or difference actually exists in the population. The beta level is the size of the this error that will be tolerated. (*See:* statistical power)

U

Unfamiliarity Effect A decision making bias in which the perception of the probability of an event is altered by the degree of familiarity or experience that an individual has with the phenomenon or its potential outcome(s).

Univariable Analysis Statistical analysis in which there is one dependent variable and no independent variable.

Universal testing Screening for disease or risk factors in an entire population even among those without risk factors such as testing all those above a certain age for HIV or hypertension.

User Perspective Perspective that takes into account the impacts of benefits, harms, and cost as they affect a particular user of the decision-making investigation. May include payer, provider, and patient perspectives.

Utility A measure of the value of a particular health state measured on a scale of 0 to 1. Measured on the same scale as probabilities in order to multiply this measurement times the probability. A variety of methods exist for measuring this factor, including the rating scale, time trade-off, and reference gamble methods.

V

Valid Measures what it intends to measure. In this book, this criteria is considered fulfilled if the measurement is appropriate for the question being addressed and is accurate, precise, complete and unaffected by observation. (see internal validity)

Validation Procedures used in the development of prediction and decision rules rules and for other purposes that aim to determine if the formulae derived from one population is able to predict outcome in other populations.

Validation Cohort A different subset of the same population that was used to derive the prediction and decision rule is used as the initial population for evaluating the prediction and decision rule

Variable Often used to refers to a characteristic for which measurements are made in a study. In strict statistical terminology, it is the representation of these characteristics in an analysis. When using nominal data with more than two categories more than one of these is needed to represent the characteristic.

Verification Bias A bias in testing that may occur when participants are chosen because they have previously undergone the index test and agree to subsequently undergo the reference standard test.

W

Weighting A method used in statistical procedures to take into account the relative importance of a specific stratum.

Willingness to Pay An approach to converting effectiveness into monetary terms that uses past choices made in specific situations to estimate how much society is willing to pay to obtain a specific outcome.

Note: Page numbers followed by f, t and n indicate figures, tables and footnotes, respectively.

S